WORLD REPORT ON DISABILITY

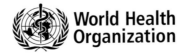

World Health
Organization

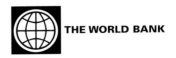

THE WORLD BANK

WHO Library Cataloguing-in-Publication Data

World report on disability 2011.

1.Disabled persons - statistics and numerical data. 2.Disabled persons - rehabilitation. 3.Delivery of health care. 4.Disabled children. 5.Education, Special. 6.Employment, Supported. 7.Health policy. I.World Health Organization.

ISBN 978 92 4 156418 2   (NLM classification: HV 1553)
ISBN 978 92 4 068521 5 (PDF)
ISBN 978 92 4 068636 6 (ePUB)
ISBN 978 92 4 068637 3 (Daisy)

Printed in Malta

Contents

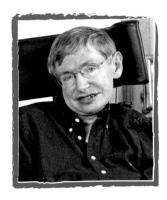

Foreword

Disability need not be an obstacle to success. I have had motor neurone disease for practically all my adult life. Yet it has not prevented me from having a prominent career in astrophysics and a happy family life.

Reading the *World report on disability*, I find much of relevance to my own experience. I have benefitted from access to first class medical care. I rely on a team of personal assistants who make it possible for me to live and work in comfort and dignity. My house and my workplace have been made accessible for me. Computer experts have supported me with an assisted communication system and a speech synthesizer which allow me to compose lectures and papers, and to communicate with different audiences.

But I realize that I am very lucky, in many ways. My success in theoretical physics has ensured that I am supported to live a worthwhile life. It is very clear that the majority of people with disabilities in the world have an extremely difficult time with everyday survival, let alone productive employment and personal fulfilment.

I welcome this first *World report on disability*. This report makes a major contribution to our understanding of disability and its impact on individuals and society. It highlights the different barriers that people with disabilities face – attitudinal, physical, and financial. Addressing these barriers is within our reach.

In fact we have a moral duty to remove the barriers to participation, and to invest sufficient funding and expertise to unlock the vast potential of people with disabilities. Governments throughout the world can no longer overlook the hundreds of millions of people with disabilities who are denied access to health, rehabilitation, support, education and employment, and never get the chance to shine.

The report makes recommendations for action at the local, national and international levels. It will thus be an invaluable tool for policy-makers, researchers, practitioners, advocates and volunteers involved in disability. It is my hope that, beginning with the *Convention on the Rights of Persons with Disabilities*, and now with the publication of the *World report on disability*, this century will mark a turning point for inclusion of people with disabilities in the lives of their societies.

Professor Stephen W Hawking

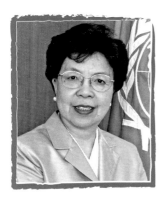 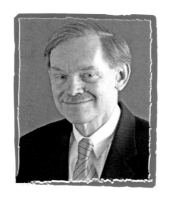

Preface

More than one billion people in the world live with some form of disability, of whom nearly 200 million experience considerable difficulties in functioning. In the years ahead, disability will be an even greater concern because its prevalence is on the rise. This is due to ageing populations and the higher risk of disability in older people as well as the global increase in chronic health conditions such as diabetes, cardiovascular disease, cancer and mental health disorders.

Across the world, people with disabilities have poorer health outcomes, lower education achievements, less economic participation and higher rates of poverty than people without disabilities. This is partly because people with disabilities experience barriers in accessing services that many of us have long taken for granted, including health, education, employment, and transport as well as information. These difficulties are exacerbated in less advantaged communities.

To achieve the long-lasting, vastly better development prospects that lie at the heart of the 2015 Millennium Development Goals and beyond, we must empower people living with disabilities and remove the barriers which prevent them participating in their communities; getting a quality education, finding decent work, and having their voices heard.

As a result, the World Health Organization and the World Bank Group have jointly produced this *World Report on Disability* to provide the evidence for innovative policies and programmes that can improve the lives of people with disabilities, and facilitate implementation of the United Nations Convention on the Rights of Persons with Disabilities, which came into force in May 2008. This landmark international treaty reinforced our understanding of disability as a human rights and development priority.

The *World Report on Disability* suggests steps for all stakeholders – including governments, civil society organizations and disabled people's organizations – to create enabling environments, develop rehabilitation and support services, ensure adequate social protection, create inclusive policies and programmes, and enforce new and existing standards and legislation, to the benefit of people with disabilities and the wider community. People with disabilities should be central to these endeavors.

Our driving vision is of an inclusive world in which we are all able to live a life of health, comfort, and dignity. We invite you to use the evidence in this report to help this vision become a reality.

Dr Margaret Chan
Director-General
World Health Organization

Mr Robert B Zoellick
President
World Bank Group

Acknowledgements

The World Health Organization and the World Bank would like to thank the more than 370 editors, contributors, regional consultation participants, and peer reviewers to this Report from 74 countries around the world. Acknowledgement is also due to the report advisors and editors, WHO regional advisors, and World Bank and WHO staff for offering their support and guidance. Without their dedication, support, and expertise this Report would not have been possible.

The Report also benefited from the efforts of many other people, in particular, Tony Kahane and Bruce Ross-Larson who edited the text of the main report, and Angela Burton who developed the alternative text and assisted with the references. Natalie Jessup, Alana Officer, Sashka Posarac and Tom Shakespeare who prepared the final text for the summary and Bruce Ross-Larson who edited the summary report.

Thanks are also due to the following: Jerome Bickenbach, Noriko Saito Fort, Szilvia Geyh, Katherine Marcello, Karen Peffley, Catherine Sykes, and Bliss Temple for technical support on the development of the Report; Somnath Chatterji, Nirmala Naidoo, Brandon Vick, and Emese Verdes for analysis and interpretation of the World Health Survey; Colin Mathers and Rene Levalee for the analysis of the Global Burden of Disease study; and to Nenad Kostanjsek and Rosalba Lembo for the compilation and presentation of the country-reported disability data. The Report benefited from the work of Chris Black, Jean-Marc Glinz, Steven Lauwers, Jazz Shaban, Laura Sminkey, and Jelica Vesic for media and communication; James Rainbird for proofreading and Liza Furnival for indexing; Sophie Guetaneh Aguettant and Susan Hobbs for graphic design; Omar Vulpinari, Alizée Freudenthal and Gustavo Millon at Fabrica for creative direction, art direction and photographs of cover design and images for chapter title pages; Pascale Broisin and Frédérique Robin-Wahlin for coordinating the printing; Tushita Bosonet for her assistance with the cover; Maryanne Diamond, Lex Grandia, Penny Hartin for feedback on the accessibility of the Report; Melanie Lauckner for the production of the Report in alternative formats; and Rachel Mcleod-Mackenzie for her administrative support and for coordinating the production process.

For assistance in recruiting narrative contributors, thanks go to the Belize Council for the Visually Impaired, Shanta Everington, Fiona Hale, Sally Hartley, Julian Hughes, Tarik Jasarevic, Natalie Jessup, Sofija Korac, Ingrid Lewis, Hamad Lubwama, Rosamond Madden, Margie Peden, Diane Richler, Denise Roza, Noriko Saito Fort, and Moosa Salie.

The World Health Organization and the World Bank also wish to thank the following for their generous financial support for the development, translation, and publication of the Report: the Governments of Australia, Finland, Italy, New Zealand, Norway, Sweden, and the United Kingdom of Great Britain and Northern Ireland; CBM International; the Japan International Cooperation Agency; the multidonor trust fund, the Global Partnership on Disability and Development; and the United Nations Population Fund.

Contributors

Editorial guidance

Editorial Committee

Sally Hartley, Venus Ilagan, Rosamond Madden, Alana Officer, Aleksandra Posarac, Katherine Seelman, Tom Shakespeare, Sándor Sipos, Mark Swanson, Maya Thomas, Zhuoying Qiu.

Executive Editors

Alana Officer (WHO), Aleksandra Posarac (World Bank).

Technical Editors

Tony Kahane, Bruce Ross-Larson.

Advisory Committee

Chair of Advisory Committee: Ala Din Abdul Sahib Alwan.
Advisory Committee: Amadaou Bagayoko, Arup Banerji, Philip Craven, Mariam Doumiba, Ariel Fiszbein, Sepp Heim, Etienne Krug, Brenda Myers, Kicki Nordström, Qian Tang, Mired bin Raad, José Manuel Salazar-Xirinachs, Sha Zukang, Kit Sinclair, Urbano Stenta, Gerold Stucki, Tang Xiaoquan, Edwin Trevathan, Johannes Trimmel.

Contributors to individual chapters

Introduction

Contributors: Alana Officer, Tom Shakespeare.

Chapter 1: Understanding disability

Contributors: Jerome Bickenbach, Theresia Degener, John Melvin, Gerard Quinn, Aleksandra Posarac, Marianne Schulze, Tom Shakespeare, Nicholas Watson.
Boxes: Jerome Bickenbach (1.1), Alana Officer (1.2), Aleksandra Posarac, Tom Shakespeare (1.3), Marianne Schulze (1.4), Natalie Jessup, Chapal Khasnabis (1.5).

Chapter 2: Disability – a global picture
Contributors: Gary Albrecht, Kidist Bartolomeos, Somnath Chatterji, Maryanne Diamond, Eric Emerson, Glen Fujiura, Oye Gureje, Soewarta Kosen, Nenad Kostanjsek, Mitchell Loeb, Jennifer Madans, Rosamond Madden, Maria Martinho, Colin Mathers, Sophie Mitra, Daniel Mont, Alana Officer, Trevor Parmenter, Margie Peden, Aleksandra Posarac, Michael Powers, Patricia Soliz, Tami Toroyan, Bedirhan Üstün, Brandon Vick, Xingyang Wen.
Boxes: Gerry Brady, Gillian Roche (2.1), Mitchell Loeb, Jennifer Madans (2.2), Thomas Calvot, Jean Pierre Delomier (2.3), Matilde Leonardi, Jose Luis Ayuso-Mateos (2.4), Xingyang Wen, Rosamond Madden (2.5).

Chapter 3: General health care
Contributors: Fabricio Balcazar, Karl Blanchet, Alarcos Cieza, Eva Esteban, Michele Foster, Lisa Iezzoni, Jennifer Jelsma, Natalie Jessup, Robert Kohn, Nicholas Lennox, Sue Lukersmith, Michael Marge, Suzanne McDermott, Silvia Neubert, Alana Officer, Mark Swanson, Miriam Taylor, Bliss Temple, Margaret Turk, Brandon Vick.
Boxes: Sue Lukersmith (3.1), Liz Sayce (3.2), Jodi Morris, Taghi Yasamy, Natalie Drew (3.3), Paola Ayora, Nora Groce, Lawrence Kaplan (3.4), Sunil Deepak, Bliss Temple (3.5), Tom Shakespeare (3.6).

Chapter 4: Rehabilitation
Contributors: Paul Ackerman, Shaya Asindua, Maurice Blouin, Debra Cameron, Kylie Clode, Lynn Cockburn, Antonio Eduardo DiNanno, Timothy Elliott, Harry Finkenflugel, Neeru Gupta, Sally Hartley, Pamela Henry, Kate Hopman, Natalie Jessup, Alan Jette, Michel Landry, Chris Lavy, Sue Lukersmith, Mary Matteliano, John Melvin, Vibhuti Nandoskar, Alana Officer, Rhoda Okin, Penny Parnes, Wesley Pryor, Geoffrey Reed, Jorge Santiago Rosetto, Grisel Roulet, Marcia Scherer, William Spaulding, John Stone, Catherine Sykes, Bliss Temple, Travis Threats, Maluta Tshivhase, Daniel Wong, Lucy Wong, Karen Yoshida.
Boxes: Alana Officer (4.1), Janet Njelesani (4.2), Frances Heywood (4.3), Donata Vivanti (4.4), Heinz Trebbin (4.5), Julia D'Andrea Greve (4.6), Alana Officer (4.7).

Chapter 5: Assistance and support
Contributors: Michael Bach, Diana Chiriacescu, Alexandre Cote, Vladimir Cuk, Patrick Devlieger, Karen Fisher, Tamar Heller, Martin Knapp, Sarah Parker, Gerard Quinn, Aleksandra Posarac, Marguerite Schneider, Tom Shakespeare, Patricia Noonan Walsh.
Boxes: Tina Minkowitz, Maths Jesperson (5.1), Robert Nkwangu (5.2), Disability Rights International (5.3).

Chapter 6: Enabling environments

Contributors: Judy Brewer, Alexandra Enders, Larry Goldberg, Linda Hartman, Jordana Maisel, Charlotte McClain-Nhlapo, Marco Nicoli, Karen Peffley, Katherine Seelman, Tom Shakespeare, Edward Steinfeld, Jim Tobias, Diahua Yu.

Boxes: Edward Steinfeld (6.1), Tom Shakespeare (6.2), Asiah Abdul Rahim, Samantha Whybrow (6.3), Binoy Acharya, Geeta Sharma, Deepa Sonpal (6.4), Edward Steinfeld (6.5), Katherine Seelman (6.6), Hiroshi Kawamura (6.7).

Chapter 7: Education

Contributors: Peter Evans, Giampiero Griffo, Seamus Hegarty, Glenda Hernandez, Susan Hirshberg, Natalie Jessup, Elizabeth Kozleski, Margaret McLaughlin, Susie Miles, Daniel Mont, Diane Richler, Thomas Sabella.

Boxes: Susan Hirshberg (7.1), Margaret McLaughlin (7.2), Kylie Bates, Rob Regent (7.3), Hazel Bines, Bliss Temple, R.A. Villa (7.4), Ingrid Lewis (7.5).

Chapter 8: Work and employment

Contributors: Susanne Bruyère, Sophie Mitra, Sara VanLooy, Tom Shakespeare, Ilene Zeitzer.

Boxes: Susanne Bruyère (8.1), Anne Hawker, Alana Officer, Catherine Sykes (8.2), Peter Coleridge (8.3), Cherry Thompson-Senior (8.4), Susan Scott Parker (8.5).

Chapter 9: The way forward: recommendations

Contributors: Sally Hartley, Natalie Jessup, Rosamond Madden, Alana Officer, Sashka Posarac, Tom Shakespeare.

Boxes: Kirsten Pratt (9.1)

Technical appendices

Contributors: Somnath Chatterji, Marleen De Smedt, Haishan Fu, Nenad Kostanjsek, Rosalba Lembo, Mitchell Loeb, Jennifer Madans, Rosamond Madden, Colin Mathers, Andres Montes, Nirmala Naidoo, Alana Officer, Emese Verdes, Brandon Vick.

Narrative contributors

The report includes narratives with personal accounts of the experiences of people with disabilities. Many people provided a narrative but not all could be included in the report. The narratives included come from Australia, Bangladesh, Barbados, Belize, Cambodia, Canada, China, Egypt, Haiti, India, Japan, Jordan, Kenya, the Netherlands, Palestinian Self-Rule Areas, Panama, the Russian Federation, the Philippines, Uganda, the United Kingdom of Great Britain and Northern Ireland, and Zambia. Only the first name of each narrative contributor has been provided for reasons of confidentiality.

Peer reviewers

Kathy Al Ju'beh, Dele Amosun, Yerker Anderson, Francesc Aragal, Julie Babindard, Elizabeth Badley, Ken Black, Johannes Borg, Vesna Bosnjak, Ron Brouillette, Mahesh Chandrasekar, Mukesh Chawla, Diana Chiriacescu, Ching Choi, Peter Coleridge, Ajit Dalal, Victoria de Menil, Marleen De Smedt, Shelley Deegan, Sunil Deepak, Maryanne Diamond, Steve Edwards, Arne Eide, James Elder-Woodward, Eric Emerson, Alexandra Enders, John Eriksen, Haishan Fu, Marcus Fuhrer, Michelle Funk, Ann Goerdt, Larry Goldberg, Lex Grandia, Pascal Granier, Wilfredo Guzman, Manal Hamzeh, Sumi Helal, Xiang Hiuyun, Judith Hollenweger, Mosharraf Hossain, Venus Ilagan, Deborah Iyute, Karen Jacobs, Olivier Jadin, Khandaker Jarulul Alam, Jennifer Jelsma, Steen Jensen, Nawaf Kabbara, Lissa Kauppinen, Hiroshi Kawamura, Peter Kercher, Chapal Khasnabis, Ivo Kocur, Johannes Koettl, Kalle Könköllä, Gloria Krahn, Arvo Kuddo, Gaetan Lafortune, Michel Landry, Stig Larsen, Connie Lauren-Bowie, Silvia Lavagnoli, Axel Leblois, Matilde Leonardi, Clayton Lewis, Anna Lindström, Gwynnyth Lleweyllyn, Mitchell Loeb, Michael Lokshin, Clare MacDonald, Jennifer Madans, Richard Madden, Thandi Magagula, Dipendra Manocha, Charlotte McClain-Nhlapo, John Melvin, Cem Mete, Susie Miles, Janice Miller, Marilyn Moffat, Federico Montero, Andres Montes, Asenath Mpatwa, Ashish Mukerjee, Barbara Murray, David Newhouse, Penny Norgrove, Helena Nygren Krug, Japheth Ogamba Makana, Thomas Ongolo, Tanya Packer, Trevor Parmenter, Donatella Pascolini, Charlotte Pearson, Karen Peffley, Debra Perry, Poul Erik Petersen, Immaculada Placencia-Porrero, Adolf Ratzka, Suzanne Reier, Diane Richler, Wachara Riewpaiboon, Tom Rikert, Alan Roulstone, Amanda Rozani, Moosa Salie, Mohammad Sattar Dulal, Duranee Savapan, Shekhar Saxena, Walton Schlick, Marguerite Schneider, Marianne Schultz, Kinnon Scott, Tom Seekins, Samantha Shann, Owen Smith, Beryl Steeden, Catherine Sykes, Jim Tobias, Stefan Trömel, Chris Underhill, Wim Van Brakel, Derek Wade, Nicholas Watson, Ruth Watson, Mark Wheatley, Taghi Yasamy, Nevio Zagaria, Ilene Zeitzer, Ruth Zemke, Dahong Zhuo.

Additional contributors

Regional consultants

WHO African Region/Eastern Mediterranean Region

Alice Nganwa Baingana, Betty Babirye Kwagala, Moussa Charafeddine, Kudakwashe Dube, Sally Hartley, Syed Jaffar Hussain, Deborah Oyuu Iyute, Donatilla Kanimba, Razi Khan, Olive Chifefe Kobusingye, Phitalis Were Masakhwe, Niang Masse, Quincy Mwya, Charlotte McClain-Nhlapo, Catherine Naughton, William Rowland, Ali Hala Ibrahim Sakr, Moosa Salie, Alaa I. Sebeh, Alaa Shukrallah, Sándor Sipos, Joe Ubiedo.

WHO Region of the Americas

Georgina Armstrong, Haydee Beckles, Aaron Bruma, Jean-Claude Jalbert, Sandy Layton, Leanne Madsen, Paulette McGinnis, Tim Surbey, Corey Willet, Valerie Wolbert, Gary L. Albrecht, Ricardo Restrepo Arbelaez, Martha Aristizabal, Susanne Bruyere, Nixon Contreras, Roberto Del Águila, Susan Hirshberg, Federico Montero, Claudia Sánchez, Katherine Seelman, Sándor Sipos, Edward Steinfeld, Beatriz Vallejo, Armando Vásquez, Ruth Warick, Lisbeth Barrantes, José Luís Di Fabio, Juan Manuel Guzmán, John Stone.

WHO South-East Asia Region/Western Pacific Region

Tumenbayar Batdulam, Amy Bolinas, Kylie Clode, David Corner, Dahong Zhuo, Michael Davies, Bulantrisna Djelantik, Mohammad Abdus Sattar Dulal, Betty Dy-Mancao, Fumio Eto, Anne Hawker, Susan Hirshberg, Xiaolin Huang, Venus Ilagan, Yoko Isobe, Emmanuel Jimenez, Kenji Kuno, Leonard Li, Rosmond Madden, Charlotte McClain-Nhlapo, Anuradha Mohit, Akiie Ninomiya, Hisashi Ogawa, Philip O'Keefe, Grant Preston, Wachara Riewpaiboon, Noriko Saito, Chamaiparn Santikarn, Mary Scott, Sándor Sipos, Catherine Sykes, Maya Thomas, Mohammad Jashim Uddin, Zhuoying Qiu, Filipinas Ganchoon, Geetika Mathur, Miriam Taylor, John Andrew Sanchez.

The WHO Regional Office for European Region

Viveca Arrhenius, Jerome Bickenbach, Christine Boldt, Matthias Braubach, Fabrizio Cassia, Diana Chiriacescu, Marleen De Smedt, Patrick Devlieger, Fabrizio Fea, Federica Francescone, Manuela Gallitto, Denise Giacomini, Donato Greco, Giampiero Griffo, Gunnar Grimby, Ahiya Kamara, Etienne Krug, Fiammetta Landoni, Maria G. Lecce, Anna Lindström, Marcelino Lopez, Isabella Menichini, Cem Mete, Daniel Mont, Elisa Patera, FrancescaRacioppi, Adolf Ratzka, Maria Pia Rizzo, Alan Roulstone, Tom Shakespeare, Sándor Sipos, Urbano Stenta, Raffaele Tangorra, Damjan Tatic, Donata Vivanti, Mark Wheatley.

None of the experts involved in the development of this Report declared any conflict of interest.

Introduction

Many people with disabilities do not have equal access to health care, education, and employment opportunities, do not receive the disability-related services that they require, and experience exclusion from everyday life activities. Following the entry into force of the United Nations *Convention on the Rights of Persons with Disabilities* (CRPD), disability is increasingly understood as a human rights issue. Disability is also an important development issue with an increasing body of evidence showing that persons with disabilities experience worse socioeconomic outcomes and poverty than persons without disabilities.

Despite the magnitude of the issue, both awareness of and scientific information on disability issues are lacking. There is no agreement on definitions and little internationally comparable information on the incidence, distribution and trends of disability. There are few documents providing a compilation and analysis of the ways countries have developed policies and responses to address the needs of people with disabilities.

In response to this situation, the World Health Assembly (resolution 58.23 on *"Disability, including prevention, management and rehabilitation"*) requested the World Health Organization (WHO) Director-General to produce a *World report on disability* based on the best available scientific evidence. The *World report on disability* has been produced in partnership with the World Bank, as previous experience has shown the benefit of collaboration between agencies for increasing awareness, political will and action across sectors.

The *World report on disability* is directed at policy-makers, practitioners, researchers, academics, development agencies, and civil society.

Aims

The overall aims of the Report are:
- To provide governments and civil society with a comprehensive description of the importance of disability and an analysis of the responses provided, based on the best available scientific information.
- Based on this analysis, to make recommendations for action at national and international levels.

Scope of the Report

The Report focuses on measures to improve accessibility and equality of opportunity; promoting participation and inclusion; and increasing respect for the autonomy and dignity of persons with disabilities. Chapter 1 defines terms such as disability, discusses prevention and its ethical considerations, introduces the *International Classification of Functioning, Disability and Health* (ICF) and the CRPD, and discusses disability and human rights, and disability and development. Chapter 2 reviews the data on disability prevalence and the situation of people with disabilities worldwide. Chapter 3 explores access to mainstream health services for people with disabilities. Chapter 4 discusses rehabilitation, including therapies and assistive devices. Chapter 5 investigates support and assistance services. Chapter 6 explores inclusive environments, both in terms of physical access to buildings, transport, and so on, but also access to the virtual environments of information and communication technology. Chapter 7 discusses education, and Chapter 8 reviews employment for people with disabilities. Each chapter includes recommendations, which are also drawn together to provide broad policy and practice considerations in Chapter 9.

Process

The development of this Report has been led by an Advisory Committee and an Editorial Board, and has taken over three years. WHO and the World Bank acted as secretariat throughout this process. Based on outlines prepared by the Editorial Board, each chapter was written by a small number of authors, working with a wider group of experts from around the world. Wherever possible, people with disabilities were involved as authors and experts. Nearly 380 contributors from various sectors and all the regions of the world wrote text for the report.

The drafts of each chapter were reviewed following input from regional consultations organized by WHO Regional Offices, which involved local academics, policy-makers, practitioners, and people with disabilities. During these consultations, experts had the opportunity to propose overall recommendations (see Chapter 9). The complete chapters were revised by editors on the basis of human rights standards and best available evidence, subjected to external peer review, which included representatives of disabled people's organizations. The text was finally reviewed by the World Bank and WHO.

It is anticipated that the recommendations in this Report will remain valid until 2021. At that time, the Department of Violence and Injury Prevention and Disability at WHO headquarters in Geneva will initiate a review of the document.

Moving forward

This *World report on disability* charts the steps that are required to improve participation and inclusion of people with disabilities. The aspiration of WHO, the World Bank, and all the authors and editors of this *World report on disability* is that it contributes to concrete actions at all levels and across all sectors, and thus helps to promote social and economic development and the achievement of the human rights of persons with disabilities across the world.

Chapter 1

Understanding disability

"I am a black woman with a disability. Some people make a bad face and don't include me. People don't treat me well when they see my face but when I talk to them sometimes it is better. Before anyone makes a decision about someone with a disability they should talk to them."

Haydeé

"Can you imagine that you're getting up in the morning with such severe pain which disables you from even moving out from your bed? Can you imagine yourself having a pain which even requires you to get an assistance to do the very simple day to day activities? Can you imagine yourself being fired from your job because you are unable to perform simple job requirements? And finally can you imagine your little child is crying for hug and you are unable to hug him due to the pain in your bones and joints?"

Nael

"My life revolves around my two beautiful children. They see me as 'Mummy', not a person in a wheelchair and do not judge me or our life. This is now changing as my efforts to be part of their life is limited by the physical access of schools, parks and shops; the attitudes of other parents; and the reality of needing 8 hours support a day with my personal care…I cannot get into the houses of my children's friends and must wait outside for them to finish playing. I cannot get to all the classrooms at school so I have not met many other parents. I can't get close to the playground in the middle of the park or help out at the sporting events my children want to be part of. Other parents see me as different, and I have had one parent not want my son to play with her son because I could not help with supervision in her inaccessible house."

Samantha

"Near the start of the bus route I climb on. I am one of the first passengers. People continue to embark on the bus. They look for a seat, gaze at my hearing aids, turn their glance quickly and continue walking by. Only when people with disabilities will really be part of the society; will be educated in every kindergarten and any school with personal assistance; live in the community and not in different institutions; work in all places and in any position with accessible means; and will have full accessibility to the public sphere, people may feel comfortable to sit next to us on the bus."

Ahiya

1

Understanding disability

Disability is part of the human condition. Almost everyone will be temporarily or permanently impaired at some point in life, and those who survive to old age will experience increasing difficulties in functioning. Most extended families have a disabled member, and many non-disabled people take responsibility for supporting and caring for their relatives and friends with disabilities (*1–3*). Every epoch has faced the moral and political issue of how best to include and support people with disabilities. This issue will become more acute as the demographics of societies change and more people live to an old age (*4*).

Responses to disability have changed since the 1970s, prompted largely by the self-organization of people with disabilities (*5, 6*), and by the growing tendency to see disability as a human rights issue (*7*). Historically, people with disabilities have largely been provided for through solutions that segregate them, such as residential institutions and special schools (*8*). Policy has now shifted towards community and educational inclusion, and medically-focused solutions have given way to more interactive approaches recognizing that people are disabled by environmental factors as well as by their bodies. National and international initiatives – such as the United Nations *Standard Rules on the Equalization of Opportunities of Persons with Disabilities* (*9*) – have incorporated the human rights of people with disabilities, culminating in 2006 with the adoption of the United Nations *Convention on the Rights of Persons with Disabilities* (CRPD).

This *World report on disability* provides evidence to facilitate implementation of the CRPD. It documents the circumstances of persons with disabilities across the world and explores measures to promote their social participation, ranging from health and rehabilitation to education and employment. This first chapter provides a general orientation about disability, introducing key concepts – such as the human rights approach to disability, the intersection between disability and development, and the *International Classification of Functioning, Disability and Health* (ICF) – and explores the barriers that disadvantage persons with disabilities.

What is disability?

Disability is complex, dynamic, multidimensional, and contested. Over recent decades, the disabled people's movement (*6, 10*) – together with numerous researchers from the social and health sciences (*11, 12*) – have identified the role of social and physical barriers in disability. The transition from an individual, medical perspective to a structural, social perspective has been described as the shift from a "medical model" to a "social model" in which people are viewed as being disabled by society rather than by their bodies (*13*).

The medical model and the social model are often presented as dichotomous, but disability should be viewed neither as purely medical nor as purely social: persons with disabilities can often experience problems arising from their health condition (*14*). A balanced approach is needed, giving appropriate weight to the different aspects of disability (*15, 16*).

The ICF, adopted as the conceptual framework for this *World report on disability*, understands functioning and disability as a dynamic interaction between health conditions and contextual factors, both personal and environmental (see **Box 1.1**) (*17*). Promoted as a "bio-psycho-social model", it represents a workable compromise between medical and social models. Disability is the umbrella term for impairments, activity limitations and participation restrictions, referring to the negative aspects of the interaction between an individual (with a health condition) and that individual's contextual factors (environmental and personal factors) (*19*).

The Preamble to the CRPD acknowledges that disability is "an evolving concept", but also stresses that "disability results from the interaction between persons with impairments and attitudinal and environmental barriers that hinder their full and effective participation in society on an equal basis with others". Defining disability as an interaction means that "disability" is not an attribute of the person. Progress on improving social participation can be made by addressing the barriers which hinder persons with disabilities in their day to day lives.

Environment

A person's environment has a huge impact on the experience and extent of disability. Inaccessible environments create disability by creating barriers to participation and inclusion. Examples of the possible negative impact of the environment include:

- a Deaf individual without a sign language interpreter
- a wheelchair user in a building without an accessible bathroom or elevator
- a blind person using a computer without screen-reading software.

Health is also affected by environmental factors, such as safe water and sanitation, nutrition, poverty, working conditions, climate, or access to health care. As the World Health Organization (WHO) Commission on Social Determinants of Health has argued, inequality is a major cause of poor health, and hence of disability (*20*).

The environment may be changed to improve health conditions, prevent impairments, and improve outcomes for persons with disabilities. Such changes can be brought about by legislation, policy changes, capacity building, or technological developments leading to, for instance:

- accessible design of the built environment and transport;
- signage to benefit people with sensory impairments;
- more accessible health, rehabilitation, education, and support services;
- more opportunities for work and employment for persons with disabilities.

Environmental factors include a wider set of issues than simply physical and information access. Policies and service delivery systems, including the rules underlying service provision, can also be obstacles (*21*). Analysis of public health service financing in Australia, for

Box 1.1. New emphasis on environmental factors

The *International Classification of Functioning, Disability and Health* (ICF) (*17*) advanced the understanding and measurement of disability. It was developed through a long process involving academics, clinicians, and – importantly – persons with disabilities (*18*). The ICF emphasizes environmental factors in creating disability, which is the main difference between this new classification and the previous *International Classification of Impairments, Disabilities, and Handicaps* (ICIDH). In the ICF, problems with human functioning are categorized in three interconnected areas:

- **impairments** are problems in body function or alterations in body structure – for example, paralysis or blindness;
- **activity limitations** are difficulties in executing activities – for example, walking or eating;
- **participation restrictions** are problems with involvement in any area of life – for example, facing discrimination in employment or transportation.

Disability refers to difficulties encountered in any or all three areas of functioning. The ICF can also be used to understand and measure the positive aspects of functioning such as body functions, activities, participation and environmental facilitation. The ICF adopts neutral language and does not distinguish between the type and cause of disability – for instance, between "physical" and "mental" health. "**Health conditions**" are diseases, injuries, and disorders, while "impairments" are specific decrements in body functions and structures, often identified as symptoms or signs of health conditions.

Disability arises from the interaction of health conditions with contextual factors – environmental and personal factors as shown in the figure below.

....

Representation of the International Classification of Functioning, Disability and Health

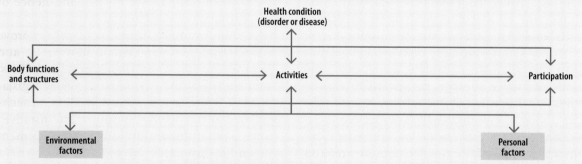

The ICF contains a classification of **environmental factors** describing the world in which people with different levels of functioning must live and act. These factors can be either facilitators or barriers. Environmental factors include: products and technology; the natural and built environment; support and relationships; attitudes; and services, systems, and policies.

The ICF also recognizes **personal factors**, such as motivation and self-esteem, which can influence how much a person participates in society. However, these factors are not yet conceptualized or classified. It further distinguishes between a person's **capacities** to perform actions and the actual **performance** of those actions in real life, a subtle difference that helps illuminate the effect of environment and how performance might be improved by modifying the environment.

The ICF is universal because it covers all human functioning and treats disability as a continuum rather than categorizing people with disabilities as a separate group: disability is a matter of more or less, not yes or no. However, policy-making and service delivery might require thresholds to be set for impairment severity, activity limitations, or participation restriction.

It is useful for a range of purposes – research, surveillance, and reporting – related to describing and measuring health and disability, including: assessing individual functioning, goal setting, treatment, and monitoring; measuring outcomes and evaluating services; determining eligibility for welfare benefits; and developing health and disability surveys.

instance, found that reimbursement of health providers did not account for the additional time often required to provide services to persons with disabilities; hospitals that treated patients with a disability were thus disadvantaged by a funding system that reimbursed them a fixed amount per patient (*22*).

Analysis of access to health care services in Europe found organizational barriers – such as waiting lists, lack of a booking system for appointments, and complex referral systems – that are more complicated for persons with disabilities who may find it difficult to arrive early, or wait all day, or who cannot navigate complex systems (*23, 24*). While discrimination is not intended, the system indirectly excludes persons with disabilities by not taking their needs into account.

Institutions and organizations also need to change – in addition to individuals and environments – to avoid excluding people with disabilities. The 2005 Disability Discrimination Act in the United Kingdom of Great Britain and Northern Ireland directed public sector organizations to promote equality for persons with disability: by instituting a corporate disability equality strategy, for example, and by assessing the potential impact of proposed policies and activities on disabled people (*25*).

Knowledge and attitudes are important environmental factors, affecting all areas of service provision and social life. Raising awareness and challenging negative attitudes are often first steps towards creating more accessible environments for persons with disabilities. Negative imagery and language, stereotypes, and stigma – with deep historic roots – persist for people with disabilities around the world (*26–28*). Disability is generally equated with incapacity. A review of health-related stigma found that the impact was remarkably similar in different countries and across health conditions (*29*). A study in 10 countries found that the general public lacks an understanding of the abilities of people with intellectual impairments (*30*). Mental health conditions are particularly stigmatized, with commonalities

in different settings (*31*). People with mental health conditions face discrimination even in health care settings (*24, 32*).

Negative attitudes towards disability can result in negative treatment of people with disabilities, for example:

- children bullying other children with disabilities in schools
- bus drivers failing to support access needs of passengers with disabilities
- employers discriminating against people with disabilities
- strangers mocking people with disabilities.

Negative attitudes and behaviours have an adverse effect on children and adults with disabilities, leading to negative consequences such as low self-esteem and reduced participation (*32*). People who feel harassed because of their disability sometimes avoid going to places, changing their routines, or even moving from their homes (*33*).

Stigma and discrimination can be combated, for example, through direct personal contact and through social marketing (see Box 1.2) (*37–40*). World Psychiatric Association campaigns against stigmatizing schizophrenia over 10 years in 18 countries have demonstrated the importance of long-term interventions, broad multisectoral involvement, and of including those who have the condition (*41*). Evidence from Norway showed that knowledge about psychosis among the general population improved after a year of information campaigns, and that the duration of untreated psychosis fell from 114 weeks in 1997 to 20 weeks in 1999 due to greater recognition and early intervention with patients (*42*).

Community-based rehabilitation (CBR) programmes can challenge negative attitudes in rural communities, leading to greater visibility and participation by people with disabilities. A three-year project in a disadvantaged community near Allahabad, India, resulted in children with disabilities attending school for the first time, more people with disabilities participating in community forums, and more people

Box 1.2. **Eliminating leprosy, improving lives**

The diagnosis and treatment of leprosy is easy and effective. The best way of preventing disabilities associated with it, as well as preventing further transmission, lies in early diagnosis and treatment. Since 1983 the disease has been curable with multidrug therapy, and since 1985 this therapy has been made available by the World Health Organization (WHO) free of charge around the world. WHO estimates that early detection and treatment with multidrug therapy have prevented about 4 million people from being disabled (*34*).

To eliminate the disease, access to information, diagnosis, and treatment with multidrug therapy are crucial (*34*). The greatest barriers to eliminating the disease are ignorance and stigma. Information campaigns about leprosy in endemic areas are of supreme importance so that people affected by leprosy and their families – historically ostracized from their communities – come forward and receive treatment. Reducing stigma also improves the quality of life of people affected by leprosy and their families by improving people's mobility, interpersonal relationships, employment, leisure, and social activities (*35*).

In India, home to two thirds of the world's people affected by leprosy, the BBC World Service Trust – in partnership with two Indian broadcasters Doordarshan TV and All-India Radio – launched a 16-month campaign on leprosy in 1999 (*36*). The campaign stressed that leprosy is curable, that drugs to cure it are available free throughout India, and that people affected by leprosy should not be excluded from society. The central messages of the campaign were:

- leprosy is not hereditary
- leprosy is not caused by bad deeds in a previous life
- leprosy is not spread by touch.

The campaign used 50 television and 213 radio programmes in 20 languages, and 85 000 information posters. More than 1700 live drama shows, 2746 mobile video screenings, and 3670 public events or competitions were performed in remote areas. Independent market surveys conducted before, during, and after the campaign found:

- **Reach of media campaign**. The radio and TV spots were seen by 59% of respondents, or 275 million people.
- **Transmissibility and curabilit**y. The proportion of people who believed leprosy was transmitted by touch fell from 52% to 27%. The proportion believing that people with leprosy who take multidrug therapy are still infectious fell from 25% to 12%. Those who knew that leprosy was curable rose from 84% to 91%.
- **Symptoms**. Awareness that loss of sensation could be a possible symptom of leprosy rose from 65% to 80%. Awareness of pale reddish patches as a possible symptom remained unchanged at 86%. Awareness of non-itchy patches as a possible symptom rose from 37% to 55%.
- **Therapies**. The awareness rate in control villages (not covered in the campaign) that multidrug therapy was a cure for leprosy was only 56%, but in villages that had been shown live drama it was 82%. In rural areas awareness that the treatment was free was 89% among those exposed to the poster campaign, against 20% in those not exposed.
- **Stigma**. The proportion of people saying they would be willing to sit next to a person affected by leprosy was 10% higher in villages where drama shows had been used than in those without. Similarly, the proportion of those claiming they would be willing to eat food served by somebody affected by leprosy was 50% in villages covered by the campaign, against 32% in those not covered.

Sources (*34–36*).

bringing their children with disabilities for vaccination and rehabilitation (*43*).

The diversity of disability

The disability experience resulting from the interaction of health conditions, personal factors, and environmental factors varies greatly. Persons with disabilities are diverse and heterogeneous, while stereotypical views of disability emphasize wheelchair users and a few other "classic" groups such as blind people and deaf people (*44*). Disability encompasses the child born with a congenital condition such as cerebral palsy or the young soldier who loses his leg to a land-mine, or the middle-aged woman with severe arthritis, or the older person with dementia, among many others. Health conditions can be visible or invisible; temporary or long term; static, episodic, or degenerating; painful or inconsequential. Note that many people with disabilities do not consider themselves to be unhealthy (45). For example, 40% of people with severe or profound disability who responded to the 2007–2008 Australian National Health Survey rated their health as good, very good, or excellent (46).

Generalizations about "disability" or "people with disabilities" can mislead. Persons with disabilities have diverse personal factors with differences in gender, age, socioeconomic status, sexuality, ethnicity, or cultural heritage. Each has his or her personal preferences and responses to disability (47). Also while disability correlates with disadvantage, not all people with disabilities are equally disadvantaged. Women with disabilities experience the combined disadvantages associated with gender as well as disability, and may be less likely to marry than non-disabled women (48, 49). People who experience mental health conditions or intellectual impairments appear to be more disadvantaged in many settings than those who experience physical or sensory impairments (50). People with more severe impairments often experience greater disadvantage, as shown by evidence ranging from rural Guatemala (51) to employment data from Europe (52). Conversely, wealth and status can help overcome activity limitations and participation restrictions (52).

Prevention

Prevention of health conditions associated with disability is a development issue. Attention to environmental factors – including nutrition, preventable diseases, safe water and sanitation, safety on roads and in workplaces – can greatly reduce the incidence of health conditions leading to disability (53).

A public health approach distinguishes:

- **Primary prevention** – actions to avoid or remove the cause of a health problem in an individual or a population before it arises. It includes health promotion and specific protection (for example, HIV education) (54).
- **Secondary prevention** – actions to detect a health problem at an early stage in an individual or a population, facilitating cure, or reducing or preventing spread, or reducing or preventing its long-term effects (for example, supporting women with intellectual disability to access breast cancer screening) (55).
- **Tertiary prevention** – actions to reduce the impact of an already established disease by restoring function and reducing disease-related complications (for example, rehabilitation for children with musculoskeletal impairment) (56).

Article 25 of the CRPD specifies Access to Health as an explicit right for people with disabilities, but primary prevention of health conditions does not come within its scope. Accordingly, this Report considers primary prevention only in so far as people with disabilities require equal access to health promotion and screening opportunities. Primary prevention issues are extensively covered in other WHO and World Bank publications, and both organizations consider primary prevention as crucial to improved overall health of countries' populations.

Viewing disability as a human rights issue is not incompatible with prevention of health conditions as long as prevention respects the rights and dignity of people with disabilities, for example, in the use of language and imagery (57, 58). Preventing disability should be regarded as a multidimensional strategy that includes prevention of disabling barriers as well as prevention and treatment of underlying health conditions (59).

Disability and human rights

Disability is a human rights issue (7) because:

- People with disabilities experience inequalities – for example, when they are denied equal access to health care, employment, education, or political participation because of their disability.
- People with disabilities are subject to violations of dignity – for example, when they are subjected to violence, abuse, prejudice, or disrespect because of their disability.
- Some people with disability are denied autonomy – for example, when they are subjected to involuntary sterilization, or when they are confined in institutions against their will, or when they are regarded as legally incompetent because of their disability.

A range of international documents have highlighted that disability is a human rights issue, including the *World Programme of Action Concerning Disabled People* (1982), the *Convention on the Rights of the Child* (1989), and the *Standard Rules on the Equalisation of Opportunities for People with Disabilities* (1993). More than 40 nations adopted disability discrimination legislation during the 1990s (60). The CRPD – the most recent, and the most extensive recognition of the human rights of persons with disabilities – outlines the civil, cultural, political, social, and economic rights of persons with disabilities (61). Its purpose is to "promote, protect, and ensure the full and equal enjoyment of all human rights and fundamental freedoms by people with disabilities and to promote respect for their inherent dignity".

The CRPD applies human rights to disability, thus making general human rights specific to persons with disabilities (62), and clarifying existing international law regarding disability. Even if a state does not ratify the CRPD, it helps interpret other human rights conventions to which the state is party.

Article 3 of the CRPD outlines the following general principles:

1. respect for inherent dignity, individual autonomy including the freedom to make one's own choices, and independence of persons;
2. non-discrimination;
3. full and effective participation and inclusion in society;
4. respect for difference and acceptance of persons with disabilities as part of human diversity and humanity;
5. equality of opportunity;
6. accessibility;
7. equality between men and women;
8. respect for the evolving capacities of children with disabilities and respect for the right of children with disabilities to preserve their identities.

States ratifying the CRPD have a range of general obligations. Among other things, they undertake to:

- adopt legislation and other appropriate administrative measures where needed;
- modify or repeal laws, customs, or practices that discriminate directly or indirectly;
- include disability in all relevant policies and programmes;
- refrain from any act or practice inconsistent with the CRPD;
- take all appropriate measures to eliminate discrimination against persons with disabilities by any person, organization, or private enterprise.

States must consult with people with disabilities and their representative organizations when developing laws, policies, and programmes to implement the CRPD. The Convention also requires public and private bodies to make "reasonable accommodation" to the situation of people with disabilities. And it is accompanied by an Optional Protocol that, if ratified, provides for a complaints procedure and an inquiry procedure, which can be lodged with the committee monitoring the treaty.

The CRPD advances legal disability reform, directly involving people with disabilities and using a human rights framework. Its core message is that people with disabilities should not be considered "objects" to be managed, but "subjects" deserving of equal respect and enjoyment of human rights.

Disability and development

Disability is a development issue, because of its bidirectional link to poverty: disability may increase the risk of poverty, and poverty may increase the risk of disability (63). A growing body of empirical evidence from across the world indicates that people with disabilities and their families are more likely to experience economic and social disadvantage than those without disability.

The onset of disability may lead to the worsening of social and economic well-being and poverty through a multitude of channels including the adverse impact on education, employment, earnings, and increased expenditures related to disability (64).

- Children with disabilities are less likely to attend school, thus experiencing limited opportunities for human capital formation and facing reduced employment opportunities and decreased productivity in adulthood (65–67).
- People with disabilities are more likely to be unemployed and generally earn less even when employed (67–72). Both employment and income outcomes appear to worsen with the severity of the disability (52, 73). It is harder for people with disabilities to benefit from development and escape from poverty (74) due to discrimination in employment, limited access to transport, and lack of access to resources to promote self-employment and livelihood activities (71).
- People with disabilities may have extra costs resulting from disability – such as costs associated with medical care or assistive devices, or the need for personal support and assistance – and thus often require more resources to achieve the same outcomes as non-disabled people. This is what Amartya Sen has called "conversion handicap" (75). Because of higher costs, people with disabilities and their households are likely to be poorer than non-disabled people with similar incomes (75–77).
- Households with a disabled member are more likely to experience material hardship – including food insecurity, poor housing, lack of access to safe water and sanitation, and inadequate access to health care (29, 72, 78–81).

Poverty may increase the risk of disability. A study of 56 developing countries found that the poor experienced worse health than the better off (82). Poverty may lead to the onset of a health conditions associated with disability including through: low birth weight, malnutrition (83, 84), lack of clean water or adequate sanitation, unsafe work and living conditions, and injuries (20, 85–87). Poverty may increase the likelihood that a person with an existing health condition becomes disabled, for example, by an inaccessible environment or lack of access to appropriate health and rehabilitation services (88) (see **Box 1.3**).

Amartya Sen's capabilities approach (91, 92) offers a helpful theoretical underpinning to understanding development, which can be of particular value for the disability human rights field (93) and is compatible with both the ICF (94) and the social model of disability (76). It moves beyond traditional economic measures such as GDP, or concepts of utility, to emphasize human rights and "development as freedom" (91), promoting the understanding that the poverty of people with disabilities – and other disadvantaged peoples – comprises social exclusion and disempowerment, not just lack of material resources. It emphasizes the diversity of aspirations and choices that different people with disabilities might hold in different cultures (95). It also resolves the paradox that many people with disabilities express that they

Box 1.3. Safety net interventions for people with disabilities

The United Nations *Convention on the Rights of Persons with Disabilities* (CRPD) states that people with disabilities have an equal right to social protection. Safety nets are a type of social protection intervention that target vulnerability and poverty.

Many countries provide safety nets to poor people with disabilities and their households, either through specific disability-targeted programmes or more commonly through general social assistance programmes.

While systematic evidence is lacking, anecdotal evidence suggests that persons with disabilities may face barriers to accessing safety nets when, for example, information is inadequate or inaccessible, the welfare offices are physically inaccessible, or the programmes' design features do not take into account specific needs of disabled people. Thus, special measures may be needed to ensure that safety nets are inclusive of disabled people. For example:

- information about programmes should be accessible and reach the intended recipients. This may require targeted outreach;
- proxies designated by persons with disabilities should be allowed to conduct many of the transactions in accessing programmes;
- the welfare offices, as well as the transport system, need to be accessible;
- programmes' eligibility criteria may need to specifically include disability;
- means testing mechanisms may need to take into account the extra costs of disability;
- cash transfers might provide higher payments to beneficiaries with disabilities to help with extra costs of living with a disability;
- conditional cash transfers may need to be adjusted to specific circumstances of children with disabilities;
- workfare can introduce quotas and be sensitive to disability;
- labour activation measures should be sensitive to disability.

Some countries, such as Albania, Bangladesh, Brazil, China, Romania, and the Russian Federation also have specific programmes targeted at people with disabilities. The design of these programmes varies. In some cases they cover all disabled people, in other cases they are means tested, or targeted at children with disabilities.

Administration of disability benefits requires assessment of disability. Many formal assessment processes still use predominantly medical criteria, though there has been a move towards adopting a more comprehensive assessment approach focusing on functioning and using the *International Classification of Functioning, Disability and Health* framework. More research is needed to better understand what works with regards to disability assessment and to identify good practice.

Evidence on the impact of safety nets on people with disabilities is limited. While they may improve health and economic status, it is less clear whether access to education also improves. For safety nets to be effective in protecting disabled people, many other public programmes need to be in place, such as health, rehabilitation, education and training and environmental access. More research is needed to better understand what works in providing safety nets to people with disabilities and their households.

Source (*89, 90*).

have a good quality of life (*96*), perhaps because they have succeeded in adapting to their situation. As Sen has argued, this does not mean that it is not necessary to address what can be objectively assessed as their unmet needs.

The capabilities approach also helps in understanding the obligations that states owe to individuals to ensure that they flourish, exercise agency, and reach their potential as human beings (*97*). The CRPD specifies these obligations to persons with disabilities, emphasizing development and measures to promote the participation and well-being of people with disabilities worldwide. It stresses the need to address disability in all programming rather than as a stand-alone thematic issue. Moreover, its Article 32 is the only international human rights treaty article promoting measures for international cooperation that include, and are accessible to, persons with disabilities.

Box 1.4. The Millennium Development Goals and disability

The Millennium Development Goals (MDGs) – agreed on by the international community in 2000 and endorsed by 189 countries – are a unified set of development objectives addressing the needs of the world's poorest and most marginalized people, and are supposed to be achieved by 2015. The goals are:

1. eradicate extreme poverty and hunger
2. achieve universal primary education
3. promote gender equality and empower women
4. reduce child mortality
5. improve maternal health
6. combat HIV/AIDS, malaria, and other diseases
7. ensure environmental sustainability
8. develop a global partnership for development.

The MDGs are a compact between developing and developed nations. They recognize the efforts that must be taken by developing countries themselves, as well as the contribution that developed countries need to make through trade, development assistance, debt relief, access to essential medicines, and technology transfer.

While some of the background documents explicitly mention people with disabilities, they are not referred to in the MDGs, or in the material generated as part of the process to achieve them.

The 2010 *MDG report* is the first to mention disabilities, noting the limited opportunities facing children with disabilities, and the link between disability and marginalization in education. The Ministerial Declaration of July 2010 recognizes disability as a cross-cutting issue essential for the attainment of the MDGs, emphasizing the need to ensure that women and girls with disabilities are not subject to multiple or aggravated forms of discrimination, or excluded from participation in the implementation of the MDGs (*101*). The United Nations General Assembly has highlighted the invisibility of persons with disabilities in official statistics (*102*).

The General Assembly concluded its High Level Meeting on the MDGs in September 2010 by adopting the resolution "Keeping the promise: united to achieve the Millennium Development Goals," which recognizes that "policies and actions must also focus on persons with disabilities, so that they benefit from progress towards achieving the MDGs" (*103*).

Despite the widely acknowledged interconnection between disability and poverty, efforts to promote development and poverty reduction have not always adequately included disability (*76, 98–100*). Disability is not explicitly mentioned in the eight Millennium Development Goals (MDGs), or the 21 targets, or the 60 indicators for achieving the goals (see Box 1.4).

People with disabilities can benefit from development projects; examples in this Report show that the situation for people with disabilities in low-income countries can be improved. But disability needs to be a higher priority, successful initiatives need to be scaled up, and a more coherent response is needed. In addition, people with disabilities need to be included in development efforts, both as beneficiaries and in the design, implementation, and monitoring of interventions (*104*). Despite the role of CBR (see Box 1.5), and many other promising initiatives by national governments or national and international NGOs, systematic removal of barriers and social development has not occurred, and disability still is often considered in the medical component of development (*104*).

Responses to disability have undergone a radical change in recent decades: the role of environmental barriers and discrimination in contributing to poverty and exclusion is now well understood, and the CRPD outlines the measures needed to remove barriers and promote participation. Disability is a development issue, and it will be hard to improve the lives of the most disadvantaged people in the world

Box 1.5. **Community-based rehabilitation**

Since the 1970s community-based rehabilitation (CBR) has been an important strategy to respond to the needs of people with disabilities, particularly in developing countries. CBR was initially promoted to deliver rehabilitation services in countries with limited resources. Field manuals such as *Training in the community for people with disabilities (105)* provided family members and community workers with practical information about how to implement basic rehabilitation interventions.

More than 90 countries around the world continue to develop and strengthen their CBR programmes. Through an ongoing evolutionary process CBR is shifting from a medical-focused, often single-sector approach, to a strategy for rehabilitation, equalization of opportunities, poverty reduction, and social inclusion of people with disabilities (*106*). Increasingly, CBR is implemented through the combined efforts of people with disabilities, their families, organizations, and communities, and the relevant government and nongovernmental services (*106*).

In Chamarajnagar, one of the poorest districts of Karnataka, India, many community members did not have access to basic sanitation facilities, putting their health at risk. The Indian government offered grants to families living in these areas to construct toilets. The total cost to construct one toilet was estimated to be US$ 150. Funding the remaining amount was difficult for most people, particularly people with disabilities. A local nongovernmental organization – Mobility India – assisted people with disabilities and their families to construct accessible toilets. Using existing community-based networks and self-help groups, Mobility India organized street plays and wall paintings to raise awareness about hygiene and the importance of proper sanitation.

As people became interested and motivated, Mobility India – with financial support from MIBLOU, Switzerland, and local contributions – facilitated access to basic sanitation. The group members selected poor households with disabled family members who had the greatest need for a toilet, and they coordinated the construction work in partnership with families and ensured proper use of funds. As a result of the pilot project, 50 accessible toilets were constructed in one year. Many people with disabilities no longer need to crawl or be carried long distances for their toileting needs. They have become independent and, importantly, been able to reclaim their dignity. Their risk of developing health conditions associated with poor sanitation has also been significantly reduced.

Evidence for the effectiveness of CBR varies, but research and evaluation are increasingly being conducted (*107–110*), and information sharing is increasing through regional networks such as the CBR Africa Network, the CBR Asia-Pacific Network, and the CBR American and Caribbean Network.

The recent publication of the *CBR guidelines (111)* joins the development and human rights aspects of disability. The guidelines:

- promote the need for inclusive development for people with disabilities in the mainstream health, education, social, and employment sectors;
- emphasize the need to promote the empowerment of people with disabilities and their family members;
- through the provision of practical suggestions, position CBR as a tool that countries can use to implement the *Convention on the Rights of Persons with Disabilities*.

without addressing the specific needs of persons with disabilities.

This *World report on disability* provides a guide to improving the health and well-being of persons with disabilities. It seeks to provide clear concepts and the best available evidence, to highlight gaps in knowledge and stress the need for further research and policy. Stories of success are recounted, as are those of failure and neglect. The ultimate goal of the Report and of the CRPD is to enable all people with disabilities to enjoy the choices and life opportunities currently available to only a minority by minimizing the adverse impacts of impairment and eliminating discrimination and prejudice.

People's capabilities depend on external conditions that can be modified by government action. In line with the CRPD, this Report shows how the capabilities of people with disabilities can be expanded; their well-being, agency, and freedom improved; and their human rights realized.

References

1. Zola IK. Toward the necessary universalizing of a disability policy. *The Milbank Quarterly*, 1989,67:Suppl 2 Pt 2401-428. doi:10.2307/3350151 PMID:2534158

2. Ferguson PM. Mapping the family: disability studies and the exploration of parental response to disability. In: Albrecht G, Seelman KD, Bury M, eds. *Handbook of Disability Studies*. Thousand Oaks, Sage, 2001:373–395.

3. Mishra AK, Gupta R. Disability index: a measure of deprivation among the disabled. *Economic and Political Weekly*, 2006,41:4026-4029.

4. Lee R. The demographic transition: three centuries of fundamental change. *The Journal of Economic Perspectives*, 2003,17:167-190. doi:10.1257/089533003772034943

5. Campbell J, Oliver M. *Disability politics: understanding our past, changing our future*. London, Routledge, 1996.

6. Charlton J. *Nothing about us without us: disability, oppression and empowerment*. Berkeley, University of California Press, 1998

7. Quinn G, Degener T. A survey of international, comparative and regional disability law reform. In: Breslin ML, Yee S, eds. *Disability rights law and policy - international and national perspectives*. Ardsley, Transnational, 2002a.

8. Parmenter TR. The present, past and future of the study of intellectual disability: challenges in developing countries. *Salud Pública de México*, 2008,50:Suppl 2s124-s131. PMID:18470339

9. *Standard rules on the equalization of opportunities of persons with disabilities*, New York, United Nations, 2003.

10. Driedger D. *The last civil rights movement*. London, Hurst, 1989.

11. Barnes C. *Disabled people in Britain and discrimination*. London, Hurst, 1991.

12. McConachie H et al. Participation of disabled children: how should it be characterised and measured? *Disability and Rehabilitation*, 2006,28:1157-1164. doi:10.1080/09638280500534507 PMID:16966237

13. Oliver M. *The politics of disablement*. Basingstoke, Macmillan and St Martin's Press, 1990.

14. Thomas C. *Female forms: experiencing and understanding disability*. Buckingham, Open University Press, 1999.

15. Shakespeare T. *Disability rights and wrongs*. London, Routledge, 2006.

16. Forsyth R et al. Participation of young severely disabled children is influenced by their intrinsic impairments and environment. *Developmental Medicine and Child Neurology*, 2007,49:345-349. doi:10.1111/j.1469-8749.2007.00345.x PMID:17489807

17. The International Classification of Functioning. *Disability and Health*. Geneva, World Health Organization, 2001.

18. Bickenbach JE, Chatterji S, Badley EM, Ustün TB. Models of disablement, universalism and the international classification of impairments, disabilities and handicaps. *Social science & medicine (1982)*, 1999,48:1173-1187. doi:10.1016/S0277-9536(98)00441-9 PMID:10220018

19. Leonardi M et al. MHADIE ConsortiumThe definition of disability: what is in a name? *Lancet*, 2006,368:1219-1221. doi:10.1016/S0140-6736(06)69498-1 PMID:17027711

20. Commission on Social Determinants of Health. *Closing the gap in a generation: Health equity through action on the social determinants of health*. Geneva, World Health Organization, 2008.

21. Miller P, Parker S, Gillinson S. *Disablism: how to tackle the last prejudice*. London, Demos, 2004.

22. Smith RD. Promoting the health of people with physical disabilities: a discussion of the financing and organization of public health services in Australia. *Health Promotion International*, 2000,15:79-86. doi:10.1093/heapro/15.1.79

23. Scheer JM, Kroll T, Neri MT, Beatty P. Access barriers for persons with disabilities: the consumers perspective. *Journal of Disability Policy Studies*, 2003,13:221-230. doi:10.1177/104420730301300404

24. *Quality in and equality of access to healthcare services*. Brussels, European Commission, Directorate General for Employment, Social Affairs and Equal Opportunities, 2008.

25. *Improving the life chances of disabled people: final report*. London, Prime Minister's Strategy Unit, 2005.

26. Ingstad B, Whyte SR, eds. *Disability and culture*. Berkley, University of California Press, 1995.

27. Yazbeck M, McVilly K, Parmenter TR. Attitudes towards people with intellectual disabilities: an Australian perspective. *Journal of Disability Policy Studies*, 2004,15:97-111. doi:10.1177/10442073040150020401

28. *People with disabilities in India: from commitments to outcomes*. Washington, World Bank, 2009.

29. Van Brakel WH. Measuring health-related stigma–a literature review. *Psychology, Health & Medicine*, 2006,11:307-334. doi:10.1080/13548500600595160 PMID:17130068

30. Siperstein GN, Norins J, Corbin S, Shriver T. *Multinational study of attitudes towards individuals with intellectual disabilities*. Washington, Special Olympics Inc, 2003.

31. Lauber C, Rössler W. Stigma towards people with mental illness in developing countries in Asia. *International Review of Psychiatry (Abingdon, England)*, 2007,19:157-178. PMID:17464793

32. Thornicroft G, Rose D, Kassam A. Discrimination in health care against people with mental illness. *International Review of Psychiatry (Abingdon, England)*, 2007,19:113-122. PMID:17464789

33. *Hate crime against disabled people in Scotland: a survey report*, Edinburgh, Capability Scotland and Disability Rights Commission, 2004.

34. *Fact sheet: leprosy*. Geneva, World Health Organization, 2009 (http://www.who.int/mediacentre/factsheets/fs101/en/index.html, accessed 29 January 2009).

35. Wong ML. Guest editorial: designing programmes to address stigma in leprosy: issues and challenges. *Asia and Pacific Disability Rehabilitation Journal*, 2004,15:3-12.

36. *India: leprosy awareness*. London, BBC World Service Trust, n.d. (http://www.bbc.co.uk/worldservice/trust/news/story/2003/09/010509_leprosy.shtml accessed 1 February 2011).

37. Cross H. Interventions to address the stigma associated with leprosy: a perspective on the issues. *Psychology, Health & Medicine*, 2006,11:367-373. doi:10.1080/13548500600595384 PMID:17130073

38. Sartorius N, Schulze H. *Reducing the stigma of mental illness: a report from a global programme of the World Psychiatric Association*. Cambridge, Cambridge University Press, 2005.

39. Sartorius N. Lessons from a 10-year global programme against stigma and discrimination because of an illness. *Psychology, Health & Medicine*, 2006,11:383-388. doi:10.1080/13548500600595418 PMID:17130075

40. Thornicroft G, Brohan E, Kassam A, Lewis-Holmes E. Reducing stigma and discrimination: Candidate interventions. *International Journal of Mental Health Systems*, 2008,2:3- doi:10.1186/1752-4458-2-3 PMID:18405393

41. *International programme to fight stigma and discrimination because of schizophrenia*. Geneva, World Psychiatric Association., n.d. (www.openthedoors.com, accessed 14 October 2010).

42. Joa I et al. The key to reducing duration of untreated first psychosis: information campaigns. *Schizophrenia Bulletin*, 2007, doi:10.1093/schbul/sbm09510.1093/schbul/sbm095

43. Dalal AK. Social interventions to moderate discriminatory attitudes: the case of the physically challenged in India. *Psychology, Health & Medicine*, 2006,11:374-382. doi:10.1080/13548500600595392 PMID:17130074

44. Park A et al. *British social attitudes survey 23rd report*. London, Sage, 2007.

45. Watson N. Well, I know this is going to sound very strange to you, but I don't see myself as a disabled person: identity and disability. *Disability & Society*, 2002,17:509-527. doi:10.1080/09687590220148496

46. *National Health Survey 2007–8: summary of results*. Canberra, Australian Bureau of Statistics, 2009.

47. *Learning lessons: defining, representing and measuring disability*. London, Disability Rights Commission, 2007.

48. Nagata KK. Gender and disability in the Arab region: the challenges in the new millennium. *Asia Pacific Disability Rehabilitation Journal*, 2003,14:10-17.

49. Rao I. *Equity to women with disabilities in India*. Bangalore, CBR Network, 2004 (http://v1.dpi.org/lang-en/resources/details.php?page=90, accessed 6 August 2010).

50. Roulstone A, Barnes C, eds. *Working futures? Disabled people, policy and social inclusion*. Bristol, Policy Press, 2005.

51. Grech S. Living with disability in rural Guatemala: exploring connections and impacts on poverty. *International Journal of Disability, Community and Rehabilitation*, 2008, 7(2) (http://www.ijdcr.ca/VOL07_02_CAN/articles/grech.shtml, accessed 4 August 2010).

52. Grammenos S. *Illness, disability and social inclusion*. Dublin, European Foundation for the Improvement of Living and Working Conditions, 2003 (http://www.eurofound.europa.eu/pubdocs/2003/35/en/1/ef0335en.pdf, accessed 6 August 2010).

53. Caulfield LE et al. Stunting, wasting and micronutrient deficiency disorders. In: Jamison DT et al., eds. *Disease control priorities in developing countries*. Washington, Oxford University Press and World Bank, 2006:551–567.

54. Maart S, Jelsma J. The sexual behaviour of physically disabled adolescents. *Disability and Rehabilitation*, 2010,32:438-443. doi:10.3109/09638280902846368 PMID:20113191

55. McIlfatrick S, Taggart L, Truesdale-Kennedy M. Supporting women with intellectual disabilities to access breast cancer screening: a healthcare professional perspective. *European Journal of Cancer Care*, 2011,20:412-20. doi:10.1111/j.1365-2354.2010.01221.x PMID:20825462

56. Atijosan O et al. The orthopaedic needs of children in Rwanda: results from a national survey and orthopaedic service implications. *Journal of Pediatric Orthopedics*, 2009,29:948-951. PMID:19934715

57. Wang CC. Portraying stigmatized conditions: disabling images in public health. *Journal of Health Communication*, 1998,3:149-159. doi:10.1080/108107398127436 PMID:10977251

58. Lollar DJ, Crews JE. Redefining the role of public health in disability. *Annual Review of Public Health*, 2003,24:195-208. doi:10.1146/annurev.publhealth.24.100901.140844 PMID:12668756

59. Coleridge P, Simonnot C, Steverlynck D. *Study of disability in EC Development Cooperation*. Brussels, European Commission, 2010.

60. Quinn G et al. The current use and future potential of United Nations human rights instruments in the context of disability. New York and Geneva, United Nations, 2002b (http://www.icrpd.net/ratification/documents/en/Extras/Quinn%20Degener%20study%20for%20OHCHR.pdf, accessed 21 Sept 2010).

61. *Convention on the Rights of Persons with Disabilities*. Geneva, United Nations, 2006 (http://www2.ohchr.org/english/law/disabilities-convention.htm, accessed 16 May 2009).

62. Megret F. The disabilities convention: human rights of persons with disabilities or disability rights? *Human Rights Quarterly*, 2008,30:494-516.

63. Sen A. *The idea of justice*. Cambridge, The Belknap Press of Harvard University Press, 2009.

64. Jenkins SP, Rigg JA. *Disability and disadvantage: selection, onset and duration effects*. London, London School of Economics, Centre for Analysis of Social Exclusion, 2003 (CASEpaper 74).

65. Filmer D. Disability, poverty and schooling in developing countries: results from 14 household surveys. *The World Bank Economic Review*, 2008,22:141-163. doi:10.1093/wber/lhm021

66. Mete C, ed. *Economic implications of chronic illness and disability in Eastern Europe and the Former Soviet Union*. Washington, World Bank, 2008.

67. Burchardt T. *The education and employment of disabled young people: frustrated ambition*. Bristol, Policy Press, 2005.

68. *Sickness, disability and work: breaking the barriers. A synthesis of findings across OECD countries*. Paris, Organisation for Economic Co-operation and Development, 2010.

69. Houtenville AJ, Stapleton DC, Weathers RR 2nd, Burkhauser RV, eds. *Counting working-age people with disabilities. What current data tell us and options for improvement*. Kalamazoo, WE Upjohn Institute for Employment Research, 2009.

70. Contreras DG, Ruiz-Tagle JV, Garcez P, Azocar I. *Socio-economic impact of disability in Latin America: Chile and Uruguay*. Santiago, Universidad de Chile, Departemento de Economia, 2006.

71. Coleridge P. Disabled people and 'employment' in the majority world: policies and realities. In: Roulstone A, Barnes C, eds. *Working futures? Disabled people, policy and social inclusion*. Bristol, Policy Press, 2005.

72. Mitra S, Posarac A, Vick B. *Disability and poverty in developing countries: a snapshot from the world health survey*. Washington, Human Development Network *Social Protection*, forthcoming

73. Emmett T. Disability, poverty, gender and race. In: Watermeyer B et al., eds. *Disability and social change: a South African agenda*. Cape Town, HSRC Press, 2006.

74. Thomas P. *Disability, poverty and the Millennium Development Goals*. London, Disability Knowledge and Research, 2005 (www.disabilitykar.net/docs/policy_final.doc, accessed 20 July 2010).

75. Zaidi A, Burchardt T. Comparing incomes when needs differ: equivalization for the extra costs of disability in the UK. *Review of Income and Wealth*, 2005,51:89-114. doi:10.1111/j.1475-4991.2005.00146.x

76. Braithwaite J, Mont D. Disability and poverty: a survey of World Bank poverty assessments and implications. *ALTER – European Journal of Disability Research / Revue Européenne de Recherche sur le Handicap*, 2009,3:219-232. doi:10.1016/j.alter.2008.10.002

77. Cullinan J, Gannon B, Lyons S. Estimating the extra cost of living for people with disabilities. *Health Economics*, 2010, doi:10.1002/hec.1619 PMID:20535832

78. Beresford B, Rhodes D. *Housing and disabled children*. York, Joseph Rowntree Foundation, 2008.

79. Loeb M, Eide H. *Living conditions among people with activity limitations in Malawi: a national representative study*. Oslo, SINTEF, 2004 (http://www.safod.org/Images/LCMalawi.pdf).

80. Eide A, van Rooy G, Loeb M. *Living conditions among people with activity limitations in Namibia: a representative national survey*. Oslo, SINTEF, 2003 (http://www.safod.org/Images/LCNamibia.pdf, accessed 15 February 2011).

81. Eide A, Loeb M. *Living conditions among people with activity limitations in Zambia: a national representative study*. Oslo, SINTEF, 2006 (http://www.sintef.no/upload/Helse/Levek%C3%A5r%20og%20tjenester/ZambiaLCweb.pdf, accessed 15 February 2011).

82. Gwatkin DR et al. *Socioeconomic differences in health, nutrition, and population within developing countries*. Washington, World Bank, 2007 (Working Paper 30544).

83. Maternal and child undernutrition [special series]. *Lancet*, January2008,

84. *Monitoring child disability in developing countries: results from the multiple indicator cluster surveys*. United Nations Children's Fund, Division of Policy and Practice, 2008.

85. Emerson E et al. Socio-economic position, household composition, health status and indicators of the well-being of mothers of children with and without intellectual disabilities. *Journal of Intellectual Disability Research: JIDR*, 2006,50:862-873. doi:10.1111/j.1365-2788.2006.00900.x PMID:17100947

86. Emerson E, Hatton C. The socio-economic circumstances of children at risk of disability in Britain. *Disability & Society*, 2007,22:563-580. doi:10.1080/09687590701560154

87. Rauh VA, Landrigan PJ, Claudio L. Housing and health: intersection of poverty and environmental exposures. *Annals of the New York Academy of Sciences*, 2008,1136:276-288. doi:10.1196/annals.1425.032 PMID:18579887

88. Peters DH et al. Poverty and access to health care in developing countries. *Annals of the New York Academy of Sciences*, 2008,1136:161-171. doi:10.1196/annals.1425.011 PMID:17954679

89. Grosh M, del Ninno C, Tesliuc E, Ouerghi A. *For protection and promotion: the design and implementation of effective safety nets*. Washington, World Bank, 2008.

90. Marriott A, Gooding K. *Social assistance and disability in developing countries*. Haywards Heath, Sightsavers International, 2007.

91. Sen A. *Development as freedom*. New York, Knopf, 1999.

92. Sen A. *Inequality reexamined*. New York and Cambridge, Russell Sage and Harvard University Press, 1992.

93. Dubois JL, Trani JF. Extending the capability paradigm to address the complexity of disability. *Alter*, 2009,3:192-218.

94. Mitra S. The capability approach and disability. *Journal of Disability Policy Studies*, 2006,16:236-247. doi:10.1177/10442073 060160040501

95. Clark DA. The capability approach. In: Clark DA, ed. The Elgar companion to development studies. Cheltenham, Edward Elgar, 2006.

96. Albrecht GL, Devlieger PJ. The disability paradox: high quality of life against all odds. *Social Science & Medicine (1982)*, 1999,48:977-988. doi:10.1016/S0277-9536(98)00411-0 PMID:10390038

97. Stein MA, Stein PJS. Beyond disability civil rights. *The Hastings Law Journal*, 2007,58:1203-1240.

98. Fritz D et al. Making poverty reduction inclusive: experiences from Cambodia, Tanzania and Vietnam. *Journal of International Development*, 2009,21:673-684. doi:10.1002/jid.1595

99. Mwendwa TN, Murangira A, Lang R. Mainstreaming the rights of persons with disabilities in national development frameworks. *Journal of International Development*, 2009,21:662-672. doi:10.1002/jid.1594

100. Riddell RC. Poverty, disability and aid: international development cooperation. In Barron T, Ncube JM, eds. *Poverty and Disability*. London, Leonard Cheshire Disability, 2010.

101. Implementing the internationally agreed goals and commitments in regard to gender equality and empowerment of women. New York, United Nations, Economic and Social Council, 2010 (E/2010/L.8, OP 9).

102. Realizing the MDGs for persons with disabilities. New York, United Nations, General Assembly, 2010 (A/RES/64/131).

103. Draft outcome document of the high-level plenary meeting of the General Assembly on the Millennium Development Goals. New York, United Nations, General Assembly, 2010 (A/RES/64/299, OP 28).

104. Kett M, Lang R, Trani JF. Disability, development and the dawning of a new Convention: a cause for optimism? *Journal of International Development*, 2009,21:649-661. doi:10.1002/jid.1596

105. *Training in the community for people with disabilities*. Geneva, World Health Organization, 1989.

106. CBR. *a strategy for rehabilitation, equalization of opportunities, poverty reduction and social inclusion of people with disabilities: joint position paper*. Geneva, World Health Organization, 2004.

107. Mitchell R. The research base of community-based rehabilitation. *Disability and Rehabilitation*, 1999,21:459-468. doi:10.1080/096382899297251 PMID:10579666

108. Mannan H, Turnbull A. A review of community based rehabilitation evaluations: Quality of life as an outcome measure for future evaluations. *Asia Pacific Disability Rehabilitation Journal*, 2007,64:1231-1241.

109. Kuipers P, Wirz S, Hartley S. Systematic synthesis of community-based rehabilitation (CBR) project evaluation reports for evidence-based policy: a proof-of-concept study. *BMC International Health and Human Rights*, 2008,8:3- doi:10.1186/1472-698X-8-3 PMID:18325121

110. Finkenflügel H, Wolffers I, Huijsman R. The evidence base for community-based rehabilitation: a literature review. *International Journal of Rehabilitation Research. Internationale Zeitschrift fur Rehabilitationsforschung. Revue Internationale de Recherches de Réadaptation*, 2005,28:187-201. PMID:16046912

111. World Health Organization, United Nations Educational, Scientific and Cultural Organization, International Labour Organization, International Disability and Development Consortium. *Community-based rehabilitation: CBR guidelines*. Geneva, World Health Organization, 2010.

Chapter 2

Disability – a global picture

"I lost my leg by landmine when I was 5 years old, at that time I went to the rice field with my mother to get firewood. Unfortunately I stepped on a mine. After the accident I was very sad when I saw the other children playing or swimming in the river because I have no leg. I used to stand with my crutch made of wood and I wish I could play freely like the other children too. And when I walked to school some children they called me *kombot*, meaning disabled person, and [the discrimination] make me feel shy and cry and disappointed. So I want all people to have equal rights and not discriminate against each other."

Song

"At the age of 9, I became deaf as a result of a bout with meningitis. In 2002, I went for Voluntary Counseling and Testing (VCT). The results showed that I was HIV+. I become devastated and lost hope to live because I thought that being HIV+ was the end of world for me. Later, I met a disabled person who spiritually encouraged me to accept my status. Now I have confidence to be able to speak out on HIV/AIDS openly. I have been interviewed widely by print and electronic media and I have been invited to speak in public meetings. I am creating awareness on the importance of VCT and encouraging people to know their status. My work is limited by lack of money. Deaf people living in rural areas have no information on HIV/AIDS. I would like to break the barriers by going to visit them right where they live."

Susan

"What makes me to feel not included in this school is because my parents are poor, they can't provide me with enough books. This makes my life difficult in the school. They also can't buy me everything which I am supposed to have, like clothes. Being in school without books and pens also makes me feel not included, because teachers used to send me out because I don't have books to write in."

Jackline

2

Disability – a global picture

Robust evidence helps to make well informed decisions about disability policies and programmes. Understanding the numbers of people with disabilities and their circumstances can improve efforts to remove disabling barriers and provide services to allow people with disabilities to participate. Collecting appropriate statistical and research data at national and international levels will help parties to the United Nations *Convention on the Rights of Persons with Disabilities* (CRPD) formulate and implement policies to achieve internationally agreed development goals (*1*).

This chapter offers a picture of disability that succeeding chapters build on. It presents estimates of the prevalence of disability; factors affecting trends in disability (demographic, health, environmental); the socioeconomic circumstances of people with disabilities, need and unmet needs, and the costs of disability. It proposes steps for improving data at national and international levels.

The evidence here is based on national (such as the census, population surveys and administrative data registries) and international data sets and a large number of recent studies. Each source has its purposes, strengths, and weaknesses. The data here are, to varying degrees, in accord with the definition of disability outlined in Chapter 1. Additional data and methodological explanations are in the Technical appendices (A, B, C, and D).

Measuring disability

Disability, a complex multidimensional experience (see Chapter 1), poses several challenges for measurement. Approaches to measuring disability vary across countries and influence the results. Operational measures of disability vary according to the purpose and application of the data, the conception of disability, the aspects of disability examined – impairments, activity limitations, participation restrictions, related health conditions, environmental factors – the definitions, question design, reporting sources, data collection methods, and expectations of functioning.

Impairment data are not an adequate proxy for disability information. Broad "groupings" of different "types of disability" have become part of the language of disability, with some surveys seeking to determine the prevalence of different "types of disability" based directly or indirectly on assessments and classifications. Often, "types of disability" are defined using only one aspect of disability, such as impairments – sensory, physical, mental, intellectual – and at other times they conflate health conditions with disability. People with chronic health conditions, communication difficulties, and other impairments may not be included in these estimates, despite encountering difficulties in everyday life.

There is an implicit assumption that each "type of disability" has specific health, educational, rehabilitation, social, and support needs. However, diverse responses may be required – for example, two individuals with the same impairment may have very different experiences and needs. While countries may need information on impairments – for instance, to help design specific services or to detect or prevent discrimination – the usefulness of such data is limited, because the resulting prevalence rates are not indicative of the entire extent of disability.

Data on all aspects of disability and contextual factors are important for constructing a complete picture of disability and functioning. Without information on how particular health conditions in interaction with environmental barriers and facilitators affect people in their everyday lives, it is hard to determine the scope of disability. People with the same impairment can experience very different types and degrees of restriction, depending on the context. Environmental barriers to participation can differ considerably between countries and communities. For example, many children drop out of school in Brazil because of a lack of reading glasses, widely available in most high-income countries (*2*). Stigma attached to impairments as diverse as missing limbs and anxiety, can result in similar limits on a person's participation in work. This was shown in a recent comparison between two surveys in the United States of America that focused on the work limitations of individuals and on actual work performance (*3*).

Disability can be conceptualized on a continuum from minor difficulties in functioning to major impacts on a person's life. Countries are increasingly switching to a continuum approach to measurement, where estimates of prevalence of disability – and functioning – are derived from assessing levels of disability in multiple domains (*4–8*). Estimates vary according to where the thresholds on the continuum of disability are set, and the way environmental influences are taken into account. Disaggregating these data further by sex, age, income, or occupation is important for uncovering patterns, trends, and other information about "subgroups" of people experiencing disability.

The data collection method also influences results. Censuses and surveys take varying approaches to measuring disability, and the use of these approaches to data collection in the same country often report different rates of disability (see **Box 2.1**). Censuses cover entire populations, occur at long intervals, and by their nature can incorporate only a few disability-relevant questions. While considerable socioeconomic data, such as employment rates and marital status, are available from censuses, they can provide only limited information about participation. On the other hand, censuses tend to be carried out regularly and so can also give information on trends over a certain period. Surveys have the possibility of providing richer information through more comprehensive questions including on institutionalized populations. In developed countries, for example, survey questions identify people with disabilities for impairments in body function and structure, but also increasingly for activities, participation, and environmental factors. Some surveys also provide information on the origins of impairments, the degree of assistance provided, service accessibility, and unmet needs.

Countries reporting a low disability prevalence rate – predominantly developing countries – tend to collect disability data through censuses or use measures focused exclusively on a narrow choice of impairments (*10–12*). Countries reporting higher disability prevalence tend to collect their data through surveys and apply a measurement approach that records activity limitations and participation restrictions in

Box 2.1. The Irish census and the disability survey of 2006

In April 2006 the Central Statistics Office in Ireland carried out a population census that included two questions on disability relating the presence of a long-term health condition and the impact of that condition on functioning. It found that 393 785 people in Ireland were disabled, a rate of 9.3%. Later in 2006 the Central Statistics Office's National Disability Survey (NDS) followed up with a sample of those who had reported a disability in the census, plus a group of people in private households who had not reported a disability. The NDS used a broader definition of disability than the census, with more domains, including pain and breathing, and a measure of severity. Completed questionnaires were received from 14 518 people who had reported a disability in the census and from 1551 who had not done so.

There was a high degree of consistency between the responses to the census and the NDS:

- of those in private households who reported a disability in the census, 88% also reported a disability in the NDS;
- of those in non-private households who reported a disability in the census, 97% also reported a disability in the NDS;
- of those in private households who did not report a disability in the census, 11.5% were found to have a disability in the NDS.

Extrapolating the NDS findings to the whole population produced an overall national disability rate of 18.5%. The differences in the disability rates obtained in the census and the NDS may result from the following:

- The NDS used face-to-face interviews, while the census forms were self-completed.
- The census was a large survey designed for a range of purposes. The NDS focused solely on disability defined as difficulties in functioning in any of the following domains: seeing, hearing, speech, mobility and dexterity, remembering and concentrating, intellectual and learning, emotional, psychological, and mental health, and pain and breathing.
- The inclusion of a pain domain in the NDS resulted in a significantly higher disability rate, with 46% of those not reporting disabilities in the census reporting pain in the NDS.
- Those who only reported a disability in the NDS had a lower level of difficulty and were more likely to have only a single disability, rather than disabilities in several domains.
- More children reported a disability in the NDS than in the census, perhaps because of the more detailed questions in the NDS.

This example shows that prevalence estimates can be affected by the number and type of questions, the level-of-difficulty scale, the range of explicit disabilities, and the survey methodology. The differences between the two measures are mainly due to the domains included and the threshold of the definition of disability. If the domain coverage is narrow (for example, pain is excluded) many people experiencing difficulties in functioning may be excluded. Where resources permit, specific surveys on disability, with comprehensive domain coverage, should be carried out in addition to a census. They provide more comprehensive data, across age groups, for policy and programmes.

Note: The actual questions used in the two surveys are available in the published reports.

Sources (5, 9).

addition to impairments. If institutionalized populations are included in a survey, prevalence rates will also be higher (13). These factors influence comparability at the national and international levels and the relevance of the data to a wider set of users. While progress is being made – as with activity limitation studies in Lesotho, Malawi, Mozambique, Zambia, and Zimbabwe – accurate data on disability are mostly lacking for developing countries.

The question design and reporting source can affect estimates. The underlying purpose of a survey – whether a health or general survey, for instance – will affect how people respond (14). Several studies have found differences in "prevalence" between self-reported and measured aspects of disability (15–18). Disability is interpreted in relation to what is considered normal functioning, which can vary based on the context, age group, or even income group

(2). For example, older persons may not self-identify as having a disability, despite having significant difficulties in functioning, because they consider their level of functioning appropriate for their age.

Where children are involved, there are further complexities. Parents or caregivers – the natural proxy responders in surveys – may not accurately represent the experience of the child (19). Questions in surveys developed for adults but used for children may also skew results. Imprecise or off-putting wording in the questions – such as using the word "disabled" when asking about difficulty with an activity (20, 21) – can also result in under-reporting (2).

Comparisons across populations must take these factors into account. Ideally, comparisons should adjust the data for differences in certain methodological effects – such as interviews and examination surveys – where such adjustments are soundly based.

A primary goal of collecting population data on people with disabilities is to identify strategies to improve their well-being. Comprehensive and systematic documentation of all aspects of functioning of the population can support the design and monitoring of interventions. For instance, such data would enable policy-makers to assess the potential benefit of assistance programmes to help people with mobility limitations get to work or to assess interventions to reduce depression (2). Data on prevalence and need should be population-based and relevant to policy, but at the same time not dependent on policy. If data are dependent on policy, estimated prevalence rates can suddenly change if, for example, the benefit system changed and people switched from an unemployment benefit to a disability benefit. With population data and administrative and service data based on the same basic concepts and frameworks, a strong integrated national information database can be developed.

International standards on data and standardized question sets can improve harmonization across the various approaches. There have been attempts in recent years to standardize disability surveys (see Technical appendix B) (22, 23). But the definitions and methodologies used vary so greatly between countries that international comparisons still remain difficult. This also makes it hard for signatories of the CRPD to monitor their progress in implementing the Convention against a common set of indicators.

Data gathered need to be relevant at the national level and comparable at the global level – both of which can be achieved by basing design on international standards, like the *International Classification of Functioning, Disability and Health* (ICF).

International frameworks and resources are important in these efforts.
- Policy frameworks and agreed principles are set out in the CRPD.
- Information-related standards are provided by the ICF (24, 25).
- Attempts to harmonize and standardize question sets for assessment of health status and disability at population level are in progress (see Technical appendix B for information on European Statistical System, United Nations Washington Group on Disability Statistics, United Nations Economic and Social Commission for Asia and the Pacific (UNESCAP), WHO Regional Office for the Americas/Pan American Health Organization/Budapest Initiative).
- A training manual on disability statistics, prepared by WHO and UNESCAP, provides useful guidance on how countries can enhance their national statistics (26).

Prevalence of disability – difficulties in functioning

In examining the prevalence of disability in the world today, this Report presents country-reported estimates of disability prevalence, as well as prevalence estimates based on two large data sources: the WHO *World Health Survey* of 2002–2004, from 59 countries, and the WHO

Global Burden of Disease study, 2004 update. These sources can be used to examine the prevalence of disability, but they are not directly comparable because they use different approaches to estimating and measuring disability.

Country-reported disability prevalence

More countries have been collecting prevalence data on disability through censuses and surveys, with many having moved from an "impairment" approach to a "difficulties in functioning" approach. Estimated prevalence rates vary widely across and within countries (*2, 11, 27*). Box 2.1 shows variations between two sources of disability data in Ireland. Technical appendix A gives an idea of the variation across countries in conceptual framework, method, and prevalence – from under 1% of the population to over 30% – and illustrates the difficulties surrounding the comparison of existing national data sets. As discussed previously, most developing countries report disability prevalence rates below those reported in many developed countries, because they collect data on a narrow set of impairments, which yield lower disability prevalence estimates.

A growing number of countries are using the ICF framework and related question sets in their national surveys and censuses (*5–8, 28–30*). Experience in Zambia that makes use of the Washington Group's six questions for census is outlined in Box 2.2. These efforts by countries – together with global and regional initiatives (see technical appendices A and B for details) – will eventually lead to more standardized and thus more comparable estimates of country disability prevalence.

Global estimates of disability prevalence

The two sources of statistical information to estimate global disability prevalence in this Report, the *World Health Survey* and the *Global Burden of Disease*, both have limitations with regard to disability. So the prevalence estimates presented here should be taken not as definitive but as reflecting current knowledge and available data.

Estimates based on the WHO World Health Survey

The *World Health Survey*, a face-to-face household survey in 2002–2004, is the largest multinational health and disability survey ever using a single set of questions and consistent methods to collect comparable health data across countries. The conceptual framework and functioning domains for the *World Health Survey* came from the ICF (*24, 32*). The questionnaire covered the health of individuals in various domains, health system responsiveness, household expenditures, and living conditions (*33*). A total of 70 countries were surveyed, of which 59 countries, representing 64% of the world population, had weighted data sets that were used for estimating the prevalence of disability of the world's adult population aged 18 years and older (*33*). The countries in the survey were chosen based on several considerations:

- the need to fill data gaps in geographical regions where data were most lacking, such as sub-Saharan Africa;
- a spread of countries that would include high-income, middle-income, and low-income countries with a focus on low-income and middle-income countries;
- inclusion of countries with large adult populations.

The samples were drawn from each country's sampling frame at the time of the *World Health Survey*, using a stratified, multistage cluster. The survey used a consistent conceptual framework to identify measurement domains.

The choice of domains to include in the *World Health Survey* was informed by analysis of WHO's MultiCountry Survey Study (MCSS). To arrive at the most parsimonious set of domains that would explain most of the variance in the valuation of health and functioning, the domains of affect, cognition, interpersonal relationships, mobility, pain, sleep and energy, self-care, and vision were included. Although hearing impairment is the most common of sensory impairments and markedly increases with age, reporting biases in general population surveys, low-endorsement rates in the general population, and the domain of hearing not contributing significantly to explaining the variance led to this domain being dropped from the *World Health Survey* (*15, 34*).

Possible self-reported responses to the questions on difficulties in functioning included: no difficulty, mild difficulty, moderate difficulty, severe difficulty, and extreme difficulty. These were scored, and a composite disability score calculated, ranging from 0 to 100, where 0 represented "no disability" and 100 was "complete disability". This process produced a continuous score range. To divide the population into "disabled" and "not disabled" groups it was necessary to create a threshold value (cut-off point). A threshold of 40 on the scale 0–100 was set to include within estimates of disability, those experiencing significant

---

Box 2.2. Using the Washington Group questions to understand disability in Zambia

The Washington Group on Disability Statistics was set up by the United Nations Statistical Commission in 2001 as an international, consultative group of experts to facilitate the measurement of disability and the comparison of data on disability across countries. The Washington Group applies an ICF-based approach to disability and follows the principles and practices of national statistical agencies as defined by the United Nations Statistical Commission. Its questions cover six functional domains or basic actions: seeing, hearing, mobility, cognition, self-care, and communication. The questions asking about difficulties in performing certain activities because of a health problem are as follows.

1. Do you have difficulty seeing, even if wearing glasses?
2. Do you have difficulty hearing, even if using a hearing aid?
3. Do you have difficulty walking or climbing steps?
4. Do you have difficulty remembering or concentrating?
5. Do you have difficulty with self-care, such as washing all over or dressing?
6. Using your usual (customary) language, do you have difficulty communicating (for example, understanding or being understood by others)?

Each question has four types of response, designed to capture the full spectrum of functioning, from mild to severe: no difficulty, some difficulty, a lot of difficulty and unable to do it at all.

This set of Washington Group questions was included in a 2006 survey of living conditions in Zambia. They had screened people with conditions, which had lasted or were expected to last for six months or more. The prevalence of difficulty in each of the six domains could be calculated from the responses (see table below).

Prevalence of disability by domain and degree of difficulty, Zambia 2006

Core domains	Degree of difficulty		
	At least some difficulty (%)	At least a lot of difficulty (%)	Unable to do it at all (%)
Seeing	4.7	2.6	0.5
Hearing	3.7	2.3	0.5
Mobility	5.1	3.8	0.8
Cognition	2.0	1.5	0.3
Self-care	2.0	1.3	0.4
Communication	2.1	1.4	0.5

Note: *n* = 28 010; 179 missing.
Source (*31*).

continues ...

... continued

Within each degree of difficulty, problems encountered with mobility were the most prevalent, followed by seeing and hearing difficulties. The results in the table were not mutually exclusive, and many individuals had a disability that covered more than one domain.

Measures that reflect the multidimensionality of disability, constructed from the results of the Washington Group questions, are in the table below.

Measures reflecting multidimensionality of disability, Zambia 2006

	Number	Percent
At least one domain is scored "some difficulty" (or higher)	4053	14.5
At least one domain is scored "a lot of difficulty" (or higher). This measure excludes those with the mildest degrees of difficulty.	2368	8.5
At least one domain is scored "cannot do it at all". This measure focuses on the most severe levels of difficulty.	673	2.4
More than one domain is scored "some difficulty" (or higher). This measure focuses on difficulties with multiple actions.	1718	6.1

Note: $n = 28\,010$.
Source (*31*).

As in the first table, higher prevalence rates are associated with definitions of disability that include milder or lesser degrees of difficulty. The relatively low overall prevalence rates for disability reported in many low-income countries (such as the figure of 2.7% in Zambia in 2000) may correspond more closely to rates of severe disability in these countries.

difficulties in their everyday lives. A threshold of 50 was set to estimate the prevalence of persons experiencing very significant difficulties. A full account of the survey method and the process of setting the threshold is in Technical appendix C.

Across all 59 countries the average prevalence rate in the adult population aged 18 years and over derived from the *World Health Survey* was 15.6% (some 650 million people of the estimated 4.2 billion adults aged 18 and older in 2004 (*35*)) (see Table 2.1) ranging from 11.8% in higher income countries to 18.0% in lower income countries. This figure refers to adults who experienced significant functioning difficulties in their everyday lives (see Technical appendix C). The average prevalence rate for adults with very significant difficulties was estimated at 2.2% or about 92 million people in 2004.

If the prevalence figures are extrapolated to cover adults 15 years and older, around 720 million people have difficulties in functioning with around 100 million experiencing very significant difficulties.

These estimates do not directly indicate the need for specific services. Estimating the size of the target group for services requires more specific information about the aims of services and the domain and extent of disability.

Across all countries, vulnerable groups such as women, those in the poorest wealth quintile, and older people had higher prevalences of disability. For all these groups the rate was higher in developing countries. The prevalence of disability in lower income countries among people aged 60 years and above, for instance, was 43.4%, compared with 29.5% in higher income countries.

Several limitations or uncertainties surrounding the *World Health Survey* data, described further in Technical appendix C, need to be noted. These include the valid debate regarding how best to set the threshold for disability, and the still unexplained variations across countries in self-reported difficulties in functioning, and the influence of cultural differences in expectations about functional

Table 2.1. Disability prevalence rates for thresholds 40 and 50 derived from multidomain functioning levels in 59 countries, by country income level, sex, age, place of residence, and wealth

Population subgroup	Threshold of 40			Threshold of 50		
	Higher income countries (standard error)	Lower income countries (standard error)	All countries (standard error)	Higher income countries (standard error)	Lower income countries (standard error)	All countries (standard error)
Sex						
Male	9.1 (0.32)	13.8 (0.22)	12.0 (0.18)	1.0 (0.09)	1.7 (0.07)	1.4 (0.06)
Female	14.4 (0.32)	22.1 (0.24)	19.2 (0.19)	1.8 (0.10)	3.3 (0.10)	2.7 (0.07)
Age group						
18–49	6.4 (0.27)	10.4 (0.20)	8.9 (0.16)	0.5 (0.06)	0.8 (0.04)	0.7 (0.03)
50–59	15.9 (0.63)	23.4 (0.48)	20.6 (0.38)	1.7 (0.23)	2.7 (0.19)	2.4 (0.14)
60 and over	29.5 (0.66)	43.4 (0.47)	38.1 (0.38)	4.4 (0.25)	9.1 (0.27)	7.4 (0.19)
Place of residence						
Urban	11.3 (0.29)	16.5 (0.25)	14.6 (0.19)	1.2 (0.08)	2.2 (0.09)	2.0 (0.07)
Rural	12.3 (0.34)	18.6 (0.24)	16.4 (0.19)	1.7 (0.13)	2.6 (0.08)	2.3 (0.07)
Wealth quintile						
Q1(poorest)	17.6 (0.58)	22.4 (0.36)	20.7 (0.31)	2.4 (0.22)	3.6 (0.13)	3.2 (0.11)
Q2	13.2 (0.46)	19.7 (0.31)	17.4 (0.25)	1.8 (0.19)	2.5 (0.11)	2.3 (0.10)
Q3	11.6 (0.44)	18.3 (0.30)	15.9 (0.25)	1.1 (0.14)	2.1 (0.11)	1.8 (0.09)
Q4	8.8 (0.36)	16.2 (0.27)	13.6 (0.22)	0.8 (0.08)	2.3 (0.11)	1.7 (0.08)
Q5(richest)	6.5 (0.35)	13.3 (0.25)	11.0 (0.20)	0.5 (0.07)	1.6 (0.09)	1.2 (0.07)
Total	11.8 (0.24)	18.0 (0.19)	15.6 (0.15)	2.0 (0.13)	2.3 (0.09)	2.2 (0.07)

Note: Prevalence rates are standardized for age and sex. Countries are divided between low-income and high-income according to their 2004 gross national income (GNI) per capita (*36*). The dividing point is a GNI of US$ 3255. Source (*37*).

requirements and other environmental factors, which the statistical methods could not adjust for.

Estimates based on the WHO Global Burden of Disease study

The second set of estimates of the global disability prevalence is derived from the *Global Burden of Disease* study, 2004 update. The first *Global Burden of Disease* study was commissioned in 1990 by the World Bank to assess the relative burden of premature mortality and disability from different diseases, injuries, and risk factors (*38, 39*).

In response to criticisms of disability-adjusted life-years (DALYs) in the original *Global Burden of Disease* study (*10, 40–42*), the concept has been further developed – for example, the use of population-based health state valuations in preference to expert opinion and better methods for cross-national comparability of survey data on health states (*43, 44*). The disability weights – years lived with disability (YLD) – used in the DALYs attempt to quantify the functional status of individuals in terms of their capacities and ignore environmental factors. The YLD uses a set of core health domains including mobility, dexterity, affect, pain, cognition, vision, and hearing.

In recent years the WHO has reassessed the *Global Burden of Disease* for 2000–2004, drawing on available data sources to produce estimates of incidence, prevalence, severity, duration, and mortality for more than 130 health conditions for 17 subregions of the world (*45, 46*). The *Global Burden of Disease* study starts with the prevalence of diseases and injuries and distributions of limitations in functioning – where available – in different regions of the world, and then estimates the severity of related disability (*46*).

The analysis of the *Global Burden of Disease* 2004 data for this Report estimates that 15.3% of the world population (some 978 million people of the estimated 6.4 billion in 2004 (*35*)) had "moderate or severe disability", while 2.9% or about 185 million experienced "severe disability" (see Table 2.2). Among those aged 0–14 years, the figures were 5.1% and 0.7%, or 93 million and 13 million children, respectively. Among those 15 years and older, the figures were 19.4% and 3.8%, or 892 million and 175 million, respectively.

The *Global Burden of Disease* study has given considerable attention to the internal consistency and comparability of estimates across populations for specific diseases and causes of injury, severity, and distributions of limitations in functioning. But it is not appropriate to infer the overall picture of disability from health conditions and impairments alone. There is substantial uncertainty about the *Global Burden of Disease* estimates – particularly for regions of the world and for conditions where the data are scarce or of poor quality – and about assessments of the average severity of related disability, whether based on published studies or expert opinion (see Technical appendix D).

About the prevalence estimates

National survey and census data cannot be compared directly with the *World Health Survey* or *Global Burden of Disease* estimates, because there is no consistent approach across countries to disability definitions and survey questions.

In 2004, the latest year for which data are available from surveys and burden of disease

estimates, the *World Health Survey* and *Global Burden of Disease* results based on very different measurement approaches and assumptions, give global prevalence estimates among the adult population of 15.6% and 19.4% respectively. The *World Health Survey* gives the prevalence of adults with very significant difficulties in functioning at 2.2%, while the *Global Burden of Disease* data indicate that 3.8% of the adult population is estimated to have "severe disability" – the equivalent of disability inferred for conditions such as quadriplegia, severe depression, or blindness.

Based on 2010 population estimates – 6.9 billion with 5.04 billion 15 years and over and 1.86 billion under 15 years – and 2004 disability prevalence estimates (*World Health Survey* and *Global Burden of Disease*) there were around 785 (15.6%) to 975 (19.4%) million persons 15 years and older living with disability. Of these, around 110 (2.2%) to 190 (3.8%) million experienced significant difficulties in functioning. Including children, over a billion people (or about 15% of the world's population) were estimated to be living with disability.

This is higher than WHO estimates from the 1970s, which suggested a global prevalence of around 10% (*47*). The *World Health Survey* estimate includes respondents who reported significant difficulties in everyday functioning. Against this, the *Global Burden of Disease* estimates result from setting a cut-off based on average disability weights that corresponds to the disability weights for typical health states associated with such conditions as low vision, arthritis, and angina. From these two sources, only the *Global Burden of Disease* provides data on prevalence of disability in children – see the section below on factors affecting disability prevalence for a broader discussion on childhood disability.

The overall prevalence rates from both the *World Health Survey* and *Global Burden of Disease* analyses are determined by the thresholds chosen for disability. Different choices of thresholds result in different overall prevalence rates, even if fairly similar approaches are used

Table 2.2. Estimated prevalence of moderate and severe disability, by region, sex, and age, Global Burden of Disease estimates for 2004

Sex/age group	Percent							
	World	High-income countries	Low-income and middle-income countries, WHO region					
			African	Americas	South-East Asia	European	Eastern Mediterranean	Western Pacific
Severe disability								
Males								
0–14 years	0.7	0.4	1.2	0.7	0.7	0.9	0.9	0.5
15–59 years	2.6	2.2	3.3	2.6	2.7	2.8	2.9	2.4
≥ 60 years	9.8	7.9	15.7	9.2	11.9	7.3	11.8	9.8
Females								
0–14 years	0.7	0.4	1.2	0.6	0.7	0.8	0.8	0.5
15–59 years	2.8	2.5	3.3	2.6	3.1	2.7	3.0	2.4
≥ 60 years	10.5	9.0	17.9	9.2	13.2	7.2	13.0	10.3
All people								
0–14 years	0.7	0.4	1.2	0.6	0.7	0.8	0.9	0.5
15–59 years	2.7	2.3	3.3	2.6	2.9	2.7	3.0	2.4
≥ 60 years	10.2	8.5	16.9	9.2	12.6	7.2	12.4	10.0
≥ 15 years	3.8	3.8	4.5	3.4	4.0	3.6	3.9	3.4
All ages	2.9	3.2	3.1	2.6	2.9	3.0	2.8	2.7
Moderate and severe disability								
Males								
0–14 years	5.2	2.9	6.4	4.6	5.3	4.4	5.3	5.4
15–59 years	14.2	12.3	16.4	14.3	14.8	14.9	13.7	14.0
≥ 60 years	45.9	36.1	52.1	45.1	57.5	41.9	53.1	46.4
Females								
0–14 years	5.0	2.8	6.5	4.3	5.2	4.0	5.2	5.2
15–59 years	15.7	12.6	21.6	14.9	18.0	13.7	17.3	13.3
≥ 60 years	46.3	37.4	54.3	43.6	60.1	41.1	54.4	47.0
All people								
0–14 years	5.1	2.8	6.4	4.5	5.2	4.2	5.2	5.3
15–59 years	14.9	12.4	19.1	14.6	16.3	14.3	15.5	13.7
≥ 60 years	46.1	36.8	53.3	44.3	58.8	41.4	53.7	46.7
≥ 15 years	19.4	18.3	22.0	18.3	21.1	19.5	19.1	18.1
All ages	15.3	15.4	15.3	14.1	16.0	16.4	14.0	15.0

Note: High-income countries are those with a 2004 gross national income (GNI) per capita of US$ 10 066 or more in 2004, as estimated by the World Bank. Low-income and middle-income countries are grouped according to WHO region and are those with a 2004 GNI per capita of less than US$ 10 066 in 2004, as estimated by the World Bank. Severe disability comprises classes VI and VII, moderate and severe disability, classes III and above.
Source (36).

in setting the threshold. This methodological point needs to be borne in mind when considering these new estimates of global prevalence.

The *World Health Survey* and *Global Burden of Disease* results appear reasonably similar in Fig. 2.1, which shows average prevalence for countries by income band. But the sex ratio for disability differs greatly between the *World Health Survey* and the *Global Burden of Disease* (see Table 2.1 and Table 2.2). At the global level, the *Global Burden of Disease* estimates of moderate and severe disability prevalence are 11% higher for females than males, reflecting somewhat higher age-specific prevalences in females, but also the greater number of older women in the population than older men. But the *World Health Survey* estimates give a female prevalence of disability nearly 60% higher than that for males. It is likely that the differences between females and males in the *World Health Survey* study result to some extent from differences in the use of response categories.

The average prevalences from country surveys and censuses, calculated from population-weighted average prevalences in Technical appendix A, are much lower in low-income and middle-income countries than in high-income countries, and much lower than prevalences derived from the *World Health Survey* or *Global Burden of Disease* (see Fig. 2.1). This probably reflects the fact that most developing countries tend to focus on impairment questions in their surveys, while some developed country surveys are more concerned with broader areas of participation and the need for services. The *World Health Survey* results show variation across countries within each income band, possibly reflecting cross-country and within-country differences in the interpretation of categories by people with the same levels of difficulty in functioning. The variation across countries in the *Global Burden of Disease* results is smaller, but this is due to some extent to the extrapolation of country estimates from regional analyses.

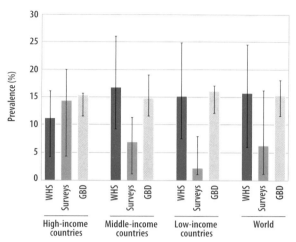

Fig. 2.1. Global disability prevalence estimates from different sources

Note: This figure compares the population-weighted average prevalence of disability for high-income, middle-income, and low-income countries from multiple sources. The solid grey bars show the average prevalence based on available data, the range lines indicate the 10th and 90th percentiles for available country prevalence within each income group. The data used for this figure are not age standardized and cannot be directly compared with Table 2.1 and Table 2.3. WHS = *World Health Survey*; GBD = the *Global Burden of Disease*, 2004 update; Surveys = Technical appendix A.
Sources (*37, 46*).

While the prevalence data in this Report draw on the best available global data sets, they are not definitive estimates. There is an urgent need for more robust, comparable, and complete data collection. Generally, a better knowledge base is required on the prevalence, nature, and extent of disability—both at a national level where policies are designed and implemented, but also in a globally comparable manner, with changes monitored over time. In the quest for more reliable and comprehensive national and international data on disability, the ICF provides a common platform for measurement and data collection. The ICF is neither a measurement tool nor a survey instrument, but a classification that can provide a standard for health and disability statistics and help in the difficult task of harmonizing approaches towards estimating disability prevalence.

Disability prevalence is the result of a complex and dynamic relationship between health conditions and contextual factors, both personal and environmental.

Health conditions

The relationship between health conditions and disabilities is complicated. Whether a health condition, interacting with contextual factors, will result in disability is determined by interrelated factors.

Often the interaction of several conditions rather than a single one contributes to the relationship between health conditions and disability. Co-morbidity, associated with more severe disability than single conditions, has implications for disability. Also the presence of multiple health problems can make the management of health care and rehabilitation services more difficult (48–50). Chronic health problems often occur together. For example, one chronic physical health condition, such as arthritis, significantly increases the likelihood of another physical health condition and mental health conditions (51, 52). So the aspect of disability that may be reported as primarily associated with one health condition may often be related to several coexisting conditions.

It is not possible to produce definitive global statistics on the relationship between disability and health conditions. Studies that try to correlate health conditions and disability without taking into account environmental effects are likely to be deficient.

The evidence suggests that the two main approaches to dealing with disability and associated health conditions yield different results. These approaches:

- Estimate disability and then look at associated health conditions – as in population surveys such as those mentioned under the section on noncommunicable diseases,

which can contribute to developing an empirical base.
- Estimate the prevalence of health conditions and then apportion disability – as in the synthetic estimates derived from the *Global Burden of Disease* study (see Technical appendix D) (46).

Trends in health conditions associated with disability

A growing body of statistical evidence presents a complex picture of shifting risk factors for different age and socioeconomic groups, with a pronounced increase in the prevalence of chronic conditions in the general population. Discussed here are trends in three broad categories of health conditions – infectious diseases, chronic conditions, and injuries.

Infectious diseases

Infectious diseases, may create, or be defined in terms of impairments. They are estimated to account for 9% of the years lived with disability in low-income and middle-income countries (46). Prominent among them are lymphatic filariasis, tuberculosis, HIV/AIDS, and other sexually transmitted diseases. Less prominent are diseases with neurological consequences, such as encephalitis (53, 54), meningitis (55, 56), and childhood cluster diseases – such as measles, mumps, and poliomyelitis (57).

Some of the trends in significant infectious diseases associated with disability:

- At the end of 2008 an estimated 33.4 million people worldwide – about 0.5% of the world population – were living with HIV. Between 2000 and 2008 the number of people living with HIV rose by 20%, but the annual global incidence of HIV infection is estimated to have declined by 17%. Sub-Saharan Africa remains the region most affected (58).
- Malaria is endemic in 109 countries, compared with 140 in the 1950s. In 7 of 45 African countries or territories with smaller populations, malaria cases

and deaths fell by at least 50% between 2000 and 2006. In 22 countries in other regions, malaria cases also fell by at least 50% (*59*).

- Polio cases fell more than 99% in 18 years, from an estimated 350 000 cases in 1988, to 1604 in 2009 (*60*). In 2010 only four countries – Afghanistan, India, Nigeria, and Pakistan – remain polio-endemic, down from more than 125 in 1988 (*60, 61*).
- The elimination of leprosy, to less than 1 per 10 000 population, was attained at the global level by 2000. At the beginning of 2003 the number of leprosy patients in the world was around 530 000, as reported by 106 countries. The number of countries with prevalence rates above 1 per 10 000 population fell from 122 in 1985 to 12 in 2002. Brazil, India, Madagascar, Mozambique, and Nepal are the most endemic countries (*62*).
- Trachoma, once endemic in many countries, is now largely confined to the poorest population groups in 40 developing countries, affecting about 84 million people, 8 million of them visually impaired (*63*). The prevalence of trachoma-related visual impairment has fallen considerably over the past two decades due to disease control and socioeconomic development (*64*).

Noncommunicable chronic diseases

The increase in diabetes, cardiovascular diseases (heart disease and stroke), mental disorders, cancer, and respiratory illnesses, observed in all parts of the world, will have a profound effect on disability (*65–73*). They are estimated to account for 66.5% of all years lived with disability in low-income and middle-income countries (*46*).

National surveys present a more detailed picture of the types of health conditions associated with disabilities:

- In a 1998 population survey in Australia of people (of all ages) with disabilities, the most common disability-related health conditions reported were: arthritis, back problems, hearing disorders, hypertension, heart disease, asthma, and vision disorders, followed by noise-induced hearing loss, speech problems, diabetes, stroke, depression, and dementia (*74*). The pattern varied with age and the extent of disability (*74*).
- In Canada, for adults aged 15 years and over with disabilities, a 2006 study found that the most common health conditions related to disability were arthritis, back problems, and hearing disorders. Other conditions included heart disease, soft tissue disorders such as bursitis and fibromyalgia, affective disorders, asthma, vision disorders, and diabetes. Among children aged 0–14 years, many of the most common health conditions were related to difficulties in learning. They included learning disabilities, specifically autism and attention deficit (with and without hyperactivity), as well as high levels of asthma and hearing problems. Other health conditions found in young people included speech problems, dyslexia, cerebral palsy, vision disorders, and congenital abnormalities (*75*).
- A 2001 OECD study in the United States of the top 10 conditions associated with disability found rheumatism to be the leading cause among elderly people, accounting for 30% of adults aged 65 years or older who reported limitations in their "activities of daily living". Heart problems were second, accounting for 23%. The other main disabling conditions were hypertension, back or neck problems, diabetes, vision disorders, lung and breathing problems, fractures, stroke, and hearing problems (*76*).

It is projected that there will continue to be large increases in non-communicable disease-related YLDs in rapidly developing regions (*65, 77, 78*). Several factors help explain the upward trend: population ageing, reduction in infectious conditions, lower fertility, and changing lifestyles related to tobacco, alcohol, diet, and physical activity (*39, 65, 79, 80*).

Box 2.3. Assistance for people with disabilities in conflict situations

Armed conflict generates injuries and trauma that can result in disabilities. For those incurring such injuries, the situation is often exacerbated by delays in obtaining emergency health care and longer-term rehabilitation. In 2009 in Gaza an assessment found such problems as (*81*):

- complications and long-term disability from traumatic injuries, from lack of appropriate follow-up;
- complications and premature mortality in individuals with chronic diseases, as a result of suspended treatment and delayed access to health care;
- permanent hearing loss caused by explosions, stemming from the lack of early screening and appropriate treatment;
- long-term mental health problems from the continuing insecurity and the lack of protection.

As many as half of the 5000 men, women, and children injured over the first three weeks of the conflict could have permanent impairments, aggravated by the inability of rehabilitation workers to provide early intervention (*82*).

In situations of conflict, those with disabilities are entitled to assistance and protection. Humanitarian organizations do not always respond to the needs of people with disabilities promptly, and gaining access to persons with disabilities who are scattered among affected communities can be difficult. A variety of measures can reduce the vulnerability of persons with disabilities including:

- effective planning to meet disability needs by humanitarian organizations before crises;
- assessments of the specific needs of people with disabilities;
- provisions of appropriate services;
- referral and follow-up services where necessary.

These measures may be carried out directly or through mainstreaming. The needs of families and carers must also be taken into account, both among the displaced population and in the host communities. In emergencies linked to conflicts, the measures need to be flexible and capable of following the target population, adjusting quickly as the situation evolves.

Injuries

Road traffic injury, occupational injury, violence, and humanitarian crises have long been recognized as contributors to disability (see Box 2.3). However, data on the magnitude of their contribution are very limited. Injury surveillance tends to focus exclusively on near-term outcomes such as mortality or the acute-care consequences of injury (*83*). For example, between 1.2 million and 1.4 million people die every year as a result of road traffic crashes. A further 20 to 50 million more are injured (*84–86*). The number of people disabled as a result of these crashes is not well documented.

A recent systematic review of the risk of disability among motor vehicle drivers surviving crashes showed substantial variability in derived estimates. Prevalence estimates of post-crash disability varied from 2% to 87%, largely a result of the methodological difficulties in measuring the non-fatal outcomes

following injuries (*87*). In Belgium a study using the country's Official Disability Rating Scale (a tool insurance companies use to assess disability rates among specific patients) found that 11% of workers injured in a road traffic crash on their way to or from work sustained a permanent disability (*88*). In Sweden 10% of all car occupants with an Abbreviated Injury Scale of 1 (the lowest injury score) sustained a permanent impairment (*89*).

Road traffic injuries are estimated to account for 1.7% of all years lived with disability – violence and conflict, for an additional 1.4% (*46*).

Demographics

Older persons

Global ageing has a major influence on disability trends. The relationship here is straightforward: there is higher risk of disability at older

Fig. 2.2. Age-specific disability prevalence, derived from multidomain functioning levels in 59 countries, by country income level and sex

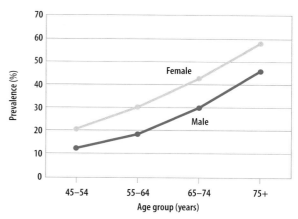

Source (*37*).

ages, and national populations are ageing at unprecedented rates.

Higher disability rates among older people reflect an accumulation of health risks across a lifespan of disease, injury, and chronic illness (*74*). The disability prevalence among people 45 years and older in low-income countries is higher than in high-income countries, and higher among women than among men.

Older people are disproportionately represented in disability populations (see Fig. 2.2). They make up 10.7% of the general population of Australia and 35.2% of Australians with disabilities (*29*). In Sri Lanka, 6.6% of the general population are 65 years or older representing 22.5% of people with disabilities. Rates of disability are much higher among those aged 80 to 89 years, the fastest-growing age cohort worldwide, increasing at 3.9% a year (*90*) and projected to account for 20% of the global population 60 years or older by 2050 (*91*). See Fig. 2.3 for the contribution of ageing to the disability prevalence in selected countries.

The ageing population in many countries is associated with higher rates of survival to an older age and reduced fertility (*99*). Despite differences between developing and developed nations, median ages are projected to increase markedly in all countries (*99*). This is an historically important demographic transition, well

under way in high-income nations, and projected to become more marked across the globe throughout the 21st century (see Table 2.3) (*90, 99, 100*).

Studies report contradictory trends in the prevalence of disability among older age groups in some countries, but the growing proportions of older people in national populations and the increased numbers of the "oldest old" most at risk of disability are well documented (*76, 101*). The Organisation for Economic Co-operation and Development (OECD) has concluded that it would be unwise for policy-makers to expect

Fig. 2.3. Distribution of ages within disability populations

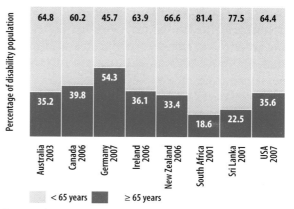

Sources (*5, 92–98*).

35

Table 2.3. Global ageing trends: median age by country income

Country income level	Median Age (years)			
	1950	1975	2005	2050
High-income countries	29.0	31.1	38.6	45.7
Middle-income countries	21.8	19.6	26.6	39.4
Low-income countries	19.5	17.6	19.0	27.9
World	23.9	22.4	28.0	38.1

Note: Middle estimate.
Source (*91*).

that reductions in severe disability among older people will offset increased demands for long-term care (*76*).

Children

Estimates of the prevalence of children with disabilities vary substantially depending on the definition and measure of disability. As presented above, the *Global Burden of Disease* estimates the number of children aged 0–14 years experiencing "moderate or severe disability" at 93 million (5.1%), with 13 million (0.7%) children experiencing severe difficulties (*46*). In 2005 the United Nations Children's Fund (UNICEF) estimated the number of children with disabilities under age 18 at 150 million (*102*). A recent review of the literature in low- and middle-income countries reports child disability prevalence from 0.4% to 12.7% depending on the study and assessment tool (*103*). A review in low-income countries pointed to the problems in identifying and characterizing disability as a result of the lack of cultural and language-specific tools for assessment (*104*). This may account in part for the variation in prevalence figures and suggests that children with disabilities are not being identified or receiving needed services.

The functioning of a child should be seen not in isolation but in the context of the family and the social environment. Children under age 5 in developing countries are exposed to multiple risks, including poverty, malnutrition, poor health, and unstimulating home environments, which can impair cognitive, motor, and social-emotional development (*105*). Children screening positive for increased risk of disability are less likely to have been breastfed or to have received a vitamin A supplement. As the severity of stunting and being underweight increases, so does the proportion of children screening positive for risk of disability (*106*). An estimated 200 million children under age 5 fail to reach their potential in cognitive and social-emotional development (*105*).

In its Multiple Indicator Cluster Surveys (MICS), for ages 2–9, UNICEF used 10 questions to screen children for risk of disability (*106*). These studies were found to lead to a large number of false positives – an overestimate of the prevalence of disability (*107*). Clinical and diagnostic evaluation of children who screen positive is required to obtain more definitive data on the prevalence of child disability. The MICS were administered in 19 languages to more than 200 000 children in 20 participating countries. Between 14% and 35% of children screened positive for risk of disability in most countries. Some authors argue that the screening was less able to identify children at risk of disabilities related to mental health conditions (*108, 109*). Also data from selected countries indicated that children in ethnic minority groups were more likely than other children to screen positive for disability. There was also evidence of regional variation within countries. Children who screened positive for increased risk of disability were also more likely than others:

- to come from poorer households;

- to face discrimination and restricted access to social services, including early-childhood education;
- to be underweight and have stunted growth;
- to be subject to severe physical punishment from their parents (*106*).

The environment

The effects of environmental factors on disability are complex.

Health conditions are affected by environmental factors

For some environmental factors such as low birth weight and a lack of essential dietary nutrients, such as iodine or folic acid, the impact on the incidence and prevalence of health conditions associated with disability is well established in the epidemiological literature (*106, 110, 111*). But the picture differs greatly because exposure to poor sanitation, malnutrition, and a lack of access to health care (say, for immunization) are all highly variable around the world,

often associated with other social phenomena such as poverty, which also represents a risk for disability (see Table 2.4) (*80*).

People's environments have a huge effect on the prevalence and extent of disability. Major environmental changes, such as those caused by natural disasters or conflict situations, will also affect the prevalence of disability not only by changing impairments but also by creating barriers in the physical environment. By contrast, campaigns to change negative attitudes towards persons with disabilities and large-scale changes to improve accessibility in the transport system or to public infrastructure will reduce barriers to activities and participation for many persons with disabilities. Other environmental changes include assistance provided by another person or an adapted or specially designed tool, device, or vehicle, or any form of environmental modification to a room, home, or workplace.

Measuring these interactions can provide useful information on whether to target the individual (providing an assistive device), the society (implementing anti-discrimination laws), or both (see Box 2.4) (*118*).

Table 2.4. Selected risk trends in selected countries

Country	Access to adequate sanitation (%)		Households consuming iodine (%)[a]		Infants with low birth weight (%)[a]		One-year-olds with DTP immunization (%)[b]	
	1990	2006	1992–1996	1998–2005	1990–1994	1998–2005	1997–1999	2005
Argentina	81	91	90	90[c]	7	8	86	90
Bangladesh	26	36	44	70	50	36	69	96
China	48	65	51	93	9	4	85	95
Egypt	50	66	0	78	10	12	94	98
Ghana	6	10	10	28	7	16	72	88
Iran	83	–	82	94	9	7[c]	100	97
Mexico	56	81	87	91	8	8	87	99
Thailand	78	96	50	63	13	9	97	99

a. Data refer to the most recent year available during the period specified in the column heading.
b. DTP = Diphtheria, tetanus, and pertussis.
c. Data refer to years or periods other than those specified in the column heading, differ from the standard definition, or refer to only part of a country.
Sources (*112–115*).

Box 2.4. **Measuring the effect of environment on disability**

The ICF model of disability provides a tool for measuring the effect of changes in the environment on the prevalence and severity of disability. It uses capacity and performance to assess the influence of the environment on disability. These constructs are as follows:

- **Capacity** indicates what a person can do in a standardized environment, often a clinical setting, without the barriers or facilitators of the person's usual environment;
- **Performance** indicates what a person does in the current or usual environment, with all barriers and facilitators in place.

Using these notions provides one way of identifying the effect of the environment and judging how a person's performance might be improved by modifying the environment.

Data were collected from a range of settings (research, primary care, rehabilitation) in the Czech Republic, Germany, Italy, Slovenia, and Spain on 1200 individuals with bipolar disorder, depression, low back pain, migraine, multiple sclerosis, other musculoskeletal conditions (including chronic widespread pain, rheumatoid arthritis and osteoarthritis), osteoporosis, Parkinson disease, stroke, or traumatic brain injury (116). Participants were rated on a five-point scale by interviewers using the ICF checklist recording levels of problems across all dimensions (117). Activity and participation items were scored using both the capacity and the performance constructs. Data were reported using a 0–100 score, with higher scores representing greater difficulties, and a composite score was created (see accompanying figure).

Mean and 95% confidence interval of the overall scores of capacity and performance in selected health conditions.

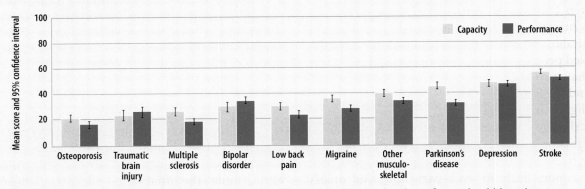

Note: Score 0 = no problems; score 100 = maximum problems. The data in the above figure should be taken not as necessarily representative of these conditions at large, but as an indication that a consistent conceptual framework can be applied in clinical settings to a wide range of health conditions.
Source (116).

Capacity scores were worst in people with stroke, depression, and Parkinson disease, while individuals with osteoporosis had the fewest limitations. Performance scores tended to be better than capacity scores, except for individuals with bipolar disorder or traumatic brain injury. This suggests that most individuals had supportive environments that promoted their functioning at or above the level of their intrinsic ability – something that applied particularly for multiple sclerosis and Parkinson disease. For people with conditions such as bipolar disorder and traumatic brain injury, the environmental factors hindered optimal performance. The data suggest that it is possible in clinical settings to disentangle aspects of disability that are particular to the individual (the capacity score) from the effects of a person's physical environment (the difference between capacity and performance).

Disability and poverty

Empirical evidence on the relation between disability and poverty in its various dimensions (income and non-income) differs greatly between developed and developing countries with most of the evidence from developed countries. But longitudinal data sets to establish the causal relation between disability and poverty are seldom available, even in developed countries.

Developed countries

Persons with disabilities experience worse educational and labour market outcomes and are more likely to be poor than persons without disabilities (*119–129*). A 2009 OECD study covering 21 upper-middle and high-income countries shows higher poverty rates among working-age people with disabilities than among working-age people without disability in all but three countries (Norway, Slovakia, and Sweden) (*130*). The relative poverty risk (poverty rate of working-age disabled relative to that of working-age non-disabled people) was shown to be the highest – more than two times higher – in Australia, Ireland, and the Republic of Korea, and the lowest – only slightly higher than for nondisabled people – in Iceland, Mexico, and the Netherlands. Working-age people with disabilities were found to be twice as likely to be unemployed. When employed, they are more likely to work part-time. And unless they were highly educated and have a job, they had low incomes.

Most studies provide a snapshot of the labour market outcomes and poverty situation of working-age persons with disabilities. Few studies provide information about people's socioeconomic status before the onset of disability and what has happened after it. A study using the British Household Panel Survey between 1991 and 1998 found that having less education, or not being in paid work, was a "selection" factor for disability (*131*). The study also found that employment rates fell with the onset of disability, and continue to fall with the duration of disability – indicating that people left the workforce early if they became disabled. Average income fell sharply with onset, but recovered subsequently, though not to pre-disability levels (*131*).

Some studies have attempted to estimate poverty rates among households with disability taking into account the extra cost of living with disabilities. A United Kingdom study found that in the late 1990s, the poverty rate among households with disabled people, depending on the assumptions used, was 20% to 44% higher after equalizing for disability (using 60% median income threshold) (*124*).

Developing countries

Quantitative research on the socioeconomic status of persons with disabilities in developing countries, while small, has recently grown. As with developed countries, descriptive data suggest that persons with disabilities are at a disadvantage in educational attainment and labour market outcomes. The evidence is less conclusive for poverty status measured by asset ownership, living conditions, and income and consumption expenditures.

The majority of studies find that persons with disability have lower employment rates and lower educational attainment than persons without disability (*31, 132–143*). In Chile and Uruguay the situation is better for younger persons with disabilities than older cohorts, as younger cohorts may have better access to education, through the allocation of additional resources (*133*). Most of the cross-section data for education suggests that children with disabilities tend to have lower school attendance rates (*30, 31, 133–136, 139, 142–146*).

An analysis of the *World Health Survey* data for 15 developing countries suggests that households with disabled members spend relatively more on health care than households without disabled members (for 51 *World Health Survey* countries, see Chapter 3 of this Report) (*132*).

A study on Sierra Leone found that households with persons with severe or very severe disabilities spent on average 1.3 times more on health care than did non-disabled respondents (*147*). While many studies find that households with disabled members generally have fewer assets (*31, 132, 134, 139, 143, 146, 147*) and worse living conditions compared with households without a disabled member (*134, 139, 146*) some studies found no significant difference in assets (*30, 140*) or living conditions (*30, 31*).

Data for income and household consumption expenditures are less conclusive. For example households with disabilities in Malawi and Namibia have lower incomes (*139, 146*) while households in Sierra Leone, Zambia, and Zimbabwe do not (*30, 31, 147*). In South Africa research suggests that, as a result of the provision of disability grants, households with a disabled member in the Eastern Cape Province had higher income than households without a disabled member (*136*).

Evidence on poverty as measured by per capita consumption expenditures is also mixed. An analysis of 14 household surveys in 13 developing countries found that adults with disabilities as a group were poorer than average households (*144*). However, a study of 15 developing countries, using *World Health Survey* data, found that households with disabilities experienced higher poverty as measured by nonhealth per capita consumption expenditures in only 5 of the countries (*132*).

Data in developing countries on whether having a disability increases the probability of being poor are mixed. In Uruguay disability has no significant effect on the probability of being poor except in households headed by severely disabled persons. By contrast, in Chile disability is found to increase the probability of being poor by 3–4 percent (*133*). In a cross-country study of 13 developing countries disability is associated with a higher probability of being poor in most countries – when poverty is measured by belonging to the two lowest quintiles in household expenditures or asset ownership. But this association disappears in most of the countries when controls for schooling are introduced (*144*).

One study attempted to account for the extra cost of disability in poverty estimates in two developing countries: Viet Nam and Bosnia and Herzegovina. Before the adjustments, the overall poverty rate in Viet Nam was 13.5% and the poverty rate among households with disability was 16.4%. The extra cost of disability was estimated at 9.0% resulting in an increase in the poverty rate among households with disability to 20.1% and in the overall poverty rate to 15.7%. In Bosnia and Herzegovina the overall poverty rate was estimated at 19.5% and among households with disability at 21.2%. The extra cost of disability was estimated at 14%, resulting in an increase in the poverty rate among households with disability to 30.8% and in the overall poverty rate to 22.4% (*148*).

Very few studies have looked at the prevalence of disability among the poor, or across the distribution of a particular welfare indicator (income, consumption, assets), or across education status. A study of 20 countries found that children in the poorest three quintiles of households in most countries are at greater risk of disability than the others (*106*). Disability across expenditure and asset quintiles in 15 developing countries, using several disability measures suggests higher prevalence in lower quintiles, but the difference is statistically significant in only a few countries (*132*).

Needs for services and assistance

People with disabilities may require a range of services – from relatively minor and inexpensive interventions to complex and costly ones. Data on the needs – both met and unmet – are important for policy and programmes. Unmet needs for support may relate to everyday activities – such as personal care, access to aids and equipment, participation in education, employment, and social activities, and modifications to the home or workplace.

In developed countries, national estimates of need are largely related to specific daily activities, rather than to types of service (*92, 149–152*). In Germany, for instance, it is estimated that 2.9% of the total population aged 8 years and older has a need for support services. In Sweden this figure has been estimated at 8.1%, solely in the 15–75 years age group (*153*). See also Box 2.5 for data on Australia.

Several developing countries have conducted national studies or representative surveys on unmet needs for broad categories of services for people with disabilities (*159–161*). Estimates of unmet needs have been included as a subcomponent in some national studies on people with disabilities in low-income and middle-income countries. The estimate of unmet needs is often based on data from a single survey and related to broad service programmes such as health, welfare, aids and equipment, education, and employment. The ICF conceptual framework has been used in the definitions of disability in most of the studies.

- In Africa national studies on living conditions of people with disabilities were conducted between 2001 and 2006 in Malawi, Namibia, Zambia, and Zimbabwe (*159*). Across the four countries the only sector that met more than 50% of reported needs for people with disabilities was health care.

The studies revealed large gaps in service provision for people with disabilities, with unmet needs particularly high for welfare, assistive devices, education, vocational training, and counselling services (see Table 2.5).

- In 2006 a national study on disability in Morocco estimated the expressed need for improved access to a range of services (*160*). People with disabilities in the study expressed a strong need for better access to health care services (55.3%), medications (21.3%), and technical devices (17.5%), and financial help for basic needs (52.5%).
- A 2006 study on unmet needs in Tonga found that 41% of people with disabilities reported a need for medical advice for their disability – more than twice the proportion of people who received such advice (*161*). Some 20% of people with disabilities needed physiotherapy, but only 6% received it.
- A 2007 national study on rehabilitation needs in China found that about 40% of people with disabilities who needed services and assistance received no help. The unmet need for rehabilitation services was particularly high for aids and equipment, rehabilitation therapy and financial support for poor people (*162*).

Box 2.5. Combining sources to better understand need and unmet need – an example from Australia

Four special national studies on unmet needs for specific disability support services were conducted in Australia over a recent decade (*154–157*). These studies relied on a combination of different data sources, especially the national population disability surveys and administrative data collections on disability services (*158*).

The use of the *International Classification of Functioning, Disability and Health* (ICF) was critical to the success of these studies; first to underpin national data standards, so as to give the maximum comparability of different sets of disability data; and second to create a framework that related data on support needs (the "demand" data from population surveys) to data on the needs for specific types of service (the "supply" data, also known as "registration data", from disability services).

An analysis of these demand and supply data combined provided an estimate of unmet needs for services. Furthermore, because the concepts were stable over time it was possible to update the estimates of unmet needs. For example, the estimate of unmet needs for accommodation and respite services was 26 700 people in 2003 and 23 800 people in 2005, after adjusting for population growth and increases in service supply during the period 2003–2005 (*157*). The users of accommodation and respite services increased from 53 722 people in 2003–2004 to 57 738 in 2004–2005, an increase of 7.5%.

....

Table 2.5. Met and unmet need for services reported by people with a disability, selected developing countries

Service	Namibia		Zimbabwe		Malawi		Zambia	
	Needed[a] (%)	Received[b] (%)	Needed[a] (%)	Received[b] (%)	Needed[a] (%)	Received[b] (%)	Needed[a] (%)	Received[b] (%)
Health services	90.5	72.9	93.7	92.0	83.4	61.0	76.7	79.3
Welfare services	79.5	23.3	76.0	23.6	69.0	5.0	62.6	8.4
Counselling for parent or family	67.4	41.7	49.2	45.4	50.5	19.5	47.3	21.9
Assistive device services	67.0	17.3	56.6	36.6	65.1	17.9	57.3	18.4
Medical rehabilitation	64.6	26.3	68.2	54.8	59.6	23.8	63.2	37.5
Counselling for disabled person	64.6	15.2	52.1	40.8	52.7	10.7	51.2	14.3
Educational services	58.1	27.4	43.4	51.2	43.9	20.3	47.0	17.8
Vocational training	47.3	5.2	41.1	22.7	45.0	5.6	35.1	8.4
Traditional healer	33.1	46.8	48.9	90.1	57.7	59.7	32.3	62.9

a. Percentage of total number of people with disabilities who expressed a need for the service.
b. Percentage of total number of people with disabilities who expressed a need for service who received the service.
Sources (*30, 31, 139, 146*).

Costs of disability

The economic and social costs of disability are significant, but difficult to quantify. They include direct and indirect costs, some borne by people with disabilities and their families and friends and employers, and some by society. Many of these costs arise because of inaccessible environments and could be reduced in a more inclusive setting. Knowing the cost of disability is important not only for making a case for investment, but also for the design of public programmes.

Comprehensive estimates of the cost of disability are scarce and fragmented, even in developed countries. Many reasons account for this situation, including:

- Definitions of disability often vary, across disciplines, different data collection instruments, and different public programmes for disability, making it difficult to compare

data from various sources, let alone compile national estimates.
- There are limited data on the cost components of disability. For instance, reliable estimates of lost productivity require data on labour market participation and productivity of persons with disabilities across gender, age, and education levels.
- There are no commonly agreed methods for cost estimation.

Progress in the technical aspects of disability cost estimates and better data are required to achieve reliable national estimates of the cost of disability – for example, the cost of productivity losses because of disability, the cost of lost taxes because of non-employment or reduced employment of disabled people, the cost of health care, social protection, and labour market programmes, and the cost of reasonable accommodation. The situation is better for data on public spending on disability benefits in cash, both contributory (social insurance benefits) and non-contributory (social assistance benefits), particularly in developed countries (*130*). But even for these programmes, consolidated data at the national level are scarce.

Direct costs of disability

Direct costs fall into two categories: additional costs that people with disabilities and their families incur to achieve a reasonable standard of living, and disability benefits, in cash and in kind, paid for by governments and delivered through various public programmes.

Extra costs of living with disability

People with disabilities and their families often incur additional costs to achieve a standard of living equivalent to that of non-disabled people (*120, 124, 148, 163*). This additional spending may go towards health care services, assistive devices, costlier transportation options, heating, laundry services, special diets, or personal assistance. Researchers have attempted to calculate these costs by asking disabled people to estimate them by pricing the goods and services that disabled people report they need, by comparing actual spending patterns of people with and without disabilities, and by using econometric techniques (*120, 124, 164*).

Several recent studies have attempted to estimate the extra cost of disability. In the United Kingdom estimates range from 11% to 69% of income (*124*). In Australia the estimated costs – depending on the degree of severity of the disability – are between 29% and 37% of income (*120*). In Ireland the estimated cost varied from 20% to 37% of average weekly income, depending on the duration and severity of disability (*164*). In Viet Nam, the estimated extra costs were 9%, and in Bosnia and Herzegovina 14% (*148*). While all studies conclude that there are extra costs related to disability, there is no technical agreement on how to measure and estimate them (*163*).

Public spending on disability programmes

Nearly all countries have some type of public programmes targeted at persons with disabilities, but in poorer countries these are often restricted to those with the most significant difficulties in functioning (*165*). They include health and rehabilitation services, labour market programmes, vocational education and training, disability social insurance (contributory) benefits, social assistance (non-contributory) disability benefits in cash, provision of assistive devices, subsidized access to transport, subsidized utilities, various support services including personal assistants and sign language interpreters, together with administrative overheads.

The cost of all programmes is significant, but no estimates of the total cost are available. For OECD countries an average of 1.2% of GDP is spent on contributory and non-contributory disability benefits, covering 6% of the working age population in 2007 (*130*). The benefits include full and partial disability benefits, as well as early retirement schemes specific to disability or reduced work capacity. The figure reaches 2% of GDP when sickness benefits are included, or almost 2.5 times the spending on unemployment benefits. The expenditure is particularly high in the Netherlands and Norway (about 5% of GDP). The cost of disability is around 10% of public social expenditure across OECD (up to 25% in some countries). At 6% of the working age population in 2007, the disability benefit recipiency rate was similar to the unemployment rate. In some countries it was close to 10%. Both the number of recipients and public spending have risen during the last two decades, creating significant fiscal concerns about affordability and sustainability of the programmes and motivating some countries, including the Netherlands and Sweden, to take steps to reduce the disability benefit dependency and to foster labour market inclusion of disabled people (*166*).

Indirect costs

Indirect economic and non-economic costs as a result of disability can be wide-ranging and substantial. The major components of economic cost are the loss of productivity from insufficient investment in educating disabled children, and exits from work or reduced work related to the onset of disability, and the loss of taxes related to the loss of productivity. Non-economic costs include social isolation and stress and are difficult to quantify.

An important indirect cost of disability is related to lost labour productivity of persons with disability and associated loss of taxes. Losses increase when family members leave employment or reduce the number of hours worked to care for family members with disabilities. The lost productivity can result from insufficient accumulation of human capital (underinvestment in human capital), from a lack of employment, or from underemployment.

Estimating disability-related loss in productivity and associated taxes is complex and requires statistical information, which is seldom available. For example, it is hard to predict the productivity that a person who has dropped out of the labour market because of disability would have if they were working. Hence, estimates of the loss of productivity are rare. One such estimate, for Canada using data from the 1998 National Population Health Survey, reports disability by type of impairment, age, and sex as well as the number of days in bed or with reduced activity. It suggests that the loss of work through short-term and long-term disability was 6.7% of GDP (*167*).

Conclusion and recommendations

Using multiple surveys from more than 100 countries, this chapter has shown that disability is a universal experience with economic and social costs to individuals, families, communities and nations.

There are around 785 (15.6% according to the *World Health Survey*) to 975 (19.4% according to the *Global Burden of Disease*) million persons 15 years and older living with disability, based on 2010 population estimates (6.9 billion with 1.86 billion under 15 years). Of these the *World Health Survey* estimates that 110 million people (2.2%) have very significant difficulties in functioning while the *Global Burden of Disease* estimates 190 million (3.8%) have "severe disability" – the equivalent of disability inferred for conditions such as quadriplegia, severe depression, or blindness. Including children, over a billion people (or about 15% of the world's population) were estimated to be living with disability.

Disability varies according to a complex mix of factors, including age, sex, stage of life, exposure to environmental risks, socioeconomic status, culture and available resources – all of which vary markedly across locations. Increasing rates of disability in many places are associated with increases in chronic health condition – diabetes, cardiovascular diseases, mental disorders, cancer, and respiratory illnesses – and injuries. Global ageing also has a major influence on disability trends because there is higher risk of disability at older ages. The environment has a huge effect on the prevalence and extent of disability, and on the disadvantage faced by persons with disabilities. Persons with disabilities and households with disabilities experience worse social and economic outcomes compared with persons without disabilities. In all settings, disabled people and their families often incur additional costs to achieve a standard of living equivalent to that of nondisabled people.

Because disability is measured on a spectrum and varies with the environment, prevalence rates are related to thresholds and context. Countries requiring estimates of the number of people needing income support, daily assistance with activities, or other services will construct their own estimates relevant to local policy.

Although the prevalence data in this Report draw on the best available global data sets, they are not definitive. Considerable and commendable efforts are being made in many countries and by major international agencies to improve disability data. Nevertheless, data quality requires further collaborative effort and there is an urgent need for more robust, comparable, and complete data collection especially in developing countries. Improving disability data may be a long-term enterprise, but it will provide essential underpinning for enhanced functioning of individuals, communities and nations. In the quest for more reliable and comprehensive national and international data on disability, the ICF provides a common platform for measurement and data collection. Improving the quality of information in this way, both nationally and internationally, is essential for monitoring progress in the implementation of the CRPD and in the achievement of internationally agreed development goals.

The following recommendations can contribute to enhancing the availability and quality of data on disability.

Adopt the ICF

Using the ICF, as a universal framework for disability data collection related to policy goals of participation, inclusion, and health will help create better data design and also ensure that different sources of data relate well to each other. The ICF is neither a measurement tool nor a survey instrument – it is a classification that can provide a standard for health and disability statistics and help in the difficult task of harmonizing approaches across sources of disability data. To achieve this, countries can:

- Base definitions and national data standards on the ICF.
- Ensure that data collection cover the broad array of ICF domains – impairments, activity limitations and participation restrictions, related health condition, environmental factors – even if a minimal set of data items is to be selected.

Improve national disability statistics

At the national level, information about people with disabilities is derived from censuses, population surveys and administrative data registries. Decisions on how and when to collect data depend on the resources available. Steps that can be taken to improve disability data, prevalence, need and unmet need, and socioeconomic status are outlined below. Disaggregating data by sex, age, and income or occupation will provide information about subgroups of persons with disabilities, such as children and older persons.

- Employ a "difficulties in functioning approach" instead of an "impairment approach" to determine prevalence of disability to better capture the extent of disability.
- As a first step national population census data can be collected in line with recommendations from the United Nations Washington Group on Disability and the United Nations statistical commission. Census data can provide an estimate of prevalence, information on socioeconomic situation, and geographical data and be used to identify populations at risk. It can also be used to screen respondents to implement more detailed follow up surveys.
- A cost-effective and efficient approach to gain comprehensive data on persons with disabilities is to add disability questions – or a disability module – to existing sample surveys such as a national household survey, national health survey, a general social survey or labour force survey.
- Dedicated disability surveys can be carried out to gain extensive information on disability and functioning – such as prevalence, health conditions associated with disability, use of and need for services, and other environmental factors, including on persons living in institutions and children.
- Data on persons with disabilities or those at particular risk of disability, including displaced persons, can also be collected through specific surveys in humanitarian crises.

- Administrative data collections can provide information on users, types and quantity of services and cost of services. In mainstream administrative data collections, standard disability identifiers can be included to monitor access to services by people with disabilities.
- Statistical linkage of various data sets can allow countries to bring together an array of information on a person from different time points, while at the same time protecting that individual's confidentiality. These linkage studies can often be conducted quickly and at relatively low cost.
- Where resources exist, collect longitudinal data that include questions on disability. Longitudinal data – the study of cohorts of people and their environments over time – allow researchers and policy-makers to understand better the dynamics of disability. Such analyses would provide better indications of what happens to individuals and their households after disability onset, how their situation is impacted by public policies aimed at improving the social and economic status of disabled people, of the causal relationship between poverty and disability, and how and when to instigate prevention programmes, modify interventions, and make environmental changes.

Improve the comparability of data

Data gathered at the national level need to be comparable at the international level.

- Standardize metadata on national disability prevalence, for example, by defining the measures of disability, purpose a measurement, indicate which aspects of disability are included, and define the cut-off on the continuum. This will facilitate the compilation of country-reported disability prevalence in international data repositories such as WHO's Global Health Observatory.
- Refine methods of generating prevalence rates using a continuous metric that measures multidomain functioning levels. This

would include more work on the various approaches for setting thresholds, including sensitivity analyses of the different thresholds and the implications for services and policies.
- Comparable definitions of disability, based on the ICF, and uniform methods for collecting data on people with disabilities need to be developed, tested across cultures, and applied consistently in surveys, censuses and administrative data.
- Extended measures of disability should be developed and tested that can be incorporated into population surveys, or used as supplements to surveys, or as the core of a disability survey as initiated by the United Nations Washington Group on Disability Statistics and the Budapest Initiative.
- Develop appropriate instruments for measuring childhood disability.
- Improve collaboration and coordination between various initiatives to measure disability prevalence at global, regional and national levels (including the Budapest Initiative, European Statistical Commission, UNESCAP, United Nations Statistical Commission, Washington Group, WHO, United States and Canada).

Develop appropriate tools and fill the research gaps

- To improve validity of estimates – further research is needed on different types of investigation, such as self-report and professional assessment.
- To gain a clearer understanding of people in their environments and their interactions – better measures of the environment and its impacts on the different aspects of disability need to be developed. These will facilitate the identification of cost-effective environmental interventions.
- To understand the lived experiences of people with disabilities, more qualitative research is required. Measures of the lived experience of disability need to be coupled

with measurements of the well-being and quality of life of people with disabilities.

- To better understand the interrelationships and develop a true epidemiology of disability – studies are needed that bring health condition (including co-morbidity) aspects of disability into a single data set describing disability, and that explore the interactions between health conditions and disability and environmental factors.
- To better understand the costs of disability – technical agreement is required on definitions and methods of calculating the extra costs of living with a disability. Data are needed on labour market participation and lost productivity due to disability as well as estimates of the cost of public spending

on disability programmes, including cost–benefit and cost–effectiveness analyses.

Data and information to inform national policies on disability should be sought in a wide range of places – including data collected by statistical agencies, administrative data collected by government agencies, reports by government bodies, international organizations, nongovernmental organizations, and disabled people's organizations – in addition to the usual academic journals. It is vital that such information – including on good practices – be shared among a wider network of countries. This will help disseminate experiences from developing countries, which are often innovative and cost-effective.

References

1. *Convention on the Rights of Persons with Disabilities*. New York, United Nations, 2006 (http://www.un.org/disabilities/documents/convention/convoptprot-e.pdf, accessed 8 June 2009).
2. Mont D. *Measuring disability prevalence*. Washington, World Bank, 2007 (SP Discussion Paper No. 0706) (http://siteresources.worldbank.org/DISABILITY/Resources/Data/MontPrevalence.pdf, accessed 9 December 2009).
3. Burkhauser RV et al. Self-reported work-limitation data: what they can and cannot tell us. *Demography*, 2002,39:541-555. doi:10.1353/dem.2002.0025 PMID:12205757
4. *Disability and social participation in Europe*. Brussels, Eurostat, 2001.
5. *National Disability Survey 2006: first results*. Dublin, Stationery Office, 2008 (http://www.cso.ie/releasespublications/nationaldisabilitysurvey06first.htm, accessed 15 November 2009).
6. *First national study on disability*. Santiago, National Fund for Disability in Chile, 2005 (http://www.ine.cl/canales/chile_estadistico/encuestas_discapacidad/pdf/estudionacionaldeladiscapacidad(ingles).pdf, accessed 2 February 2010).
7. Encuesta nacional de evaluación del desempeño, 2003 [National performance evaluation survey, 2003]. In: *Programa nacional de salud 2007–2012 [National health programme, 2007–2012]*. Mexico City, Secretaria de Salud, 2007.
8. Lerma RV. *Generating disability data in Mexico* [Estadística sobre personas con discapacidad en Centroamérica]. Managua, Inter-American Development Bank, 2004 (http://tinyurl.com/ylgft9x, accessed 3 February 2010).
9. *Census 2006, Volume 11: disability, carers and voluntary activities*. Dublin, Stationery Office, 2007 (http://www.cso.ie/census/census2006_volume_11.htm, accessed 15 November 2009).
10. Mont D. Measuring health and disability. [comment]*Lancet*, 2007,369:1658-1663. doi:10.1016/S0140-6736(07)60752-1 PMID:17499607
11. Barbotte E, Guillemin F, Chau N. Lorhandicap GroupPrevalence of impairments, disabilities, handicaps and quality of life in the general population: a review of recent literature. *Bulletin of the World Health Organization*, 2001,79:1047-1055. PMID:11731812
12. Me A, Mbogoni M. Review of practices in less developed countries on the collection of disability data. In: Barnatt SN, Altman BM, eds. *International views on disability measures: moving toward comparative measurement*. Oxford, Elesevier, 2006:63–87.
13. She P, Stapleton DC. *A review of disability data for the institutional population: research brief*. Ithaca, Rehabilitation Research and Training Center on Disability Demographics and Statistics, Cornell University, 2006.
14. Cambois E, Robine JM, Mormiche P. Une forte baisse de l'incapacité en France dans les années 1990? Discussion autour des questions de l'enquête santé. *Population*, 2007,62:363-386. doi:10.2307/20451015
15. Ikeda N, Murray CJL, Salomon JA. Tracking population health based on self-reported impairments: Trends in the prevalence of hearing loss in US adults, 1976–2006. *American Journal of Epidemiology*, 2009,170:80-87. doi:10.1093/aje/kwp097 PMID:19451176

16. Andresen EM et al. Reliability and validity of disability questions for US Census 2000. *American Journal of Public Health*, 2000,90:1297-1299. doi:10.2105/AJPH.90.8.1297 PMID:10937013

17. Doyle J, Wong LL. Mismatch between aspects of hearing impairment and hearing disability/handicap in adult/elderly Cantonese speakers: some hypotheses concerning cultural and linguistic influences. *Journal of the American Academy of Audiology*, 1996,7:442-446. PMID:8972445

18. Lane SD et al. Sociocultural aspects of blindness in an Egyptian delta hamlet: visual impairment vs. visual disability. *Medical Anthropology*, 1993,15:245-260. doi:10.1080/01459740.1993.9966093 PMID:8114621

19. Chamie M. Can childhood disability be ascertained simply in surveys? *Epidemiology (Cambridge, Mass.)*, 1994,5:273-275. PMID:7518696

20. Schneider M. The difference a word makes: responding to questions on 'disability' and 'difficulty' in South Africa. *Disability and Rehabilitation*, 2009,31:42-50. doi:10.1080/09638280802280338 PMID:19194809

21. Schneider M et al. Measuring disability in censuses: the case of South Africa. *European Journal of Disability Research*, 2009,3:245-265.

22. Altman B. The Washington Group: origin and purpose. In: Barnatt SN, Altman BM, eds. *International views on disability measures: moving toward comparative measurement*. Oxford, Elesevier, 2006:9–16.

23. *Report of the meeting of the group of experts on measurement of health status, of 14–16 November 2005*. New York, United Nations Economic and Social Council, 2006.

24. International Classification of Functioning. *Disability and Health (ICF)*. Geneva, World Health Organization, 2001.

25. *International Classification of Functioning, Disability and Health, Children and Youth Version (ICF-CY)*. Geneva, World Health Organization, 2007.

26. *Training manual on disability statistics*. Geneva, World Health Organization and Bangkok, United Nations Economic and Social Commission for Asia and the Pacific, 2008.

27. *United Nations demographic yearbook, special issue: population ageing and the situation of elderly persons*. New York, United Nations, 1993.

28. *Classifying and measuring functioning*. Washington, United States National Committee on Vital and Health Statistics, 2001.

29. *Testing a disability question for the census*. Canberra, Family and Community Statistics Section, Australian Bureau of Statistics, 2003.

30. Eide AH, van Rooy G, Loeb ME. *Living conditions among people with activity limitations in Namibia: a representative, national study*. Oslo, SINTEF, 2003 (http://www.safod.org/Images/LCNamibia.pdf, accessed 9 November 2009).

31. Eide AH, Loeb ME, eds. *Living conditions among people with activity limitations in Zambia: a national representative study*. Oslo, SINTEF, 2006 (http://www.sintef.no/upload/Helse/Levekår%20og%20tjenester/ZambiaLCweb.pdf, accessed 7 December 2009).

32. Üstün TB et al. WHO multi-country survey study on health and responsiveness 2000–2001. In: Murray CJL, Evans DB, eds. *Health systems performance assessment: debates, methods and empiricism*. Geneva, World Health Organization, 2003:761–796.

33. Üstün TB et al. The World Health Surveys. In: Murray CJL, Evans DB, eds. *Health systems performance assessment: debates, methods and empiricism*. Geneva, World Health Organization, 2003.

34. Mathers C, Smith A, Concha M. *Global burden of hearing loss in the year 2000*. Global Burden of Disease, 2000 (http://www.who.int/healthinfo/statistics/bod_hearingloss.pdf).

35. 2004 demographic yearbook- fifty-sixth issue department of Economic and Social Affairs, New York, United Nations, 2007 (http://unstats.un.org/unsd/demographic/products/dyb/dybsets/2004%20DYB.pdf, accessed??).

36. *Data and statistics: country groups*. Washington, World Bank, 2004 (http://go.worldbank.org/D7SN0B8YU0, accessed 4 January 2010).

37. *World Health Survey*. Geneva, World Health Organization, 2002–2004 (http://www.who.int/healthinfo/survey/en/, accessed 9 December 2009)

38. World Bank. *World Development Report 1993: investing in health*. New York, Oxford University Press, 1993.

39. Murray CJL, Lopez AD, eds. *The Global Burden of Disease: a comprehensive assessment of mortality and disability from diseases, injuries and risk factors in 1990 and projected to 2020*, 1st ed. Cambridge, MA, Harvard University Press, 1996.

40. Arnesen T, Nord E. The value of DALY life: problems with ethics and validity of disability adjusted life years. *BMJ (Clinical research ed.)*, 1999,319:1423-1425. PMID:10574867

41. Fox-Rushby JA. *Disability Adjusted Life Years (DALYS) for decision-making? An overview of the literature*. London, Office of Health Economics, 2002.

42. Reidpath DD et al. Measuring health in a vacuum: examining the disability weight of the DALY. *Health Policy and Planning*, 2003,18:351-356. doi:10.1093/heapol/czg043 PMID:14654511

43. Murray CJL et al. *Summary measures of population health: concepts, ethics, measurement and applications*. Geneva, World Health Organization, 2002.

44. Salomon J et al. Quantifying individual levels of health: definitions, concepts and measurement issues. In: Murray CJL, Evans D, eds. *Health systems performance assessment: debate, methods and empiricism*. Geneva, World Health Organization, 2003:301–318.

45. Mathers CD, Lopez AD, Murray CJL. The burden of disease and mortality by condition: data, methods and results for 2001. In: Lopez AD et al., eds. *Global burden of disease and risk factors*, 1st ed. Washington, Oxford University Press and World Bank, 2006:45–240.

46. *The global burden of disease: 2004 update*. Geneva, World Health Organization, 2008.

47. *Disability prevention and rehabilitation: report of the WHO expert committee on disability prevention and rehabilitation*. Geneva, World Health Organization, 1981 (Technical Report Series 668) (http://whqlibdoc.who.int/trs/WHO_TRS_668.pdf, accessed 9 December 2009).

48. Merikangas KR et al. The impact of comorbidity of mental and physical conditions on role disability in the US adult household population. *Archives of General Psychiatry*, 2007,64:1180-1188. doi:10.1001/archpsyc.64.10.1180 PMID:17909130

49. Moussavi S et al. Depression, chronic diseases, and decrements in health: results from the World Health Surveys. *Lancet*, 2007,370:851-858. doi:10.1016/S0140-6736(07)61415-9 PMID:17826170

50. Sousa RM et al. Contribution of chronic diseases to disability in elderly people in countries with low and middle incomes: a 10/66 Dementia Research Group population-based survey. *Lancet*, 2009,374:1821-1830. doi:10.1016/S0140-6736(09)61829-8 PMID:19944863

51. Croft P, Dunn KM, Von Korff M. Chronic pain syndromes: you can't have one without another. *Pain*, 2007,131:237-238. doi:10.1016/j.pain.2007.07.013 PMID:17728065

52. Gureje O et al. The relation between multiple pains and mental disorders: results from the World Mental Health Surveys. *Pain*, 2008,135:82-91. doi:10.1016/j.pain.2007.05.005 PMID:17570586

53. Kaiser R. The clinical and epidemiological profile of tick-borne encephalitis in southern Germany 1994–98: a prospective study of 656 patients. *Brain*, 1999,122:2067-2078. doi:10.1093/brain/122.11.2067 PMID:10545392

54. Lewis P, Glaser CA. Encephalitis. *Pediatrics in Review / American Academy of Pediatrics*, 2005,26:353-363.

55. Hodgson A et al. Survival and sequelae of meningococcal meningitis in Ghana. *International Journal of Epidemiology*, 2001,30:1440-1446. doi:10.1093/ije/30.6.1440 PMID:11821360

56. van de Beek D et al. Community-acquired bacterial meningitis in adults. *The New England Journal of Medicine*, 2006,354:44-53. doi:10.1056/NEJMra052116 PMID:16394301

57. Galazka AM, Robertson SE, Kraigher A. Mumps and mumps vaccine: a global review. *Bulletin of the World Health Organization*, 1999,77:3-14. PMID:10063655

58. *AIDS epidemic update, December 2009*. Geneva, Joint United Nations Programme on HIV/AIDS and World Health Organization, 2009.

59. *World malaria report 2008*. Geneva, World Health Organization, 2008.

60. *Poliomyelitis: fact sheet*. Geneva, World Health Organization, 2008d (http://www.who.int/mediacentre/factsheets/fs114/en/index.html, accessed 25 November 2009).

61. *Polio this week: wild polio virus list*. Geneva, The Global Polio Eradication Initiative, 2010 (http://www.polioeradication.org/casecount.asp, accessed 6 September 2010)

62. Daumerie D. Leprosy in the global epidemiology of infectious diseases. In: Murray C, Lopez A, Mathers C, eds. *The global epidemiology of infectious diseases [Global burden of disease and injury series, Volume IV]*. Geneva, World Health Organization, 2004.

63. *Priority eye diseases: fact sheet*. Geneva, World Health Organization, 2009 (http://www.who.int/blindness/causes/priority/en/print.html, accessed 14 December 2009).

64. Thylefors B et al. Trachoma-related visual loss. In: Murray C, Lopez A, Mathers C, eds. *The global epidemiology of infectious diseases [Global burden of disease and injury series, Volume IV]*. Geneva, World Health Organization, 2004.

65. *Preventing chronic diseases: a vital investment. WHO global report*. Geneva, World Health Organization, 2005.

66. Engelgau MM et al. The evolving diabetes burden in the United States. *Annals of Internal Medicine*, 2004,140:945-950. PMID:15172919

67. Jemal A et al. Trends in the leading causes of death in the United States, 1970–2002. *JAMA: the Journal of the American Medical Association*, 2005,294:1255-1259. doi:10.1001/jama.294.10.1255 PMID:16160134

68. Mannino DM et al. Surveillance for asthma–United States, 1980–1999. *MMWR. Surveillance summaries: Morbidity and mortality weekly report. Surveillance summaries / CDC*, 2002,51:1-13. PMID:12420904

69. Green A, Christian Hirsch N, Pramming SK. The changing world demography of type 2 diabetes. *Diabetes/Metabolism Research and Reviews*, 2003,19:3-7. doi:10.1002/dmrr.340 PMID:12592640

70. Perenboom RJM et al. Life expectancy without chronic morbidity: trends in gender and socioeconomic disparities. *Public health reports (Washington, DC: 1974)*, 2005,120:46-54. PMID:15736331

71. Sans S, Kesteloot H, Kromhout D. The burden of cardiovascular diseases mortality in Europe. *European Heart Journal*, 1997,18:1231-1248.

72. Wang L et al. Preventing chronic diseases in China. *Lancet*, 2005,366:1821-1824. doi:10.1016/S0140-6736(05)67344-8 PMID:16298221

73. *Mental health atlas*. Geneva, World Health Organization, 2005.

74. *Disability and its relationship to health conditions and other factors*. Canberra, Australian Institute of Health and Welfare, 2004 (http://www.aihw.gov.au/publications/dis/drhcf/drhcf.pdf, accessed 9 December 2009).

75. Custom tabulation of PALS 2006 data. Ottawa, Statistics Canada, 2006.

76. Lafortune G, Balestat G. *Trends in severe disability among elderly people: assessing the evidence in 12 OECD countries and the future implications* [OECD Health Working Papers No. 26]. Paris, Organisation for Economic Co-operation and Development, 2007 (http://www.oecd.org/dataoecd/13/8/38343783.pdf, accessed 9 December 2009).

77. Ezzati M et al. *Comparative quantification of health risks: global and regional burden of diseases attributable to selected major risk factors*. Geneva, World Health Organization, 2004.

78. Adeyi O, Smith O, Robles S. *Public policy and the challenge of chronic noncommunicable diseases*. Washington, International Bank for Reconstruction and Development, World Bank, 2007.

79. Lopez AD et al. *Global burden of disease and risk factors*, New York, Oxford University Press, 2006 (http://www.dcp2.org/pubs/GBD).

80. Mathers CD, Loncar D. Projections of global mortality and burden of disease from 2002 to 2030. *PLoS Medicine*, 2006,3:e442- doi:10.1371/journal.pmed.0030442 PMID:17132052

81. Gaza Strip Health Cluster Bulletin No. 2. Geneva, World Health Organization, 2009 (http://www.who.int/hac/crises/international/wbgs/sitreps/gaza_health_cluster_4feb2009/en/index.html, accessed 15 November 2009).

82. *Call for all agencies in Gaza to ensure rights for people with disabilities*. Bensheim, CBM, 2009 (http://www.cbm-nz.org.nz/NEWS/Archives/Call+for+all+agencies+in+Gaza+to+ensure+rights+for+people+with+disabilities.html, accessed 15 November 2009).

83. *Injury: a leading cause of the global burden of disease, 2000*. Geneva, World Health Organization, 2002.

84. *Global status report on road safety: time for action*. Geneva, World Health Organization, 2009 (http://www.who.int/violence_injury_prevention/road_safety_status/2009, accessed 5 January 2010).

85. *World report on road traffic injury prevention*. Geneva, World Health Organization, 2004 (http://whqlibdoc.who.int/publications/2004/9241562609.pdf, accessed 5 January 2010).

86. *World health statistics*. Geneva, World Health Organization, 2008.

87. Ameratunga SN et al. Risk of disability due to car crashes: a review of the literature and methodological issues. *Injury*, 2004,35:1116-1127. doi:10.1016/j.injury.2003.12.016 PMID:15488502

88. Levêque A, Coppieters Y, Lagasse R. Disabilities secondary to traffic accidents: what information is available in Belgium? *Injury Control and Safety Promotion*, 2002,9:113-120. doi:10.1076/icsp.9.2.113.8698 PMID:12461838

89. Malm S et al. Risk of permanent medical impairment (RPMI) in road traffic accidents. *Annals of advances in automotive medicine / Annual Scientific Conference ... Association for the Advancement of Automotive Medicine. . Scientific Conference*, 2008,52:93-100. PMID:19026226

90. Robine JM, Michel JP. Looking forward to a general theory on population aging. *The journals of gerontology. Series A, Biological sciences and medical sciences*, 2004,59:M590-597. PMID:15215269

91. *World population prospects: the 2006 revision*. New York, United Nations, Department of Economic and Social Affairs, Population Division, 2007.

92. *Disability, ageing and carers: summary of findings, 2003* (No. 4430.0). Canberra, Australian Bureau of Statistics, 2004 (http://tinyurl.com/ydr4pbh, accessed 9 December 2009).

93. *Participation and activity limitation survey 2006: tables*. Ottawa, Social and Aboriginal Statistics Division, Statistics Canada, 2007 (http://tinyurl.com/yftgvb5, accessed 9 December 2009).

94. *Statistics on severely handicapped persons*. Bonn, Federal Statistical Office, 2009 (http://www.gbe-bund.de/gbe10/abrechnung.prc_abr_test_logon?p_uid=gast&p_aid=4711&p_knoten=VR&p_sprache=E&p_suchstring=disability, accessed 15 December 2009).

95. *2006 disability survey*. Wellington, Statistics New Zealand, 2007 (http://www.stats.govt.nz/browse_for_stats/health/disabilities/disabilitysurvey2006_hotp06.aspx, accessed 18 November 2009).

96. *Prevalence of disability in South Africa census 2001*. Pretoria, Statistics South Africa, 2005.

97. *2001 Census of population and housing*. Colombo, Sri Lanka Department of Census and Statistics, 2001 (http://www.statistics.gov.lk/PopHouSat/index.asp, accessed 12 November 2009).

98. *2007 American community survey, 1-year estimates (S1801 disability characteristics)*. Washington, United States Census Bureau, 2007 (http://tinyurl.com/ydvqugn, accessed 18 November 2009).

99.   Lee R. The demographic transition: three centuries of fundamental change. *The Journal of Economic Perspectives*, 2003,17:167-190. doi:10.1257/089533003772034943

100. *Why population aging matters: a global perspective*. Bethesda, National Institute on Aging, US National Institutes of Health, 2007.

101. Manton KG, Gu XL. Changes in the prevalence of chronic disability in the United States black and nonblack population above age 65 from 1982 to 1999. *Proceedings of the National Academy of Sciences of the United States of America*, 2001,98:6354-6359. doi:10.1073/pnas.111152298 PMID:11344275

102. *The state of the world's children 2006: excluded and invisible*. New York, United Nations Children's Fund, 2005.

103. Maulik PK, Darmstadt GL. Childhood disability in low- and middle-income countries: overview of screening, prevention, services, legislation, and epidemiology. *Pediatrics*, 2007,120:Suppl 1S1-S55. doi:10.1542/peds.2007-0043B PMID:17603094

104. Hartley S, Newton CRJC. Children with developmental disabilities in the majority of the world. In: Shevell M, ed. *Neurodevelopmental disabilities: clinical and scientific foundations*. London, Mac Keith Press, 2009.

105. Grantham-McGregor S et al. International Child Development Steering GroupDevelopmental potential in the first 5 years for children in developing countries. *Lancet*, 2007,369:60-70. doi:10.1016/S0140-6736(07)60032-4 PMID:17208643

106. United Nations Children's Fund, University of Wisconsin. *Monitoring child disability in developing countries: results from the multiple indicator cluster surveys*. New York, United Nations Children's Fund, 2008.

107. *Workshop on Millennium Development Goals Monitoring*. Geneva, United Nations Statistics Division, 8–11 November 2010 (http://unstats.un.org/unsd/mdg/Host.aspx?Content=Capacity/Geneva.htm).

108. Robson C, Evans P. *Educating children with disabilities in developing countries: the role of data sets*. Huddersfield, University of Huddersfield, 2005 (http://siteresources.worldbank.org/DISABILITY/Resources/280658-1172610312075/EducatingChildRobson.pdf, accessed 23 October 2009).

109. Robertson J, Hatton C, Emerson E. *The identification of children with or at significant risk of intellectual disabilities in low and middle income countries: a review*. Lancaster, Centre for Disability Research, Lancaster University, 2009.

110. Hack M, Klein NK, Taylor HG. Long-term developmental outcomes of low birth weight infants. *The Future of children/Center for the Future of Children, the David and Lucile Packard Foundation*, 1995,5:176-196. doi:10.2307/1602514 PMID:7543353

111. Wang J et al. A ten year review of the iodine deficiency disorders program of the People's Republic of China. *Journal of Public Health Policy*, 1997,18:219-241. doi:10.2307/3343436 PMID:9238845

112. *The state of the world's children 1998*. New York, United Nations Children's Fund, 1998.

113. *Progress on drinking water and sanitation: special focus on sanitation*. New York, United Nation's Children's Fund and Geneva, World Health Organization, 2008.

114. *The state of the world's children 2001*. New York, United Nations Children's Fund, 2001.

115. *The state of the world's children 2007: child survival*. New York, United Nations Children's Fund, 2007.

116. Leonardi M et al. *MHADIE background document on disability prevalence across different diseases and EU countries*. Milan, Measuring Health and Disability in Europe, 2009 (http://www.mhadie.it/publications.aspx, accessed 21 January 2010).

117. ICF checklist: version 2.1a, clinician form: for international classification of functioning, disability and health. Geneva, World Health Organization, 2003 (http://www.who.int/classifications/icf/training/icfchecklist.pdf).

118. Schneidert M et al. The role of environment in the International Classification of Functioning, Disability and Health (ICF). *Disability and Rehabilitation*, 2003,25:588-595. doi:10.1080/0963828031000137090 PMID:12959332

119. Buddelmeyer H, Verick S. Understanding the drivers of poverty dynamics in Australian households. *The Economic Record*, 2008,84:310-321. doi:10.1111/j.1475-4932.2008.00493.x

120. Saunders P. *The costs of disability and incidence of poverty*. Sydney, Social Policy Research Centre, University of New South Wales, 2006.

121. Gannon B, Nolan B. Disability and labour market participation in Ireland *The Economic and Social Review*, 2004,35:135-155.

122. Parodi G, Sciulli D. Disability in Italian households: income, poverty and labour market participation. *Applied Economics*, 2008,40:2615-2630. doi:10.1080/00036840600970211

123. Kuklys W. *Amartya Sen's capability approach: theoretical insights and empirical applications*. Cambridge, Cambridge University, 2004.

124. Zaidi A, Burchardt T. Comparing incomes when needs differ: equivalization for the extra costs of disability in the UK. *Review of Income and Wealth*, 2005,51:89-114. doi:10.1111/j.1475-4991.2005.00146.x

125. Meyer BD, Mok WKC. Disability, earnings, income and consumption. Working paper No. 06.10. Chicago, The Harris School of Public Policy Studies, The University of Chicago, 2008.

126. Mitra S, Findley PA, Sambamoorthi U. Health care expenditures of living with a disability: total expenditures, out-of-pocket expenses, and burden, 1996 to 2004. *Archives of Physical Medicine and Rehabilitation*, 2009,90:1532-1540. doi:10.1016/j.apmr.2009.02.020 PMID:19735781

127. She P, Livermore GA. Material hardship, poverty and disability among working-age adults. *Social Science Quarterly*, 2007,88:970-989. doi:10.1111/j.1540-6237.2007.00513.x

128. She P, Livermore GA. Long term poverty and disability among working-Age Adults. *Journal of Disability Policy Studies*, 2009,19:244-256.

129. Houtenville AJ et al., eds. *Counting working-age people with disabilities: what current data tell us and options for improvement*. Kalamazoo, WE Upjohn Institute for Employment Research, 2009.

130. *Sickness, Disability and Work: Keeping on Track in the Economic Downturn*. Paris, Organisation for Economic Co-operation and Development, 2009 (Background Paper).

131. Jenkins SP, Rigg JA. *Disability and disadvantage: selection, onset and duration effects*. London, Centre for Analysis of Social Exclusion, London School of Economics, 2003 (CASEpaper 74).

132. Mitra S, Posarac A, Vick B. *Disability and poverty in developing countries: a snapshot from the world health survey*. Washington, Human Development Network *Social Protection*, forthcoming

133. Contreras DG et al. *Socio-economic impact of disability in Latin America: Chile and Uruguay*. Santiago, Universidad de Chile, Departemento de Economia, 2006.

134. Eide AH, Kamaleri Y. *Living conditions among people with disabilities in Mozambique: a national representative study*. Oslo, SINTEF, 2009 (http://www.sintef.no/upload/Helse/Levekår%20og%20tjenester/LC%20Report%20Mozambique%20-%202nd%20revision.pdf, accessed 11 April 2011).

135. Mete C, ed. *Economic implications of chronic illness and disease in Eastern Europe and the former Soviet Union*. Washington, World Bank, 2008.

136. Loeb M et al. Poverty and disability in Eastern and Western Cape provinces, South Africa. *Disability & Society*, 2008,23:311-321. doi:10.1080/09687590802038803

137. Mitra S. The recent decline in the employment of persons with disabilities in South Africa, 1998–2006. *The South African Journal of Economics*, 2008,76:480-492. doi:10.1111/j.1813-6982.2008.00196.x

138. Mitra S, Sambamoorthi U. Disability and the rural labor market in India: evidence for males in Tamil Nadu. *World Development*, 2008,36:934-952. doi:10.1016/j.worlddev.2007.04.022

139. Loeb ME, Eide AH, eds. *Living conditions among people with activity limitations in Malawi: a national representative study*. Oslo, SINTEF, 2004 (http://www.safod.org/Images/LCMalawi.pdf, accessed 9 November 2009).

140. Trani J, Loeb M. Poverty and disability: a vicious circle? Evidence from Afghanistan and Zambia. *Journal of International Development*, 2010,n/a- doi:10.1002/jid.1709

141. Zambrano S. Trabajo y Discapacidad en el Perú: laboral, políticas públicas e inclusión social. Lima, Fondo Editorial del Congreso del Perú, 2006.

142. Rischewski D et al. Poverty and musculoskeletal impairment in Rwanda. *Transactions of the Royal Society of Tropical Medicine and Hygiene*, 2008,102:608-617. doi:10.1016/j.trstmh.2008.02.023 PMID:18430444

143. *People with disabilities in India: from commitments to outcomes*. Washington, World Bank, 2009.

144. Filmer D. Disability, poverty and schooling in developing countries: results from 14 household surveys. *The World Bank Economic Review*, 2008,22:141-163. doi:10.1093/wber/lhm021

145. Trani J, VanLeit B. *Increasing inclusion of persons with disabilities: reflections from disability research using the ICF in Afghanistan and Cambodia*. London, Leonard Cheshire International, 2010.

146. Eide AH et al. *Living conditions among people with activity limitations in Zimbabwe: a representative regional survey*. Oslo, SINTEF, 2003 (http://www.safod.org/Images/LCZimbabwe.pdf, accessed 9 November 2009).

147. Trani J et al. *Disability in and around urban areas of Sierra Leone*. London, Leonard Cheshire International, 2010

148. Braithwaite J, Mont D. Disability and poverty: a survey of World Bank poverty assessments and implications. *ALTER – European Journal of Disability Research / Revue Européenne de Recherche sur le Handicap*, 2009, 3(3):219–232.

149. *Disability supports in Canada, 2001: participation and activity limitation survey*. Ottawa, Statistics Canada, 2003 (http://www.statcan.ca/english/freepub/89-580-XIE/help.htm, accessed 30 August 2007).

150. *Supports and services for adults and children aged 5–14 with disabilities in Canada: an analysis of data on needs and gaps*. Ottawa, Canadian Council on Social Development, 2004 (http://www.socialunion.ca/pwd/title.html, accessed 30 August 2007).

151. *Living with disability in New Zealand: a descriptive analysis of results from the 2001 Household Disability Survey and the 2001 Disability Survey of Residential Facilities*. Wellington, New Zealand Ministry of Health, 2004 (http://www.moh.govt.nz/moh.nsf/238fd5fb4fd051844c256669006aed57/8fd2a69286cd6715cc256f33007aade4?OpenDocument, accessed 30 August 2007).

152. Kennedy J. Unmet and under met need for activities of daily living and instrumental activities of daily living assistance among adults with disabilities: estimates from the 1994 and 1995 disability follow-back surveys. *Journal of Medical Care*, 2001,39:1305-1312. doi:10.1097/00005650-200112000-00006

153. Ratzka AD. *Independent living and attendant care in Sweden: a consumer perspective*. New York, World Rehabilitation Fund, 1986 (Monograph No. 34) (http://www.independentliving.org/docs1/ar1986spr.pdf, accessed 27 December 2007).

154. Madden R et al. *The demand for disability support services in Australia: a study to inform the Commonwealth/State Disability Agreement evaluation*. Canberra, Australian Institute of Health and Welfare, 1996.

155. *Demand for disability support services in Australia: size, cost and growth*. Canberra, Australian Institute of Health and Welfare, 1997.

156. *Unmet need for disability services: effectiveness of funding and remaining shortfall*. Canberra, Australian Institute of Health and Welfare, 2002.

157. *Current and future demand for specialist disability services*. Canberra, Australian Institute of Health and Welfare, 2007.

158. *Disability support services 2004–05: national data on services provided under the Commonwealth State/Territory Disability Agreement*. Canberra, Australian Institute of Health and Welfare, 2006.

159. Southern African Federation of the Disabled, Norwegian Federation of Disabled People, SINTEF. *Living conditions among people with activity limitation in Southern Africa: representative surveys on living conditions among people with activity limitations in Malawi, Namibia, Zambia, Zimbabwe and Mozambique*, Oslo, SINTEF, 2007.

160. *Childhood and disabled persons, Kingdom of Morocco. The national survey on disability: results synthesis, 2006*. Rabat, Secretariat of Family, Morocco, 2006.

161. *Tonga national disability identification survey*. Nuku'Alofa, Tonga Disability Action Committee, 2006.

162. Qiu ZY. *Rehabilitation need of people with disability in China: analysis and strategies* [in Chinese]. Beijing, Huaxia Press, 2007.

163. Tibble M. *Review of the existing research on the extra costs of disability*. London, Department for Work and Pensions, 2005 (Working Paper No. 21).

164. Cullinan J, Gannon B, Lyons S. Estimating the extra cost of living for people with disabilities. *Health Economics*, 2010,n/a- www.interscience.wiley.com doi:10.1002/hec.1619 PMID:20535832

165. Marriott A, Gooding K. *Social assistance and disability in developing countries*. Haywards Heath, Sightsavers International, 2007.

166. *Sickness, disability and work: breaking the barriers. A synthesis of findings across OECD countries*. Paris, Organisation for Economic Co-operation and Development, 2010.

167. *The economic burden of illness in Canada, 1998*. Ottawa, Health Canada, 2002.

Chapter 3

General health care

"My doctor is great. He is my friend and not just my doctor. He used to be my father's doctor too. When I want to see the doctor he always has time for me. He always talks to me about this, about that, before he says, "What is wrong?" I used to be on 60 mg of blood pressure medicine for my high blood pressure. But then my doctor told me that I had to get more life to help my pressure. He did not want me to twiddle my thumbs and watch soap operas seven days a week. He wanted me to move around and be active. It was a good idea. So I went and got some volunteer work. Now I have friends and I always talk to people. And I only need 20 mg of medicine!"

Jean-Claude

"You can not have a baby", those were the words of the first gynecologist I visited few months after I got married. I was so confused. Why wouldn't I be able to have a baby? I am physically disabled, but I have no medical reason not to. I faced a lot of challenges either because of bad attitude of nurses or doctors questioning my eligibility to be a mother or the inaccessible medical facilities, whether it is the entrances, bathrooms, examinations beds etc. I am now a mother of a 5 year old boy which is one of the best things that ever happened to me, but I keep thinking why did it end up to be a luxury thing while it is a right? Why was I only able to do it when I had the money to go to a better medical care system?"

Rania

"Even though during my appointments to the medical centre, doctors haven't discussed health promotion with me and they don't even have a scale to measure my body weight, I still try to engage in activities that would enhance my health and wellbeing. It's not easy as most fitness facilities and equipment are not accessible. I'm yet to find dietary advice for people with spinal cord injury or identify a dentist near my place of residence with accessible facility and equipment."

Robert

3

General health care

Health can be defined as "a state of physical, mental, and social well-being and not merely the absence of disease or infirmity" (*1*). Good health is a prerequisite for participation in a wide range of activities including education and employment. Article 25 of the United Nations *Convention on the Rights of Persons with Disabilities* (CRPD) reinforces the right of persons with disabilities to attain the highest standard of health care, without discrimination (*2*).

A wide range of factors determine health status, including individual factors, living and working conditions, general socioeconomic, cultural and environmental conditions, and access to health care services (*3, 4*). This Report shows that many people with disabilities experience worse socioeconomic outcomes than people without disabilities: they experience higher rates of poverty, lower employment rates, and have less education. They also have unequal access to health care services and therefore have unmet health care needs compared with the general population (*5–8*).

This chapter focuses on how health systems can address the health inequalities experienced by people with disabilities. It provides a broad overview of their health status, explores the main barriers to using health care, and suggests ways to overcome them.

Understanding the health of people with disabilities

This section provides a general overview of the health status of people with disabilities by looking at the different types of health conditions they may experience and several factors that may contribute to the health disparities for this population (see Box 3.1). Increasing evidence suggests that, as a group, people with disabilities experience poorer levels of health than the general population (*18*). They are often described as having a narrower or thinner margin of health (*9, 17*).

Primary health conditions

Disability is associated with a diverse range of primary health conditions: some may result in poor health and high health care needs; others do not

Box 3.1. Terminology

Primary health condition

A primary health condition is the possible starting point for impairment, an activity limitation, or participation restriction (9). Examples of primary health conditions include depression, arthritis, chronic obstructive pulmonary disease, ischaemic heart disease, cerebral palsy, bipolar disorder, glaucoma, cerebrovascular disease, and Down syndrome. A primary health condition can lead to a wide range of impairments, including mobility, sensory, mental, and communication impairments.

Secondary conditions

A secondary condition is an additional condition that presupposes the existence of a primary condition. It is distinguished from other health conditions by the lapse in time from the acquisition of the primary condition to the occurrence of the secondary condition (10). Examples include pressure ulcers, urinary tract infections, and depression. Secondary conditions can reduce functioning, lower the quality of life, increase health care costs, and lead to premature mortality (11). Many such conditions are preventable and can be anticipated from primary health conditions (12, 13).

Co-morbid conditions

A co-morbid condition is an additional condition independent of and unrelated to the primary condition (14). The detection and treatment of co-morbid conditions are often not well managed for people with disabilities and can later have an adverse affect on their health (12): for example, people with intellectual impairments and mental health problems commonly experience "diagnostic overshadowing" (15). Examples of co-morbid conditions include cancer or hypertension for a person with an intellectual impairment.

General health care needs

People with disabilities require health services for general health care needs like the rest of the population. General health needs include health promotion, preventive care (immunization, general health screening), treatment of acute and chronic illness, and appropriate referral for more specialized needs where required. These needs should all be meet through primary health care in addition to secondary and tertiary as relevant. Access to primary health care is particularly important for those who experience a thinner or narrower margin of health to achieve their highest attainable standard of health and functioning (16).

Specialist health care needs

Some people with disabilities may have a greater need for specialist health care than the general population. Specialist health care needs may be associated with primary, secondary, and co-morbid health conditions. Some people with disabilities may have multiple health conditions, and some health conditions may involve multiple body functions and structures. Assessment and treatment in these instances can be quite complex and therefore may necessitate the knowledge and skills of specialists (17).

keep people with disabilities from achieving good health (19). For example:

- A child born blind may not specifically require ongoing health care for a primary health condition and associated impairment (20).
- An adolescent with a traumatic spinal cord injury may have considerable health care needs during the acute phase of the primary condition but thereafter may require only services to maintain health – for example, to prevent secondary conditions (20).

- Adults with chronic conditions such as multiple sclerosis, cystic fibrosis, severe arthritis, or schizophrenia may have complex and continuing health care needs related to their primary health condition or associated impairments (20).

Risk of developing secondary conditions

Depression is a common secondary condition in people with disabilities (21–23). Pain has been reported in children and adults with cerebral palsy (24, 25), children with spina bifida (26), and adults with post-polio paralysis (27), neuromuscular disease (28), and traumatic brain injury (29). Osteoporosis is common in people with a spinal cord injury (30), spina bifida (31), or cerebral palsy (32, 33).

Risk of developing co-morbid conditions

People with disabilities develop the same health problems that affect the general population, such as influenza and pneumonia. Some may be more susceptible to developing chronic conditions because of the influence of behavioural risk factors such as increased physical inactivity (18). They also may experience earlier onset of these conditions (17). One study indicated that adults with developmental disabilities had a similar or greater rate of chronic health conditions such as high blood pressure, cardiovascular disease, and diabetes than people without disabilities (34). The prevalence of diabetes in people with schizophrenia is around 15%, compared with the general population rate of 2–3% (21).

Greater vulnerability to age-related conditions

The ageing process for some groups of people with disabilities begins earlier than usual. Some people with developmental disabilities show signs of premature ageing in their 40s and 50s (35) and they may experience age-related health conditions more frequently. For example, people with Down syndrome have a higher incidence of Alzheimer disease than the general population, while people with intellectual impairments (unrelated to Down syndrome) have higher rates of dementia (35). The ageing process and associated changes (presbycusis, deconditioning, loss of strength and balance, osteoporosis) may have a greater impact on people with disabilities. For example, those with existing mobility impairments

may increasingly experience functional loss as they age (9).

Increased rates of health risk behaviours

The health behaviours practiced by some adults with disabilities can differ in degree from those of the general population (12). In Australia, people with disabilities aged between 15–64 were more likely to be overweight or obese than other people (48% compared with 39%) and to smoke daily (3). Data cited from the 2001 and 2003 Behavioural Risk Factor Surveillance System in the United States of America reported similar findings. People with disabilities have higher rates of smoking (30.5% compared with 21.7%), are more likely to be physically inactive (22.4% compared with 11.9%), and are more likely to be obese (31.2% compared with 19.6%) (18). A Canadian study using a national sample showed that people with hearing impairments were more likely than the general population to report low levels of physical activity (36). A study in Rwanda reported that adults with lower limb amputations engaged in poor health-related behaviours such as smoking, alcohol consumption, recreational drug use, and a lack of exercise (37).

Greater risk of being exposed to violence

Violence is linked to health outcomes both immediate and long term, including injuries, physical and mental health problems, substance abuse, and death (38). People with disabilities are at greater risk of violence than those without disabilities. In the United States violence against people with disabilities has been reported to be 4–10 times greater than that against people without disabilities (39). The prevalence of sexual abuse against people with disabilities has been shown to be higher (40, 41), especially for institutionalized men and women with intellectual disabilities (42–44), intimate partners (40, 45), and adolescents (46).

Higher risk of unintentional injury

People with disabilities are at higher risk of nonfatal unintentional injury from road traffic crashes, burns, falls, and accidents related to assistive devices (47–51). One study found that children with developmental disabilities – including autism, attention deficit disorder, and attention deficit hyperactivity disorder – were two to three times more at risk of an injury than those without (50). Other studies conclude that children with disabilities have a significantly higher risk of falls (52), burn-related injuries (53), and injuries from crashes involving motor vehicles or bicycles (54).

Higher risk of premature death

Mortality rates for people with disabilities vary depending on the health condition. People with schizophrenia and depression have an increased risk of premature death (2.6 and 1.7 times greater, respectively) (21). An investigation in the United Kingdom of Great Britain and Northern Ireland regarding health inequalities among people with learning impairments and people with mental health disorders found that they had a lower life expectancy (see Box 3.2) (15).

In some instances mortality rates for people with disabilities have fallen in developed countries. For example, adults with cerebral palsy have lifespans close to those of people with no disability (55). Over the past few decades people with a spinal cord injury in the United Kingdom and the United States have improved survival rates during the first one to two years following injury (56, 57), but beyond this period there is no evidence of improvement (57). The data are limited on mortality rates for people with disabilities in low-income countries. A study in Bangladesh suggests that people with cerebral palsy may have higher rates of premature death (58).

Needs and unmet needs

Disabled respondents from 51 countries reported seeking more inpatient and outpatient care than people without disabilities in the WHO 2002–2004 *World Health Survey* (see Table 3.1). Women seek care more often than men, and so do respondents with disabilities in high-income countries compared with respondents in low-income countries across gender and age groups. The proportion of respondents seeking care in high-income countries increases with age; the results varied for low-income countries.

Disabled respondents reported not receiving care more than people without disabilities, across both sex and age grouping. Respondents with disabilities in low-income countries show higher rates of not receiving care (6.1–6.6) than respondents in high-income countries (3.3–4.6). Age-standardized analysis across all countries suggests that older respondents with disabilities have less unmet care needs than younger (≤ 59) respondents.

Need and unmet needs exist across the spectrum of health services – promotion, prevention, and treatment.

Health promotion and prevention

Misconceptions about the health of people with disabilities have led to assumptions that people with disabilities do not require access to health promotion and disease prevention (60).

Evidence shows that health promotion interventions such as physical activities are beneficial for people with disabilities (61–65). But health promotion activities seldom target people with disabilities, and many experience multiple barriers to participation. For example, limited access to health promotion has been documented for people with multiple sclerosis (66), stroke (67), poliomyelitis (67), intellectual impairment (15), and mental health problems (15).

While some research indicates minimal differences in immunization rates (68–70), people with disabilities are generally less likely to receive screening and preventive services. Several studies found that women with disabilities receive less screening for breast and cervical cancer compared with women without disabilities (15, 68, 69, 71–75), and men with disabilities are less likely to receive

Box 3.2. Health inequalities experienced by people with disabilities

The Disability Rights Commission in the United Kingdom formally investigated premature deaths among people with learning disabilities or mental health problems and local reports of unequal access to health care between 2004 and 2006.

People with long-term mental health problems – such as severe depression, bipolar disorder, or schizophrenia – and learning disabilities, such as autism:

- Had more chronic health conditions than the general population. They were more likely to be obese and have heart disease, high blood pressure, respiratory disease, diabetes, strokes, or breast cancer. People with schizophrenia were nearly twice as likely to have bowel cancer. Although the recording of people with learning disability in primary care settings was poor, higher rates of respiratory disease and obesity in this population were indicated.
- Developed chronic health conditions at a younger age than other people. For example, 31% of people with schizophrenia were diagnosed with heart disease under the age of 55, compared with 18% of others with heart disease.
- Died sooner following diagnosis. Five years following a diagnosis of heart disease (adjusting for age), 22% of people with schizophrenia and 15% of people with bipolar disorder had died, compared with 8% of people without serious mental health problems. The pattern was similar for stroke and chronic obstructive pulmonary disorder.

Social deprivation was a major contributor to these health inequalities, and people with mental health problems and learning disabilities were at a high risk of poverty. The lack of health promotion, service access, and equal treatment were also cited as significant barriers. Disabled people identified fear and mistrust, limited access to general practice lists, difficulty negotiating appointment systems, inaccessible information, poor communication, and diagnostic overshadowing. Service providers identified issues such as fear, ignorance, and inadequate training.

Responses to the study were positive. Prominent health care professionals endorsed the findings. The British Medical Association established training for medical students, and nongovernmental organizations ran campaigns on health inequalities. The British government introduced incentives to encourage people with learning disabilities to undergo health checks and strengthened guidance for mental health-care workers. The Health Care Commission in association with RADAR – a disability NGO – undertook further work to explore disabling factors in health care and to produce guidelines on good practice and criteria for future health care inspections.

Source (15).

screening for prostate cancer (68, 76). A United Kingdom investigation found that people with intellectual impairment and diabetes are less likely than others with just diabetes to have their weight checked, and people with schizophrenia and a high risk of coronary heart disease are less likely to receive cholesterol screening (15).

Sexual and reproductive health services

Sexual and reproductive health services include family planning, maternal health care, preventing and managing gender-based violence, and preventing and treating sexually transmitted infections including HIV/AIDS. While little information is available, it is widely thought that people with disabilities have significant unmet needs (77). Adolescents and adults with disabilities are more likely to be excluded from sex education programmes (78, 79). A national study in the United States showed that women with functional limitations were less likely to be asked about contraceptive use during visits to general practitioners (71).

Dental care

The oral health of many people with disabilities is poor, and access to dental care limited (80–86). An Australian study investigating dental treatment of children with disabilities found that the simple treatment needs of 41% of the sample were not met (81). A study of the use of oral health care services by children in Lagos, Nigeria, found that children with disabilities and children from lower socioeconomic status did not adequately use dental facilities (84).

Table 3.1. **Individual's seeking health care and not receiving needed care.**

	Percent					
	Low-income countries		**High-income countries**		**All countries**	
	Not disabled	**Disabled**	**Not disabled**	**Disabled**	**Not disabled**	**Disabled**
Male						
Sought inpatient care	13.7	22.7*	21.7	42.4*	16.5	28.5*
Sought outpatient care	49.3	58.4*	55.0	61.8*	51.1	59.5*
Needed, but did not get care	4.6	6.6*	2.8	3.3	4.1	5.8*
Female						
Sought inpatient care	16.8	21.9*	30.1	46.7*	20.9	29.0*
Sought outpatient care	49.6	59.3*	67.0	68.5	55.8	61.7*
Needed, but did not get care	4.8	6.1	1.8	4.6*	3.7	5.8*
18–49						
Sought inpatient care	13.5	23.2*	23.1	46.6*	16.1	28.1*
Sought outpatient care	48.8	58.5*	56.7	63.4*	50.9	59.3*
Needed, but did not get care	4.3	6.2*	2.3	4.1	3.8	6.0*
50–59						
Sought inpatient care	13.9	20.7*	22.1	42.9*	16.6	27.1*
Sought outpatient care	52.1	67.4*	61.4	74.9*	55.1	69.2*
Needed, but did not get care	4.2	6.7*	2.2	4.6	3.6	6.4*
60 and over						
Sought inpatient care	18.6	20.6	31.4	42.3*	23.7	29.9*
Sought outpatient care	49.9	56.7	67.9	67.6	57.3	60.8
Needed, but did not get care	5.6	6.3	2.2	3.8	4.2	5.3

Note: Estimates are weighted using WHS post-stratified weights, when available (probability weights otherwise) and age-standardized.
* *t*-test suggests significant difference from "Not disabled" at 5%.
Source (*59*).

Mental health services

Many people with mental health conditions do not receive mental health care despite the fact that effective interventions exist, including medication. A large multicountry survey supported by WHO showed that between 35% and 50% of people with serious mental disorders in developed countries, and between 76% and 85% in developing countries, received no treatment in the year before the study (*87*). A meta-analysis of 37 epidemiological studies across 32 developed and developing countries uncovered a median treatment gap between 32% and 78% for a range of mental health conditions including schizophrenia, mood disorders, anxiety disorders, and alcohol abuse or dependence (*88*).

Addressing barriers to health care

People with disabilities encounter a range of barriers when they attempt to access health care services (*7, 89, 90*). Analysis of the *World Health Survey* data showed a significant difference between men and women with disabilities and people without disabilities in terms of the attitudinal, physical, and system level barriers faced in accessing care (see Table 3.2).

Research in Uttar Pradesh and Tamil Nadu states of India found that cost (70.5%), lack of services in the area (52.3%), and transportation (20.5%) were the top three barriers to using

health facilities (*91*). These findings are supported by studies in Southern Africa that identified cost, distance, and lack of transport as reasons for not using services, along with services no longer being helpful or the individual not being satisfied by the services (*92–95*).

Table 3.2. **Reasons for lack of care**

	Percent					
	Low-income countries		High-income countries		All countries	
	Not disabled	Disabled	Not disabled	Disabled	Not disabled	Disabled
Male						
Could not afford the visit	40.2	58.8*	11.6	29.8*	33.5	53.0*
No transport	18.4	16.6	6.9	28.3*	15.2	18.1
Could not afford transport	20.1	30.6	2.1	16.9*	15.5	27.8*
Health-care provider's equipment inadequate	8.5	18.7*	5.0	27.8*	7.7	22.4*
Health-care provider's skills inadequate	5.8	14.6*	9.9	13.5	6.7	15.7*
Were previously treated badly	4.6	17.6*	7.2	39.6*	5.1	23.7*
Could not take time off	9.5	11.9	6.2	7.9	8.8	11.8
Did not know where to go	5.1	12.4	1.5	23.1*	4.3	15.1*
The person did not think he/she/his/her child was sick enough	42.6	32.2	44.1	18.0*	43.7	28.4*
Tried but was denied care	5.2	14.3*	18.7	44.3*	8.5	23.4*
Other	12.8	18.6	12.5	20.5	12.4	18.1
Female						
Could not afford the visit	35.6	61.3*	25.8	25.0	32.2	51.5*
No transport	14.0	18.1	7.9	20.4*	13.8	17.4
Could not afford transport	15.3	29.4*	4.4	15.2*	13.3	24.6*
Health-care provider's equipment inadequate	10.2	17.0	8.4	25.7*	9.8	17.0*
Health-care provider's skills inadequate	5.3	13.6*	8.9	20.6*	6.3	15.7*
Were previously treated badly	3.7	8.5*	9.3	20.1*	5.3	10.2*
Could not take time off	6.1	8.3	8.3	17.8	6.6	10.6
Did not know where to go	7.7	13.2	9.3	16.2	9.0	12.2
The person did not think he/she/his/her child was sick enough	30.7	28.2	21.3	22.6	29.3	29.3
Tried but was denied care	3.8	9.0*	19.6	54.6*	7.3	21.7*
Other	30.2	17.0*	23.0	24.0	28.5	16.4*
Could not afford the visit						
18–49						
Could not afford the visit	38.7	65.4*	14.1	27.7*	33.6	58.7*
No transport	12.7	13.7	6.6	25.1	11.3	16.0
Could not afford transport	15.0	29.5*	4.6	11.2*	12.8	25.8*

continues ...

... continued

	Percent					
	Low-income countries		High-income countries		All countries	
	Not disabled	Disabled	Not disabled	Disabled	Not disabled	Disabled
Health-care provider's equipment inadequate	9.7	17.4*	9.2	29.3	9.5	20.3*
Health-care provider's skills inadequate	6.2	15.4*	10.9	18.4	7.4	16.3*
Were previously treated badly	5.1	15.1*	6.8	17.9*	5.5	15.5*
Could not take time off	9.0	13.4	8.8	23.9	8.8	15.8
Did not know where to go	7.0	11.9	2.0	9.0*	5.9	11.8*
The person did not think he/she/his/her child was sick enough	40.2	30.6*	26.8	26.9	37.0	29.4
Tried but was denied care	5.3	12.9*	27.5	49.5*	10.5	21.4*
Other	16.0	13.5	17.5	14.4	16.2	13.3
50–59						
Could not afford the visit	49.6	67.4*	17.9	26.7	42.8	58.0
No transport	19.8	16.0	2.9	2.3	16.3	13.0
Could not afford transport	23.1	33.0	0.7	4.0	18.5	26.3
Health-care provider's equipment inadequate	8.6	14.5	4.2	29.1	7.7	15.1
Health-care provider's skills inadequate	6.5	13.3	10.0	40.9*	7.2	17.6
Were previously treated badly	6.7	12.4	7.2	31.1	6.8	14.0
Could not take time off	8.8	9.7	14.9	10.8	10.2	9.7
Did not know where to go	11.6	18.5	6.5	4.5	10.5	15.6
The person did not think he/she/his/her child was sick enough	35.4	14.5*	38.2	5.3*	36.0	13.0*
Tried but was denied care	6.4	17.9	18.0	55.3*	9.0	24.5*
Other	18.6	12.8	34.8	44.5	22.1	19.9
60 and over						
Could not afford the visit	36.8	47.7	14.4	21.1	30.6	38.7
No transport	25.1	24.3	9.5	30.3*	20.6	22.0
Could not afford transport	23.6	27.5	1.9	28.5*	18.0	24.7
Health-care provider's equipment or are inadequate	9.1	17.1	3.2	20.6	7.7	16.5
Health-care provider's skills inadequate	4.1	11.8	6.6	18.5	4.8	14.8
Were previously treated badly	1.7	6.7*	8.7	36.7*	3.7	14.1
Could not take time off	5.4	4.1	2.7	1.2	5.1	3.2
Did not know where to go	4.5	13.8	9.0	37.6*	6.1	16.5
The person did not think he/she/his/her child was sick enough	31.8	32.7	56.2	21.6*	38.9	31.2
Tried but was denied care	2.6	7.8	4.5	62.1*	3.2	25.8*
Other	27.7	25.2	12.2	35.5*	23.7	22.6

Note: Results are significant in every case according to Pearson's Chi-Square test, corrected for survey design. Estimates are weighted using WHS post-stratified weights, when available (probability weights otherwise) and age-standardized.
* *t*-test suggests significant difference from "Not disabled" at 5%.
Source (*59*).

Governments can improve health outcomes for people with disabilities by improving access to quality, affordable health care services, which make the best use of available resources. Usually several factors interact to inhibit access to health care (*96*), so reforms in all the interacting components of the health care system are required:

- reforming policy and legislation
- addressing barriers to financing and affordability
- addressing barriers to service delivery
- addressing human resource barriers
- filling gaps in data and research (*97*).

Reforming policy and legislation

International, regional, and national policy and legislation can help meet the health care needs of people with disabilities where political will, funding, and technical support accompany implementation. Policy formulated at the international level can affect national health care policies (*98*). International agreements such as the CRPD (*2*) and the Millennium Development Goals can provide countries with rationale and support to improve availability of health care for people with disabilities. The CRPD indicates the following areas for action:

- **Accessibility** – stop discrimination against people with disabilities when accessing health care, health services, food or fluid, health insurance, and life insurance. This includes making the environment accessible.
- **Affordability** – ensure that people with disabilities get the same variety, quality, and standard of free and affordable health care as other people.
- **Availability** – put early intervention and treatment services as close as possible to where people live in their communities.
- **Quality** – ensure that health workers give the same quality care to people with disabilities as to others.

Formal acknowledgement, within national health care policies, that some groups of persons with disabilities experience health inequalities is needed to remove health disparities (*11*). Countries such as Australia, Canada, the United Kingdom and the United States have published national agendas or position papers that specifically address the health problems of people with intellectual impairment (*14*). In the United States *Healthy People 2010* – a framework for preventing health conditions in the entire population – makes reference to people with disabilities (*60*).

In addition to the health sector, many other sectors can enact "disability-friendly" policies to prevent access barriers and enable those with disabilities to promote their health and actively participate in community life (*99*). Legislation and policies within the education, transport, housing, labour, and social welfare sectors can all influence the health of people with disabilities (see Chapters 5–8 for further information).

People with disabilities are most intimately familiar with and most affected by barriers to health care access, and eliminating these barriers requires input from these people (*89*). Research has shown the benefits of involving users in the design and operation of health care systems (*100*). People with diverse disabilities can contribute, including people with intellectual impairment (*101*), people with mental health conditions (*102–104*), children with disabilities (*105*), and families and caregivers (*106, 107*).

Commitment to collaboration is necessary, and input is required from health-care providers familiar with the structural, institutional, and professional challenges of providing access to quality care. The time, technical, and resource challenges of involving users must be acknowledged (*100, 106*), but the benefits are also significant. People with disabilities are frequent users of the health care system, and tend to use a wide range of services across the continuum of care, so their experiences can also help measure overall performance of the health system (*17, 89*).

Table 3.3. Overview of health expenditures, proportion of disabled and not disabled respondents

| | Percent | | | | | |
| | Low-income countries | | High-income countries | | All countries | |
	Not disabled	Disabled	Not disabled	Disabled	Not disabled	Disabled
Men						
Paid with current income	84.6	81.4*	73.3	70.1	80.9	79.1
Paid with savings	10.6	9.8	11.5	12.9	10.8	11.1
Paid with insurance	1.8	1.8	11.3	13.3	5.1	5.2
Paid by selling items	13.6	17.6*	3.3	5.3	9.9	13.6*
Family paid	15.8	23.8*	7.7	13.5*	12.9	21.3*
Paid by borrowing	13.7	25.2*	5.9	14.7*	11.0	21.6*
Paid by other means	5.3	5.1	2.6	6.5*	4.3	5.5
Women						
Paid with current income	82.9	82.8	71.5	74.9	78.5	80.3
Paid with savings	9.1	10.8	11.4	11.6	10.1	10.8
Paid with insurance	2.0	1.8	11.1	16.0*	5.7	6.2
Paid by selling items	12.0	14.2*	2.4	4.7*	8.3	10.7*
Family paid	16.7	26.6*	9.3	15.1*	13.7	22.7*
Paid by borrowing	14.0	23.5*	6.4	12.7*	11.2	19.5*
Paid by other means	6.7	5.8	2.6	3.6	4.9	5.3

Note: Estimates are weighted using WHS post-stratified weights, when available (probability weights otherwise) and age-standardized.
* *t*-test suggests significant difference from "Not disabled" at 5%.
Source (*59*).

Addressing barriers to financing and affordability

A review of the 2002–2004 *World Health Survey* reveals that affordability was the primary reason why people with disabilities, across gender and age groups, did not receive needed health care in low-income countries. For 51 countries 32–33% of nondisabled men and women cannot afford health care, compared with 51–53% of people with disabilities (see Table 3.2). Transport costs also rank high as a barrier to health care access in low-income and high-income countries, and across gender and age groups.

Health services are funded through a variety of sources including government budgets, social insurance, private health insurance, external donor funding, and private sources including nongovernmental arrangements and out-of-pocket expenses. The *World Health Survey* showed that the rate at which people with disabilities pay with current income, savings, or insurance is roughly the same as for people without disabilities, but paying with personal means varies between groups: paying with insurance is more common in high-income countries, while selling items and relying on friends and family is more common in low-income countries, and people with disabilities are more likely to sell items, borrow money, or rely on a family member (see Table 3.3).

Public health systems theoretically provide universal coverage, but this is rare (*108, 109*): no country has ensured that everybody has immediate access to all health care services (*110*). In the poorest countries only the most basic services may be available (*110*). Restrictions in public health sector expenditure are resulting in an inadequate supply of services and a significant increase in the proportion of out-of-pocket expenditure by households (*109, 111*). In many low-income countries less than 1% of health budgets are spent on mental health care, with countries relying on out-of-pocket payments as the primary financing mechanism (*112*). Some middle-income countries are moving towards private sector provision for treatments such as mental health services (*113*).

People with disabilities experience lower rates of employment, are more likely to be economically disadvantaged, and are therefore less likely to afford private health insurance (*114*). Employed people with disabilities may be excluded from private health insurance because of pre-existing conditions or be "underinsured" (*114*) because they have been denied coverage for a long period (*11*), or are excluded from claiming for treatment related to a pre-existing condition, or must pay higher premiums and out-of-pocket expenses. This has been a problem in the United States for example, but the new Affordable Care Act enacted in March 2010 will prohibit the denial of insurance to those with pre-existing conditions starting in 2014 (*115*).

Analysis from the 2002–2004 *World Health Survey* across 51 countries showed that men and women with disabilities, in high-income and low-income countries, had more difficulties than adults without disabilities in obtaining, from private health care organizations or the government, payment exemptions or the right to special rates for health care. Furthermore people with disabilities experienced more difficulties in finding out which benefits they were entitled to from health insurance and obtaining reimbursements from health insurance. This finding was most evident in the age group 18–49 with some variability in the older age groups across income settings (see Table 3.4).

Social health insurance systems are generally characterized by mandatory payroll contributions from individuals and employers (*109*). These employer-based systems may be inaccessible for many adults with disabilities because they have lower employment rates than people without disabilities. Even employed people with disabilities may not be able to afford insurance premiums associated with employer-based health insurance plans (*114*), while disabled people working in the informal sector or for small businesses are unlikely to be offered insurance (*114*).

The *World Health Survey* found that disabled respondents in 31 low-income and low middle-income countries spend 15% of total household expenditure on out-of-pocket health care costs compared with 11% for nondisabled respondents. People with disabilities were also found to be more vulnerable to catastrophic health expenditure (see Table 3.5) across gender and age groups, and for both low-income and high-income countries as defined by the World Bank. For all countries, 28–29% of all people with disabilities suffer catastrophic expenditures compared with 17–18% of nondisabled people, but low-income countries show significantly higher rates than high-income countries across sex and age groups.

Financing options

Health system financing options determine whether health services – a mix of promotion, prevention, treatment, and rehabilitation – are available and whether people are protected from financial risks associated with using them (*110, 116*). Contributions such as social insurance and copayment for health services must be affordable and fair, and take into account the individual's ability to pay. Full access will be achieved only when governments cover the cost of the available health services for disabled people who cannot afford to pay (*110*).

A range of health financing options can increase the availability of health care services to the general population, and improve access for individuals with disabilities. The *World Health Report 2010* outlines an action agenda for paying for health that does not deter people from using services including (*110*):

- raise sufficient resources for health by increasing the efficiency of revenue collection, reprioritizing government spending,

Table 3.4. **Difficulties in access to health care financing**

	Percent					
	Low-income countries		**High-income countries**		**All countries**	
	Not disabled	**Disabled**	**Not disabled**	**Disabled**	**Not disabled**	**Disabled**
Male						
Difficulties in:						
obtaining exemptions or special rates	17.7	24.1*	7.5	14.1*	15.0	22.0*
completing insurance applications	3.6	6.6	4.7	12.4*	4.3	10.1*
finding out insurance benefits/entitlements	4.0	9.0*	8.6	17.2*	6.4	13.2*
getting reimbursed from health insurance	3.3	7.4*	3.5	11.8*	3.4	8.6*
Female						
Difficulties in:						
obtaining exemptions or special rates	15.7	23.5*	5.9	16.5*	12.3	21.1*
completing insurance applications	3.3	5.2	5.1	9.3*	4.5	7.0*
finding out insurance benefits/entitlements	3.3	6.0*	8.4	15.9*	6.2	10.7*
getting reimbursed from health insurance	3.2	5.4*	3.2	5.8*	3.1	5.6*
18–49						
Difficulties in:						
obtaining exemptions or special rates	15.7	22.5*	6.3	15.8*	13.7	21.6*
completing insurance applications	4.2	6.7*	4.2	10.7*	4.1	8.3*
finding out insurance benefits/entitlements	4.6	8.0*	9.9	17.7*	7.3	12.1*
getting reimbursed from health insurance	4.2	7.1*	4.1	10.6*	4.1	8.0*
50–59						
Difficulties in:						
obtaining exemptions or special rates	17.5	24.2*	7.9	18.5*	14.9	23.1*
completing insurance applications	3.8	5.8	5.9	14.6*	5.0	10.4*
finding out insurance benefits/entitlements	5.0	7.9	9.1	19.9*	7.4	13.8*
getting reimbursed from health insurance	4.4	7.1	5.0	8.0	4.7	7.4
≥ 60						
Difficulties in:						
obtaining exemptions or special rates	18.6	25.5	6.9	14.0*	13.6	20.1*
completing insurance applications	2.1	4.4	6.0	7.8	4.7	6.7
finding out insurance benefits/entitlements	1.6	6.1*	5.8	11.7*	4.2	9.6*
getting reimbursed from health insurance	1.3	4.7	1.5	4.8*	1.5	4.7*

Note: Estimates are weighted using WHS post-stratified weights, when available (probability weights otherwise) and age-standardized.

* t-test suggests significant difference from "Not disabled" at 5%.

Source (59).

Table 3.5. **Overview of catastrophic health expenditures, proportion of disabled and not disabled respondents**

	Percent					
	Low-income countries		High-income countries		All countries	
	Not disabled	Disabled	Not disabled	Disabled	Not disabled	Disabled
Male	20.2	31.2	14.5	18.5	18.4	27.8
Female	20.0	32.6	12.7	18.7	17.4	28.7
18–49	19.9	33.4	13.2	16.1	17.9	29.2
50–59	18.2	32.6	13.0	24.7	16.4	30.1
60 and over	21.2	29.5	14.2	21.5	18.3	26.3

Note: All results are significant according to Pearson's Chi-Square test, corrected for survey design. Estimates are weighted using WHS post-stratified weights, when available (probability weights otherwise) and age-standardized. Source (*59*).

using innovative financing, and providing development assistance;
- remove financial risks and barriers to access;
- promote efficiency and eliminate waste.

While improving access to affordable, quality health care pertains to everyone, the evidence presented above suggests that people with disabilities have more health care needs and more unmet needs. This section therefore focuses specifically on financing strategies that may improve access to health services for persons with disabilities.

Provide affordable health insurance

Having insurance (public, private, or mixed) can increase disabled people's access to, and use of, health care services. Having insurance improves a variety of outcomes including an increase in the likelihood of receiving primary care, a decrease in unmet needs (including for speciality care), and a reduction in delays or in foregoing care (*117–119*). Insurance for a wide range of basic medical services can improve clinical outcomes (*120*), and can reduce the financial problems and the burden of out-of-pocket payments for families (*118*). Subsidizing health insurance can also extend coverage to persons with disabilities. In Taiwan, China the health insurance scheme pays for part of the insurance premium for people with intellectual disabilities according to their level of

disability (*121*). In Colombia subsidized health insurance increased coverage for the poorest quintile of the population (*122*), which may benefit people with disabilities because they are disproportionately represented in the bottom quintile.

Target people with disabilities who have the greatest health care needs

Some governments have targeted funding to primary care doctors and organizations to support health care of people with the greatest need. Care Plus – a primary health care initiative in New Zealand – provides an additional approximately 10% capitation funding to primary health organizations to include services such as comprehensive assessments, individual care plan development, patient education, and regular follow-ups, as well as better-coordinated and lower cost services (*123, 124*). Medicare, a United States government social insurance scheme, provides additional payment to primary care physicians for physician-patient-family-nurse conferences to facilitate communication, support lifestyle changes, and improve treatment compliance (*125*). The programme improved functioning of elderly people with heart conditions and has the potential to lower total health care expenditures (*125*). Many governments also extend financial assistance to disabled people's organizations and nongovernmental organizations for health programmes targeting people with disabilities (*91, 126, 127*).

Link income support to use of health care
Reviews of health financing mechanisms for the poor in Latin America indicate that conditional cash transfers can increase the use of preventative health services and encourage informed and active health care consumers, where effective primary health care and a mechanism to disburse payments are in place (*111, 128–131*). Conditional cash transfers, targeted at those groups of people with disabilities who typically receive fewer preventative services, may increase access to these services (*114*).

Provide general income support
Unconditional cash transfers for people with disabilities recognize the additional barriers they face in accessing health care and rehabilitation, transport, education, and working, among other things. Many countries provide income support through these transfers to poor households, including poor households with a disabled member, and directly to individuals with disabilities. Some, such as Bangladesh, Brazil, India, and South Africa, have unconditional cash transfer programmes targeted at poor people and households with a disabled member. The programmes aim at increasing the disposable income of poor households, which they spend according to their priorities – for example by buying food, enrolling children in education, or paying for health care. No best practice formula is available to guide policy, but cash transfers can exist along with other social policies and social protection programmes.

Reduce or remove out-of-pocket payments to improve access
Reduction or elimination of out-of-pocket payments for fees – whether formal or informal – can increase poor people's use of health care services, and reduce financial hardship and catastrophic health expenditure (*110, 111*). This is particularly important for people with disabilities who spend more on health than people without disabilities (see Table 3.3). Removing fees does not guarantee access, however, as even "free" health services may not get used. People with mental health conditions, for example, might not access services because of barriers such as stigma, or people with mobility impairments may face physical barriers to health care access (*72, 113*).

Provide incentives for health providers to promote access
Some people with disabilities require prolonged care and accommodations requiring additional resources to ensure effective coordination (*114*). In the United States tax credits to small practices help make up for the cost of patient accommodations (*132*). In Wales new disability access criteria for primary care doctors create incentives for general medical practices to make services more accessible to disabled people (*15*).

Addressing barriers to service delivery

Ensuring the availability of services and disabled peoples' awareness of the services, including those in rural and remote communities, is essential to improving access (see Box 3.3). Where services do exist people with disabilities may encounter a range of physical, communication, information, and coordination barriers when they attempt to access health care services.

Physical barriers may be related to the architectural design of health facilities, or to medical equipment, or transportation (*11, 69, 72, 96*).

Barriers to facilities include inaccessible parking areas, uneven access to buildings, poor signage, narrow doorways, internal steps, and inadequate bathroom facilities. A study of 41 Brazilian cities examining the architectural barriers in basic health care units found that about 60% did not allow adequate access for people with functional difficulties (*137*). Similarly, a survey carried out in Essen, Germany found that 80% of orthopaedic surgeries and 90% of neurological surgeries did not meet access

Box 3.3. **Access to mental health services**

The 2001 *World Health Report* called for adequate access to effective and humane treatment for people with mental health conditions (*133*). Access to appropriate care is problematic for many people with mental health conditions, and certain groups – such as rural populations – typically have less access to services than other groups (*134*).

In ensuring access to mental health services, one of the most important factors to consider is the extent to which services are community-based (*135*). But in most countries, care is still predominantly provided in institutions. In low-income and middle-income countries there is less than one outpatient contact or visit (0.7) per day spent in inpatient care (*136*). The move from institutional to community care is slow and uneven. A recent study of mental health systems in 42 low-income and middle-income countries (*136*) showed that resources for mental health are overwhelmingly concentrated in urban settings. A considerable number of people with mental health conditions are being hospitalized in mental hospitals in large cities. Controlling for population density, there were nearly three times as many psychiatric beds in the largest city of a country, than in the rest of the country (see figure below). In low-income countries, the imbalance was even greater with more than six times as many beds based in the largest city. A similar pattern was found for human resources: across the participating countries, the ratio per population of psychiatrists and nurses working in the largest city was more than twice that of psychiatrists and nurses working in the entire country.

Ratio of psychiatric beds located in or near the largest city to beds in the entire country

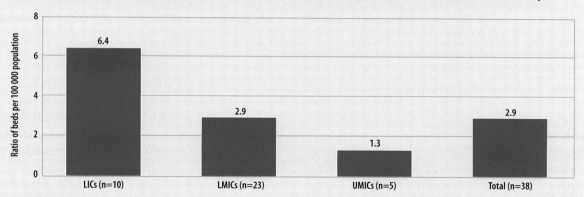

Note: Low-income countries (LICs), lower middle-income countries (LMICs), and upper middle-income countries (UMICs)
To increase access to services for people with mental health conditions, community care systems need to be strengthened. This will include greater integration into primary health care, as well as discouraging hospitalization, especially in large mental hospitals, and strengthening outpatient mental health care through follow-up care and mobile teams (*161*). Wherever delivered, mental health services need to respect the human rights of people with mental health conditions, in line with the CRPD (*162*).

standards, which limited wheelchair users from accessing their doctor of choice (*138*).

Medical equipment is often not accessible for people with disabilities, particularly those with mobility impairments. In the *World Health Survey* men with disabilities report health service provider's equipment (including medication) to be inadequate across income settings (22.4% compared with 7.7% for men without disabilities); women with disabilities in high-income countries report similar difficulties (see **Table 3.2**). For example, many women with mobility impairments are unable to access breast and cervical cancer screening because examination tables are not height-adjustable and mammography equipment only accommodates women who are able to stand (*11, 132*).

People with disabilities frequently cite transport as a barrier to accessing health care, particularly when they are located at a distance from health care facilities (see Table 3.2) (91–95). Transport for people with disabilities is often limited, unaffordable, or inaccessible (139). The majority of disabled participants in a United States study said that transportation problems were a major barrier to accessing health care (89). A study in the Republic of Korea suggested that transportation barriers were a likely factor in keeping people with severe physical and communication impairments from participating in population screenings for chronic diseases (140).

Communication difficulties between people with disabilities and service providers are regularly cited as an area of concern (79, 141, 142). Difficulties can arise when people with disabilities attempt to make appointments with service providers, provide a medical history and description of their symptoms, or try to understand explanations about diagnosis and management of health conditions. Inaccurate case histories may be provided to health-care practitioners when information is supplied by caregivers, family members, or others (143).

Service providers may feel uncomfortable communicating with people with disabilities. For example, many health-care providers have not been trained to interact with people with serious mental illness, and feel uncomfortable or ineffective in communicating with them (144). An investigation into Deaf women's access to health care in the United States found that health-care workers often turn their heads down when talking, preventing deaf women from lip-reading (141).

Failure to communicate in appropriate formats can lead to problems with compliance and attendance (145). A survey commissioned by the Zimbabwe Parents of Handicapped Children's Association found that people with disabilities were excluded from general HIV/AIDS services because counselling and testing were not offered in sign language for people with hearing impairments, and education and communication materials were not offered in Braille for people with visual impairments (146).

Some people with disabilities may have multiple or complex health needs, including rehabilitation, which require input from different service providers. These needs may extend across services in different sectors such as the education and social sectors. People with disabilities who require multiple services often receive fragmented or duplicative services (147). They may also encounter transitional difficulties when care is transferred from one service provider to another (148), such as when transitioning from child to adult services (149–151), and from adult services to elderly services (152, 153).

Lack of communication between service providers can hamper coordinated service delivery (154). Primary health-care professionals' referrals to specialists often lack sufficient information, for example. Conversely primary health-care professionals frequently receive inadequate consultation reports from specialists, and discharge summaries following hospital admission may never reach the primary care doctor (155).

Primary care consultations can take longer for people with disabilities than for people without disabilities (156). Adults with intellectual impairment often require extra time for examinations, screening, clinical procedures, and health promotion (99). Health-care practitioners are often not reimbursed for the additional consultation time they spend with people with disabilities (132, 156), and the disparities between actual cost and reimbursement can be a disincentive for service providers to provide comprehensive health care (156). Short consultations may leave little time for service providers to understand and address the sometimes complex health care needs of people with disabilities (154, 157).

Perceptions of health status may influence health behaviours, including attendance at health care services, and how health needs are communicated. A study on people with epilepsy in rural Ghana, for example, found that spiritual beliefs surrounding epilepsy influenced health and seeking of treatment (158). A study in rural areas of the Gambia reported that only 16% of 380 people with epilepsy knew that preventive treatment was possible; of the 48% of people with epilepsy who had never used treatment, 70% did not know that clinics offered treatment for seizures (*158*). People with intellectual impairment in minority ethnic communities have also been found to be less likely to use health care services (*14, 159*). An Australian study on women with mental health conditions and physical, sensory, and intellectual impairment found that self-perceptions regarding sexuality, painful past experiences associated with reproductive screening, and memories of themselves before disability were all barriers to seeking health care (*72*). In another example, people who experience disability as they age may "normalize" their symptoms as "just part of ageing" rather than seeking appropriate treatment (*160*).

Include people with disabilities in general health care services

All groups in society should have access to comprehensive, inclusive health care (*122, 163*). An international survey of health research priorities indicated that addressing the specific impairments of people with disabilities is secondary to integrating their health needs into primary health care systems (*164*). Primary care services are generally the most accessible, affordable, and acceptable for communities (*161*). For example, a systematic review of studies from six developing countries in Africa, Asia, and Latin America confirmed that local, affordable primary health care programmes were more effective than other programmes for people with mental health conditions (*165*).

Providers may have to cater to the range of needs stemming from hearing, vision, speech, mobility, and cognitive impairments to include people with disabilities in primary health care services. Table 3.6 lists examples of accommodations. While evidence on the efficacy of such accommodations is limited, they represent practical approaches, widely recommended throughout the literature and within the disability community.

Within low-income and lower middle-income settings, community-based rehabilitation (CBR) programmes can promote and facilitate access to health care services for people with disabilities and their families. As outlined in the health component of the *CBR guidelines (166)*, programmes can assist people with disabilities to overcome access barriers, train primary health care workers in disability awareness, and initiate referrals to health services.

Target interventions to complement inclusive health care

Targeted interventions can help reduce inequities in health and meet the specific needs of individuals with disabilities (*4, 17*). Groups that are difficult to reach through broad-based programmes – people with intellectual impairment, mental health conditions, or Deaf people, for example – may warrant targeted interventions. Targeted interventions may also be useful for people with disabilities with a higher risk of secondary conditions or co-morbidities, or where there are specific health needs requiring ongoing care (see Box 3.4).

Health promotion efforts targeted at people with disabilities can have a substantial impact on improving lifestyle behaviours, increasing the quality of life, and reducing medical costs (*18, 168*). Several small health promotion programmes for weight loss and fitness developed specifically for people with intellectual impairment have demonstrated some success (*169*). An intervention in the United States for adults with Down syndrome included a 12-week fitness and health education programme, which led to significantly improved fitness, strength, and endurance, and slight but significant reductions in body weight (*65*).

Improve access to specialist health services

Primary care teams require support from specialized services, organizations, and institutions (*170*) to provide comprehensive health care to people with disabilities. A survey of general

Table 3.6. Examples of reasonable accommodations

Accommodations	Suggested approaches
Structural modifications to facilities	Ensuring an accessible path of travel from the street or transit to the clinic; allocating adequate parking bays for people with disabilities; configuring the layout of examination rooms and other clinic spaces to provide access for mobility equipment or support people; installing ramps and grab rails; widening doorways; clearing hallways of equipment obstructing the path of travel; installing lifts; high contrast, large print and Braille signage; providing modified toilets and hand washing facilities; providing seating for those who cannot stand or sit on the floor to wait.
Using equipment with universal design features	Height-adjustable examination tables or availability of a lower cot or bed for examination; seated or platform scales; wheelchair accessible diagnostic equipment: for example, mammography equipment.
Communicating information in appropriate formats	Presenting health information in alternative formats such as large print, Braille, audio and picture format; speaking clearly and directly to the individual; providing information slowly to ensure comprehension; demonstrating activities rather than just describing them; sign language interpreting services; providing readers, scribes, or interpreters to assist with forms.
Making adjustments to appointment systems	Provisions for making appointments via e-mail or fax; sending text or phone appointments reminders; scheduling additional time for appointments; offering first or last appointments; clustering appointments for general health and disability needs.
Using alternative models of service delivery	Telemedicine; mobile clinic services, and house calls; involving family members and caregivers in medical consultations when appropriate and desired by the patient; assistance with transportation to health services.

Box 3.4. Preventing HIV/AIDS among young people with disabilities in Africa

In 1999 the international network Rehabilitation International began an HIV/AIDS project in Mozambique and the United Republic of Tanzania to promote the African Decade of Persons with Disabilities, and to provide HIV/AIDS leadership and human rights training. The nongovernmental organizations Miracles in Mozambique, the Disabled Organization for Legal Affairs, and Social Economic Development in the United Republic of Tanzania were local partners in the project, with support by the Swedish International Development Agency.

A baseline survey carried out with 175 disabled people aged 12–30 revealed that knowledge about HIV/AIDS was low, there was a lack of health information available in accessible formats and health facilities were also often inaccessible.

The project developed educational materials on HIV/AIDS issues and rights for youths and young adults with disabilities, as well as for outreach workers and peer educators working with this group. The materials included manuals in accessible formats such as Braille and a DVD with sign language. Project materials were widely disseminated to HIV/AIDS and disability organizations. Four training workshops, delivered in Kiswahili and Portuguese to 287 participants, were later expanded to include people with disabilities in rural areas of Mozambique. Some participants trained to serve locally as HIV/AIDS educators. At the same time, a wide-ranging campaign used mass media, the Internet, and seminars involving representatives of governments and nongovernmental organizations to educate the public.

At the conclusion of the project, it was recommended that disability issues should be mainstreamed within HIV/AIDS educational programmes. The participatory and inclusive approach proved effective in training young people with disabilities as well as peer educators and outreach workers.

Source (167).

practitioners in the Netherlands found that while they agreed that people with intellectual impairment should receive services in primary care settings, they rated access to specialist support as "important to very important" for health issues such as behavioural and psychiatric problems and epilepsy (*171*). Comprehensive health reviews in primary care settings have also been recommended for people with intellectual impairment with specialist multidisciplinary backup where required (*169*).

Good practices in mental health highlight the importance of specialists (*161*). In Uganda mental health specialists travel to primary care clinics to provide supervision and support; in Brazil visiting mental health specialists see patients together with primary care practitioners; and in Australia general practitioners are able to contact psychogeriatric nurses, psychologists, or psychiatrists as required (*161*).

Dedicated community-based services meet specialist health needs in some countries. In the United Kingdom, learning disability teams are widely available for people with intellectual impairment. These teams provide specialist treatment where general services are unable to meet needs, support primary care services to identify and meet health needs, facilitate access to general services, and provide education and advice to individuals, families, and other professionals (*172*). Outreach teams in Brazil and India follow-up on patients with spinal cord injuries to address issues such as skin care, bowel and bladder management, joint and muscle problems, and pain management (*173*).

Provide people-centred health services

Many disabled people seek more collaborative relationships with primary care providers in managing primary, secondary, and co-morbid conditions (*7*). A comprehensive health assessment programme in Australia designed to enhance interactions between adults with intellectual impairment and caregivers showed that the assessment increased general practitioners'

attention to the health needs of adults with intellectual impairment, and improved health promotion and disease prevention (*174*).

People-centred approaches should:

- Educate and support people with disabilities to manage their health. Self-management approaches have been effective in improving health outcomes and quality of life for a range of chronic conditions, and in some instances have lowered costs for the health care system (*125, 175, 176*). With appropriate training and support, and opportunities for collaborative decision-making, people with disabilities can actively improve their health (see Box 3.5). People with disabilities with more knowledge can communicate better, negotiate the health system more effectively, and are generally more satisfied with their care (*179, 180*).

- Provide time-limited, self-management courses, involving peer support to enable persons with disabilities to better manage their health (*176*). In Nicaragua, where the health system is overburdened with increasing patients with chronic disease, "chronic clubs" have been established in health centres to teach people with diabetes about risk factors, disease management, signs of complications, and healthy lifestyles (*181*). In Rwanda a study regarding the health promotion needs of individuals with lower limb amputation recommended workshops to enable people with disabilities to share experiences and motivate each other to improve health behaviours (*37*).

- Involve family members and caregivers in service delivery where appropriate. Family members and caregivers may have limited knowledge and skills. They may not understand the importance of a healthy lifestyle, or they may not be able to identify changes in a person with a disability that would be indicative of a health problem (*182*). Family members and caregivers can support the health-seeking behaviours of people with

---

Box 3.5. People with spinal cord injuries on the medical care team

In 2005 a multicountry initiative was launched to investigate how people with disabilities could play a greater role in the management of their own care. The "New Paradigm of Medical Care for Persons with Disabilities" was a joint initiative between the World Health Organization (WHO), the Associazione Italiana Amici di Raoul Follereau (AIFO), and Disabled Peoples' International (DPI). It followed an earlier WHO recommendation that health care services organized according to the traditional model of acute care were inappropriate for long-term health care because they did not give people with disabilities a sufficient role in managing their own care (*177*).

The "New Paradigm" project in Piedecuesta, Colombia, encouraged people with spinal cord injuries to meet regularly as a group to discuss their health care needs. Health care and social workers provided information on health and led interactive training sessions in practical self-care skills. Topics covered included pressure sores, urinary problems, catheter management, and issues related to sexuality.

Participants reported improved relationships with health care workers, and a better quality of life after the project started. The group decided to form an association after two years of regular meetings. Members of the association share their experiences with new people admitted to the local hospital in Piedecuesta with spinal cord injuries, making the members part of the local health care team (*178*).

---

disabilities by identifying health needs, helping obtain health care, including scheduling appointments, accompanying individuals to their appointments, and communicating information and helping to promote and maintain healthy activities (*14*). One study in the United States suggested that spouses, partners and paid caregivers were more likely than other types of caregivers to ensure the participation of people with disabilities in preventive health care services (*183*).

Coordinate services

Care coordination promotes a collaborative, interdisciplinary team approach to health care service delivery, linking people with disabilities to appropriate services and resources, and ensuring a more efficient and equitable distribution of resources (*147, 154, 184*). While perhaps increasing service delivery costs in the short-term, coordination has the potential to improve quality, efficiency, and cost–effectiveness of health care service delivery in the longer term (*184–188*). Targeting those who can benefit will help improve outcomes and reduce unnecessary coordination costs (*189*). Studies have confirmed that integrated and coordinated approaches across service

organizations – including those involved in housing and education – can reduce the use of hospitals and nursing homes for people with disabilities and improve their general health and participation in the community (*190, 191*).

Effective and efficient ways to coordinate the seamless transition of health care services for people with disabilities are still under development. But some general strategies thought to be effective include the following elements (*148, 152, 192*):

- **Identify a care coordinator.** A range of health personnel can assume the role of care coordinator. Primary care structures are probably the most efficient for coordinating care throughout the health care system (*155, 185*), and many people with disabilities see general practitioners as having the overall responsibility for their health care and being "gatekeepers" for the wide range of community-based services (*193*). Sometimes, dedicated care coordination services and health facilitators can assist people to access primary health care services (*120*), as in the United Kingdom where clinical nurse specialists coordinate health care for people with intellectual impairment (*169*).

- **Develop an individual care plan.** A customized care plan is important to bridge current and past care and for arranging future needs. A plan should be flexible enough to accommodate changes in people's needs and circumstances (*194*). Enhanced Primary Care in Australia encourages general practitioners to carry out comprehensive health assessments, multidisciplinary care plans, and case conferences with older people, people with chronic illness, and people with intellectual impairment (*169*).
- **Provide appropriate referral and effective information transfer to other services.** Timely referral can facilitate access and decrease stress, frustration, and the development of secondary conditions (*154, 195, 196*). Good communication between service providers is critical (*197*). Electronic records or client passbooks – which include information on a person's abilities, challenges, and methods of learning or communicating – can support transition between child and adult services and between multiple health care practitioners (*154*). Inventories of relevant services and community resources also may be useful.

Use information and communication technologies

Information and communication technologies can increase the capacity of health care services, improve the delivery of services and enable people to better manage their own health (*198*). Evidence on the efficacy of some technologies is limited, or shows limited effect, while other technologies promise benefits for the health care system and for improvement in individual health outcomes (*199*).

- **Electronic medical records** – shared electronic medical records can overcome common problems in care continuity (*200*).
- **Telemedicine services** – people receiving psychiatric telemedicine services, such as psychiatric evaluations and medication management, have reported high satisfaction with their care (*201*), and video conferencing also has successfully delivered self-management programmes (*202*).
- **Consumer health informatics** – internet-based, self-management programmes have helped people with chronic disease (*175, 203*). A study compared internet-based hearing screening with conventional screening to demonstrate that the former could be accomplished successfully (*204*), and internet portals can offer "e-coaching" to prepare individuals for visits to primary care physicians and to discuss chronic conditions (*180*).

Addressing human resource barriers

Common barriers include health-service providers' attitudes, knowledge and skills, and ensuring that heath practices do not conflict with the rights of persons with disabilities.

People with disabilities may be reluctant to seek health care because of stigmatization and discrimination (*205*). People with disabilities may have experienced institutionalization or other involuntary treatment, abuse, neglect and persistent devaluation. Negative experiences in the health system, including instances of insensitivity or disrespect, may result in distrust of health providers, failure to seek care, and reliance upon self diagnosis and treatment (*89, 206*). Therefore, respectful, knowledgeable and supportive responses to people with disabilities from health-care providers are vital.

However, attitudes and misconceptions among health-care providers remain barriers to health care for people with disabilities (*90, 207*). Some health-care providers may feel uncomfortable about treating people with disabilities (*157*), and clinical decision-making may be influenced by negative attitudes and assumptions. The common misconception that people with disabilities are not sexually active often leads health professionals to fail to offer sexual and reproductive health services, for example (*11, 79, 89, 208*).

Health-care workers often lack adequate knowledge and skills on primary and secondary and co-morbid conditions associated with disability and how to effectively manage the health care needs of people with disabilities (*89, 154, 209*). Service providers may be unsure how to address health needs directly related to a disability and how to distinguish between health problems related and unrelated to a disability, and may not understand the need for comprehensive health care services (*96*).

Undergraduate training programmes for health-care workers rarely address the health needs of people with disabilities, for example (*11, 145*), and general practitioners frequently indicate that a lack of training influences their ability to provide health care for people with disabilities (*143*).

Limited knowledge and understanding of disability among health-care providers often prevents timely and effective coordination of health care services (*96, 154*), sometimes leading to inadequate examinations and uncomfortable and unsafe experiences for people with disabilities (*210*). Variations in treatment can be wide where health-care providers are unsupported by research and clinical guidelines related to people with disabilities. One study found that the main reason people with spinal cord injury were not prescribed medication for osteoporosis was because general practitioners lacked evidence-based guidelines (*30*).

The presence of a particular health condition is not sufficient to determine capacity (*211*). The assumption that people with certain conditions lack capacity is unacceptable, according to Article 12 of the CRPD. Denying people with disabilities the right to exercise their legal capacity may prevent them from taking an active role in their own health care. The way forward is supported decision-making, rather than guardianship or other forms of substitute decision-making (see Box 3.6).

Education and training for health care workers about disability is an important priority to increase awareness about the health care needs of people with disabilities and improve access to services (*89, 127, 142, 143, 209, 217*). Health-care workers should be taught the causes, consequences, and treatment of disabling conditions, and of the incorrect assumptions about disabilities that result from stigmatized views about people with disabilities (*145, 150, 154*).

Box 3.6. Sexual and reproductive rights of persons with disabilities

The United Nations *Convention on the Rights of Persons with Disabilities* (CRPD) specifies that persons with disabilities enjoy legal capacity on an equal basis with others (Article 12), have the right to marry and found a family and retain their fertility (Article 23), and have access to sexual and reproductive health care (Article 25). The prejudice that people with disabilities are asexual or else that they should have their sexuality and fertility controlled is widespread (*77*). There is evidence that people with disabilities are sexually active (*212*), so access to sex education is important to promote sexual health and positive experiences of sex and relationships for all people with disabilities.

Despite legal prohibitions, there are many cases of involuntary sterilization being used to restrict the fertility of some people with a disability, particularly those with an intellectual disability, almost always women (*213–216*). Sterilization may also be used as a technique for menstrual management.

Involuntary sterilization of persons with disabilities is contrary to international human rights standards. Persons with disabilities should have access to voluntary sterilization on an equal basis with others. Furthermore, sterilization is almost never the only option for menstrual management or fertility control (*214*). Nor does it offer any protection against sexual abuse or sexually transmitted diseases. Legal frameworks and reporting and enforcement mechanisms need to be put in place to ensure that, whenever sterilization is requested, the rights of persons with disabilities are always respected above other competing interests.

A survey of general practitioners in France recommends the introduction of disability courses into medical school curriculums, relevant continuing education, and provision of adequate resources (157). In one innovative approach to education and training, people with disabilities educate students and health care providers on a wide range of disability issues, including discriminatory attitudes and practices, communication skills, physical accessibility, the need for preventive care, and the consequences of poor care coordination (145, 154). Training delivered by people with physical, sensory, and mental health impairments may improve knowledge of issues experienced by people with disabilities (142).

Integrate disability education into undergraduate training

Educators are increasingly teaching students about communicating with patients, including people with disabilities (144), and many studies have reported successful outcomes across a range of health professionals:

- A study of Australian fourth-year undergraduate medical students indicated a significant change in attitudes towards people with developmental disabilities following a three-hour communication skills workshop (218).
- In a United States study, third-year medical students reported that they felt less "awkward" and "sorry for" people with disabilities after attending a 90-minute education session (219).
- A study found that medical students educated by individuals with disabilities helped students to learn how disability affects treatment plans, and helped students reflect on, and recognize, attitudes about disability (220).
- A study of fourth-year medical students used panel presentations led by individuals with disabilities. Students reported that they valued hearing about the personal experiences of people with disabilities, and

about what worked and what did not in the medical setting and in patient-provider relationships (221).
- Introductory courses for students enrolled in the first occupational therapy and post-diploma management courses in the Russian Federation, developed and taught by the All-Russian Society of the Disabled, successfully developed positive attitudes in the students (222).
- A study to determine whether a change in curriculum affected nursing student's attitudes towards people with disabilities showed that their attitudes were more positive at the completion of their senior year (223).

Provide health-care workers with continuing education

Many health-care workers acknowledge a need for continuing education about disability (143). In one study service providers described specific educational needs, including information about how to access disability resources, coordinate care, make reasonable accommodations for people with disabilities, address sexuality and reproductive health needs, and complete forms for disability status (209). Evidence from the United Kingdom found that while practice nurses in primary health care generally had positive attitudes towards working with people with intellectual impairment, they regarded training in this area as a priority (224).

The Rehabilitation Council of India implemented a national programme (1999–2004) to educate medical officers working in primary health care centres about disability issues. Objectives included disseminating knowledge about prevention, health promotion, early identification, treatment, and rehabilitation; raising awareness about services for people with disabilities; and sensitizing officers about general disability issues such as legislation and human rights. On conclusion of the programme 18 657 medical officers from a baseline figure of 25 506 had received training (225).

Support health care workers with adequate resources

Evidence-based clinical practice guidelines can support health professionals in providing appropriate health care to people with disabilities. For example, the *Clinical guidelines and integrated care pathways for the oral health care of people with learning disabilities (226)* helps health professionals to improve the oral health of people with learning impairments. The manual *Table manners and beyond* describes and provides pictures of alternative examination positions to assist clinicians in gynaecological examinations for women with disabilities *(132)*. Resource directories can also assist health workers to refer patients to specialists, and link people with disabilities to community-based services including exercise programmes, self-help groups, and home-care agencies. Disseminated to a wide audience including health care workers, the *Directory of disability services in Malawi* details all disability-focused organizations, groups, and services in Malawi *(227)*.

Filling gaps in data and research

Evidence leads to better decisions and better health outcomes *(228, 229)*. Reliable information is essential for increasing public awareness of health issues, informing planning and policy, and allocating resources to reduce disparities *(230)*. Therefore, data and research are critical for providing information to help understand the factors that determine health status, to develop policy, to guide implementation, and to monitor health care services for people with disabilities – and in doing these things to strengthen health care systems *(231)*. A lack of data and research evidence can create a significant barrier for policy-makers and decision-makers, which in turn can influence the ability of people with disabilities to access mainstream health services.

The availability of data related to people with disabilities varies greatly between countries *(232)*. Few sources of national data are available, and information to determine the extent of health disparities experienced by people with disabilities is limited *(233)*. Surveillance systems do not often disaggregate data based on disability, and people with disabilities are also often excluded from trials that seek scientific evidence for the outcomes of a health intervention *(234, 235)*. Often, eligibility criteria prevent the participation of people with disabilities *(11)* as their primary conditions may be seen as "confounders" to research questions. Certain barriers – transport, for example – may also sometimes limit opportunities for people with disabilities to participate in research *(236)*.

A recent exercise on research priorities determined that the identification of barriers in mainstream health care, and strategies for overcoming barriers, were the highest priorities *(164)*. Other priorities included prevention of secondary conditions and early detection and referral of health problems through primary health care. Some of the relevant areas for health research and data collection are outlined below.

Health services research

Data needed to strengthen health care systems include:

- number of people with disabilities
- health status of people with disabilities *(11)*
- social and environmental factors influencing the health of people with disabilities
- responsiveness of health care systems to people with disabilities
- use of health care services by people with disabilities
- need, both met and unmet, for care *(237)*.

People with disabilities should be included in all general health care surveillance *(233)*, and data on people with disabilities should be disaggregated. A good example at the state level is the Centers for Disease Control and Prevention Behavioural Risk Factor Surveillance System (BRFSS), which includes two general disability identifier questions to ensure provision of state-specific disability data *(233)*. Research should also focus on the quality and structure of health care systems, examining, for example, reasonable accommodations needed for people with disabilities.

Research related to health conditions associated with disability

Preventing secondary conditions related to existing disabilities is an important priority. Preliminary results from a systematic review of health promotion interventions for people with disabilities indicates that research in this area is a growing field and that there is evidence of effective interventions (238). But stronger research designs require precise dosing for intervention, and research and multicentre trials will increase recruitment and the ability to generalize findings (237).

Ensuring the relevance and applicability of general clinical research to people with disabilities, given evidence of high co-morbidity rates, is also important. For example, the increased risk of people with schizophrenia for diabetes and cardiovascular disease requires monitoring and management (239), but genetic research to understand metabolic mechanisms is also recommended (240).

Relevant strategies for inclusive health research as well as improving comparability, quality, and disability research capacity include:

- Organizations funding research could routinely require researchers to include people with disabilities in their population samples. Despite challenges, randomized controlled trials with people with intellectual impairment are possible (172). Researchers should be required to justify restricted eligibility criteria on scientific grounds (11). People with intellectual disabilities, people who face communication barriers, and others with low levels of literacy may need support completing survey instruments or participating in interviews (17, 235).
- People with disabilities can actively participate in research, as researchers themselves, as participants in consultations or advisory groups, or playing a central role in

commissioning and monitoring research (99, 235, 241). In the United Kingdom the Quality Research in Dementia Network involves 180 patients and caregivers prioritizing research, allocating funds to medical research, monitoring projects, and assessing outcomes (242). Patient and public involvement can improve the quality and impact of research, but barriers to access must be removed so people with disabilities can attend health consultations or research meetings (235).

- The *International Classification of Functioning, Disability and Health* (ICF) – which uses accepted and understood terminology, language, and concepts – can ensure consistency across studies and settings, thus removing these as barriers to progress in disability and health research and public policy (9).
- A range of research methods are needed including clinical trials, observational and epidemiological studies, health services research, surveys, and social and behavioural studies. Well designed, qualitative research can be used to investigate the full range of barriers and document good practices (243).
- Capacity building, research tools, and research training on disability are needed. Good instruments are particularly important for disability outcome research given evidence that people with disabilities often perceive health status and quality of life differently than people without disabilities (243).

Conclusion and recommendations

People with disabilities experience health disparities and greater unmet needs in comparison to the general population. All countries need to work towards removing barriers and making existing health care systems more inclusive and accessible to people with disabilities.

This chapter has identified several strategies to ensure that persons with disabilities can achieve their highest attainable standard of health including: financial measures to improve coverage and affordability; measures to improve service delivery, including training of health-care personnel; measures to empower people with disabilities to improve their own health; and measures to improve research and data to monitor, evaluate, and strengthen health systems. A range of strategies are needed to close the gap in access to health care between people with and without disabilities. Given the limited evidence available on the efficacy of some of these strategies across different contexts and groups, costs and health outcomes must be carefully evaluated.

In realizing the recommendations summarized below, a broad range of stakeholders have roles to play. Governments should develop, implement, and monitor policies, regulatory mechanisms, and standards for health care provision to ensure that they include people with disabilities. Service providers should provide the highest quality of health services. Service users, disabled people's organizations, and professional organizations should increase awareness, participate in policy development, and monitor implementation of policies and services. Through international cooperation, good and promising practices can be shared and technical assistance provided to countries to strengthen existing policies, system, and services.

Policy and legislation

- Assess existing policies, systems, and services, including an analysis of the needs, experiences, and views of people with disabilities, identify gaps and priorities to reduce health inequalities and plan improvements for access and inclusion.
- Make required changes in policies, systems, and services to comply with the CRPD.

- Establish health care standards related to care of persons with disabilities and frameworks and enforcement mechanisms to ensure standards are met.
- Involve people with disabilities in audits and related development and implementation of policies and services.

Financing and affordability

- Ensure that people with disabilities benefit equally from public health care programmes.
- In countries where private health insurance dominates health care financing, ensure that people with disabilities are not denied insurance and consider measures to make the premiums affordable for people with disabilities.
- Use financial incentives to encourage health-care providers to make services accessible and provide comprehensive assessments, evidence-based treatment, and follow-ups.
- In low-income and middle-income countries, where effective primary care and mechanisms of disbursement exist, consider targeted conditional cash transfer schemes linked to the use of health care to improve affordability and the use of services.
- Consider options for reducing or removing out-of-pocket payments for people with disabilities who do not have other means of financing health care services.
- Consider providing support to meet the indirect costs associated with accessing health care, such as transport.

Service delivery

- Empower people with disabilities to maximize their health by providing information, training, and peer support. Where appropriate, include family members.
- Provide a broad range of reasonable accommodations.

- Support primary health-care workers with specialists, who may be located elsewhere.
- Explore the options for use of communication and information technologies for improving services, health care capacity, and information access to persons with disabilities.
- Identify groups who require alternative service delivery models, for example, targeted services, care coordination to improve access to health care.
- In high-income countries incorporate disability access and quality standards into contracts with public, private, and voluntary service providers.
- Promote community-based rehabilitation, specifically in less-resourced settings, to facilitate access for disabled people to existing services.

Human resources

- Integrate disability education into undergraduate and continuing education for all health care professionals.

- Involve people with disabilities as providers of education and training wherever possible.
- Provide evidence-based guidelines for assessment and treatment emphasizing patient-centred care.
- Train community workers so that they can play a role in screening and preventive health care services.

Data and research

- In health and disability related research use the ICF, to provide a consistent framework.
- Conduct more research on the needs, barriers to general health care, and health outcomes for people with specific disabilities.
- Establish monitoring and evaluation systems to assess interventions and long-term health outcomes for people with disabilities.
- Include people with disabilities in research on general health care services.
- Include people with disabilities in health care surveillance by using disability identifiers - see Chapter 2 for more information.

References

1. Constitution of the World Health Organization. Geneva, World Health Organization, 1948 (http://apps.who.int/gb/bd/PDF/bd47/EN/constitution-en.pdf, accessed 7 May 2009).
2. United Nations *Convention on the Rights of Persons with Disabilities*. Geneva, United Nations, 2006 (http://www2.ohchr.org/english/law/disabilities-convention.htm, accessed 16 May 2009).
3. *Australia's health 2010*. Canberra, Australian Institute of Health and Welfare, 2010.
4. *Closing the gap in a generation: Health equity through action on the social determinants of health.* Geneva, World Health Organization, 2008.
5. Beatty PW et al. Access to health care services among people with chronic or disabling conditions: patterns and predictors. *Archives of Physical Medicine and Rehabilitation*, 2003,84:1417-1425. doi:10.1016/S0003-9993(03)00268-5 PMID:14586907
6. VanLeit B et al. *Secondary prevention of disabilities in the Cambodian Provinces of Siem Reap and Takeo: perceptions of and use of the health system to address health conditions associated with disability in children.* Brussels, Handicap International, 2007.
7. Bowers B et al. Improving primary care for persons with disabilities: the nature of expertise. *Disability & Society*, 2003,18:443-455. doi:10.1080/0968759032000080995
8. Gulley SP, Altman BM. Disability in two health care systems: access, quality, satisfaction, and physician contacts among working-age Canadians and Americans with disabilities. *Disability and Health Journal*, 2008,1:196-208. doi:10.1016/j.dhjo.2008.07.006 PMID:21122730
9. Field MJ, Jette AM, eds. *The future of disability in America.* Washington, The National Academies Press, 2007.
10. Field MJ, Jette AM. Martin, L eds. *Workshop on disability in America: a new look.* Washington, Board of Health Sciences Policy, 2005.
11. Nosek MA, Simmons DK. People with disabilities as a health disparities population: the case of sexual and reproductive health disparities. *Californian Journal of Health Promotion*, 2007,5:68-81.
12. Drum CE et al. Health of people with disabilities: determinants and disparities. In: Drum C, Krahn G, Bersani H, eds. *Disability and Public Health*, Washington, American Public Health Association, 2009a:125–144.

13. Marge M. Secondary conditions revisited: examining the expansion of the original concept and definition. *Disability and Health Journal*, 2008,1:67-70. doi:10.1016/j.dhjo.2008.02.002 PMID:21122713

14. Krahn GL, Hammond L, Turner A. A cascade of disparities: health and health care access for people with intellectual disabilities. *Mental Retardation and Developmental Disabilities Research Reviews*, 2006,12:70-82. doi:10.1002/mrdd.20098 PMID:16435327

15. *Equality treatment: closing the gap: a formal investigation into the physical health inequalities experiences by people with learning disabilities and/or mental health problems*. London, Disability Rights Commission, 2006.

16. Drum CE et al. Recognizing and responding to the health disparities of people with disabilities. *Californian Journal of Health Promotion*, 2005,3:29-42.

17. Dejong G et al. The organization and financing of health services for persons with disabilities. *The Milbank Quarterly*, 2002,80:261-301. doi:10.1111/1468-0009.t01-1-00004 PMID:12101873

18. Rimmer JH, Rowland JL. Health promotion for people with disabilities: implications for empowering the person and promoting disability-friendly environments. *Journal of Lifestyle Medicine*, 2008,2:409-420. doi:10.1177/1559827608317397

19. Emerson E et al. *Intellectual and physical disability, social mobility, social inclusion and health*. Lancaster, Centre for Disability Research, Lancaster University, 2009.

20. Iezzoni LI. Quality of care for Medicare beneficiaries with disabilities under the age of 65 years. *Expert Review of Pharmaeconomics & Outcomes Research*, 2006,a6:261-273. doi:10.1586/14737167.6.3.261 PMID:20528520

21. Prince M et al. No health without mental health. *Lancet*, 2007,370:859-877. doi:10.1016/S0140-6736(07)61238-0 PMID:17804063

22. Khlat M et al. Lorhandicap GroupSocial disparities in musculoskeletal disorders and associated mental malaise: findings from a population-based survey in France. *Scandinavian Journal of Public Health*, 2010,38:495-501. doi:10.1177/1403494810371246 PMID:20529964

23. Ohayon MM, Schatzberg AF. Chronic pain and major depressive disorder in the general population. *Journal of Psychiatric Research*, 2010,44:454-461. doi:10.1016/j.jpsychires.2009.10.013 PMID:20149391

24. Hadden KL, von Baeyer CL. Global and specific behavioral measures of pain in children with cerebral palsy. *The Clinical Journal of Pain*, 2005,21:140-146. doi:10.1097/00002508-200503000-00005 PMID:15722807

25. Engel JM, Kartin D, Jensen MP. Pain treatment in persons with cerebral palsy: frequency and helpfulness. *American Journal of Physical Medicine & Rehabilitation/Association of Academic Physiatrists*, 2002,81:291-296. doi:10.1097/00002060-200204000-00009 PMID:11953547

26. Oddson BE, Clancy CA, McGrath PJ. The role of pain in reduced quality of life and depressive symptomology in children with spina bifida. *The Clinical Journal of Pain*, 2006,22:784-789. doi:10.1097/01.ajp.0000210929.43192.5d PMID:17057560

27. Klein MG et al. The relation between lower extremity strength and shoulder overuse symptoms: a model based on polio survivors. *Archives of Physical Medicine and Rehabilitation*, 2000,81:789-795. doi:10.1016/S0003-9993(00)90113-8 PMID:10857526

28. Guy-Coichard C et al. Pain in hereditary neuromuscular disorders and myasthenia gravis: a national survey of frequency, characteristics, and impact. *Journal of Pain and Symptom Management*, 2008,35:40-50. doi:10.1016/j.jpainsymman.2007.02.041 PMID:17981001

29. Hoffman JM et al. Understanding pain after traumatic brain injury: impact on community participation. *American Journal of Physical Medicine & Rehabilitation/Association of Academic Physiatrists*, 2007,a86:962-969. doi:10.1097/PHM.0b013e31815b5ee5 PMID:18090437

30. Morse LR et al. VA-based survey of osteoporosis management in spinal cord injury. *PM&R: the Journal of Injury, Function and Rehabilitation*, 2009,1:240-244. PMID:19627901

31. Dosa NP et al. Incidence, prevalence, and characteristics of fractures in children, adolescents, and adults with spina bifida. *The journal of spinal cord medicine*, 2007,30:Suppl 1S5-S9. PMID:17874679

32. Henderson RC et al. Bisphosphonates to treat osteopenia in children with quadriplegic cerebral palsy: a randomized, placebo-controlled clinical trial. *The Journal of Pediatrics*, 2002,141:644-651. doi:10.1067/mpd.2002.128207 PMID:12410192

33. Turk MA et al. The health of women with cerebral palsy. *Physical Medicine and Rehabilitation Clinics of North America*, 2001,12:153-168. PMID:11853034

34. Havercamp SM, Scandlin D, Roth M. Health disparities among adults with developmental disabilities, adults with other disabilities, and adults not reporting disability in North Carolina. *Public Health Reports (Washington, DC: 1974)*, 2004,119:418-426. doi:10.1016/j.phr.2004.05.006 PMID:15219799

35. *Disability and ageing: Australian population patterns and implications*. Canberra, Australian Institute of Health and Welfare, 2000.

36. Woodcock K, Pole JD. Health profile of deaf Canadians: analysis of the Canada Community Health Survey. *Canadian Family Physician Médecin de Famille Canadien*, 2007,53:2140-2141. PMID:18077753

37. Amosun SL, Mutimura E, Frantz JM. Health promotion needs of physically disabled individuals with lower limb amputation in Rwanda. *Disability and Rehabilitation*, 2005,27:837-847. doi:10.1080/09638280400018676 PMID:16096236

38. *World report on violence and health*. Geneva, World Health Organization, 2002a.

39. Marge DK, ed. *A call to action: preventing and intervening in violence against children and adults with disabilities: a report to the nation*. Syracuse, State University of New York Upstate Medical University Duplicating and Printing Services, 2003.

40. Hague G, Thaira RK, Magowan P. *Disabled women and domestic violence: making the links*. Bristol, Women's Aid Federation of England, 2007.

41. McCarthy M. *Sexuality and women with learning disabilities*. London, Jessica Kingsley Publishers, 1999.

42. Peckham NG. The vulnerability and sexual abuse of people with learning disabilities. *British Journal of Learning Disabilities*, 2007,35:131-137. doi:10.1111/j.1468-3156.2006.00428.x

43. Reichard AA et al. Violence, abuse, and neglect among people with traumatic brain injuries. *The Journal of Head Trauma Rehabilitation*, 2007,22:390-402. doi:10.1097/01.HTR.0000300234.36361.b1 PMID:18025971

44. Yoshida KK et al. Women living with disabilities and their experiences and issues related to the context and complexities of leaving abusive situations. *Disability and Rehabilitation*, 2009,31:1843-1852. doi:10.1080/09638280902826808 PMID:19479561

45. Barrett KA et al. Intimate partner violence, health status, and health care access among women with disabilities. *Women's Health Issues: official publication of the Jacobs Institute of Women's Health*, 2009,19:94-100. doi:10.1016/j.whi.2008.10.005 PMID:19272559

46. Yousafzai AK et al. HIV/AIDS information and services: the situation experienced by adolescents with disabilities in Rwanda and Uganda. *Disability and Rehabilitation*, 2005,27:1357-1363. doi:10.1080/09638280500164297 PMID:16372430

47. *Secondary injuries among individuals with disabilities*. Research summary brief. Columbus, Centre for Injury Research and Policy, Nationwide Children's Hospital, 2009.

48. Sinclair SA, Xiang H. Injuries among US children with different types of disabilities. *American Journal of Public Health*, 2008,98:1510-1516. doi:10.2105/AJPH.2006.097097 PMID:18048794

49. *World report on child injury and prevention*. Geneva, World Health Organization, 2008.

50. Lee LC et al. Increased risk of injury in children with developmental disabilities. *Research in Developmental Disabilities*, 2008,29:247-255. doi:10.1016/j.ridd.2007.05.002 PMID:17582739

51. Xiang H, Chany A-M, Smith GA. Wheelchair related injuries treated in US emergency departments. *Injury Prevention: Journal of the International Society for Child and Adolescent Injury Prevention*, 2006,a12:8-11. doi:10.1136/ip.2005.010033 PMID:16461412

52. Petridou E et al. Injuries among disabled children: a study from Greece. *Injury Prevention: Journal of the International Society for Child and Adolescent Injury Prevention*, 2003,9:226-230. doi:10.1136/ip.9.3.226 PMID:12966010

53. Chen G et al. Incidence and pattern of burn injuries among children with disabilities. *The Journal of Trauma*, 2007,62:682-686. doi:10.1097/01.ta.0000203760.47151.28 PMID:17414347

54. Xiang H et al. Risk of vehicle-pedestrian and vehicle-bicyclist collisions among children with disabilities. *Accident; Analysis and Prevention*, 2006,b38:1064-1070. doi:10.1016/j.aap.2006.04.010 PMID:16797463

55. Turk MA. Health, mortality, and wellness issues in adults with cerebral palsy. *Developmental Medicine and Child Neurology*, 2009,51:Suppl 424-29. doi:10.1111/j.1469-8749.2009.03429.x PMID:19740207

56. Frankel HL et al. Long-term survival in spinal cord injury: a fifty year investigation. *Spinal Cord*, 1998,36:266-274. doi:10.1038/sj.sc.3100638 PMID:9589527

57. Strauss DJ et al. Trends in life expectancy after spinal cord injury. *Archives of Physical Medicine and Rehabilitation*, 2006,87:1079-1085. doi:10.1016/j.apmr.2006.04.022 PMID:16876553

58. Khan NZ et al. Mortality of urban and rural young children with cerebral palsy in Bangladesh. *Developmental Medicine and Child Neurology*, 1998,40:749-753. doi:10.1111/j.1469-8749.1998.tb12343.x PMID:9881804

59. *World Health Survey*. Geneva, World Health Organization, 2002–2004 (http://www.who.int/healthinfo/survey/en/, accessed 10 September 2010).

60. *Healthy people 2010: understanding and improving health*, 2nd ed. Washington, Department of Health and Community Services, 2000.

61. Allen J et al. Strength training can be enjoyable and beneficial for adults with cerebral palsy. *Disability and Rehabilitation*, 2004,26:1121-1127. doi:10.1080/09638280410001712378 PMID:15371024

62. Durstine JL et al. Physical activity for the chronically ill and disabled. [Erratum appears in Sports Medicine 2001, 31:627] *Sports Medicine (Auckland, N.Z.)*, 2000,30:207-219. doi:10.2165/00007256-200030030-00005 PMID:10999424

63. Fragala-Pinkham MA, Haley SM, Goodgold S. Evaluation of a community-based group fitness program for children with disabilities. *Pediatric Physical Therapy: the official publication of the Section on Pediatrics of the American Physical Therapy Association*, 2006,18:159-167. doi:10.1097/01.pep.0000223093.28098.12 PMID:16735864

64. Mead GE et al. Exercise for depression. *Cochrane Database of Systematic Reviews*, 2009,3CD004366-

65. Rimmer JH et al. Improvements in physical fitness in adults with Down syndrome. *American Journal of Mental Retardation: AJMR*, 2004,109:165-174. doi:10.1352/0895-8017(2004)109<165:IIPFIA>2.0.CO;2 PMID:15000673

66. Becker H, Stuifbergen A. What makes it so hard? Barriers to health promotion experienced by people with multiple sclerosis and polio. *Family & Community Health*, 2004,27:75-85. PMID:14724504

67. Rimmer JH, Wang E, Smith D. Barriers associated with exercise and community access for individuals with stroke. *Journal of Rehabilitation Research and Development*, 2008,45:315-322. doi:10.1682/JRRD.2007.02.0042 PMID:18566948

68. Hoffman JM et al. Association of mobility limitations with health care satisfaction and use of preventive care: a survey of Medicare beneficiaries. *Archives of Physical Medicine and Rehabilitation*, 2007,88:583-588. doi:10.1016/j.apmr.2007.02.005 PMID:17466726

69. Iezzoni LI et al. Mobility impairments and use of screening and preventive services. *American Journal of Public Health*, 2000,90:955-961. doi:10.2105/AJPH.90.6.955 PMID:10846515

70. Groce NE, Ayora P, Kaplan LC. Immunization rates among disabled children in Ecuador: unanticipated findings. *The Journal of Pediatrics*, 2007,151:218-220. doi:10.1016/j.jpeds.2007.04.061 PMID:17643783

71. Chevarley FM et al. Health, preventive health care, and health care access among women with disabilities in the 1994–1995 National Health Interview Survey, Supplement on Disability. *Women's Health Issues: official publication of the Jacobs Institute of Women's Health*, 2006,16:297-312. doi:10.1016/j.whi.2006.10.002 PMID:17188213

72. Johnson K et al. Screened out: women with disabilities and preventive health. *Scandinavian Journal of Disability Research*, 2006,8:150-160. doi:10.1080/15017410600802201

73. Sullivan SG, Slack-Smith LM, Hussain R. Understanding the use of breast cancer screening services by women with intellectual disabilities. *Sozial- und Präventivmedizin*, 2004,49:398-405. doi:10.1007/s00038-004-3121-z PMID:15669440

74. Mele N, Archer J, Pusch BD. Access to breast cancer screening services for women with disabilities. *Journal of Obstetric, Gynecologic, and Neonatal Nursing: JOGNN/NAACOG*, 2005,34:453-464. doi:10.1177/0884217505276158 PMID:16020413

75. Reichard A, Stolzle H, Fox MH. Health disparities among adults with physical disabilities or cognitive limitations compared to individuals with no disabilities in the United States. *Disability and Health Journal*, 2011,4:59-67. doi:10.1016/j.dhjo.2010.05.003 PMID:21419369

76. Ramirez A et al. Disability and preventive cancer screening: results from the 2001 California Health Interview Survey. *American Journal of Public Health*, 2005,95:2057-2064. doi:10.2105/AJPH.2005.066118 PMID:16195509

77. *Promoting sexual and reproductive health for persons with disabilities*. Geneva, World Health Organization and United Nations Population Fund, 2009.

78. Rohleder P et al. HIV/AIDS and disability in Southern Africa: a review of relevant literature. *Disability and Rehabilitation*, 2009,31:51-59. doi:10.1080/09638280802280585 PMID:19194810

79. *The forgotten: HIV and disability in Tanzania*. Dar es Salaam, Tanzanian Commission for AIDS, 2009 (http://www.gtz.de/de/dokumente/gtz2009-en-hiv-and-disability-tanzania.pdf, accessed 5 April 2010).

80. Bhansali S et al. A study of the prosthodontic and oral health needs of an ageing psychiatric population. *Gerodontology*, 2008,25:113-117. doi:10.1111/j.1741-2358.2007.00209.x PMID:18282147

81. Desai M, Messer LB, Calache H. A study of the dental treatment needs of children with disabilities in Melbourne, Australia. *Australian Dental Journal*, 2001,46:41-50. doi:10.1111/j.1834-7819.2001.tb00273.x PMID:11355240

82. Jensen PM et al. Factors associated with oral health-related quality of life in community-dwelling elderly persons with disabilities. *Journal of the American Geriatrics Society*, 2008,56:711-717. doi:10.1111/j.1532-5415.2008.01631.x PMID:18284537

83. del Valle LML et al. Puerto Rican athletes with special health care needs: an evaluation of oral health status. *ASDC Journal of Dentistry for Children*, 2007,74:130-132.

84. Oredugba FA. Use of oral health care services and oral findings in children with special needs in Lagos, Nigeria. *Special Care in Dentistry: official publication of the American Association of Hospital Dentists, the Academy of Dentistry for the Handicapped, and the American Society for Geriatric Dentistry*, 2006,26:59-65. doi:10.1111/j.1754-4505.2006.tb01511.x PMID:16681240

85. Pezzementi ML, Fisher MA. Oral health status of people with intellectual disabilities in the southeastern United States. *The Journal of the American Dental Association (1939)*, 2005,136:903-912. PMID:16060471

86. De Camargo MA, Antunes JL. Untreated dental caries in children with cerebral palsy in the Brazilian context. *International journal of paediatric dentistry / the British Paedodontic Society [and] the International Association of Dentistry for Children*, 2008,18:131-138. doi:10.1111/j.1365-263X.2007.00829.x PMID:18237296

87. Demyttenaere K et al. WHO World Mental Health Survey ConsortiumPrevalence, severity, and unmet need for treatment of mental disorders in the World Health Organization World Mental Health Surveys. *JAMA: Journal of the American Medical Association*, 2004,291:2581-2590. doi:10.1001/jama.291.21.2581 PMID:15173149

88. Kohn R et al. The treatment gap in mental health care. *Bulletin of the World Health Organization*, 2004,82:858-866. PMID:15640922

89. Drainoni M-L et al. Cross-disability experiences of barriers to health-care access: consumer perspectives. *Journal of Disability Policy Studies*, 2006,17:101-115. doi:10.1177/10442073060170020101

90. McColl MA et al. Physician experiences providing primary care to people with disabilities. *Healthcare Policy = Politiques de Sante*, 2008,4:e129-e147. PMID:19377334

91. *People with disabilities in India: from commitments to outcomes*. Washington, World Bank, 2009 (http://www-wds.world-bank.org/external/default/WDSContentServer/WDSP/IB/2009/09/02/000334955_20090902041543/Rendered/PDF/502090WP0Peopl1Box0342042B01PUBLIC1.pdf, accessed, 10 September 2010).

92. Loeb ME, Eide AH, eds. *Living conditions among people with activity limitations in Malawi: a national representative study*. Oslo, SINFEF, 2004.

93. Eide AH, van Rooy G, Loeb ME. *Living conditions among people with activity limitations in Namibia: a representative national survey*. Oslo, SINTEF, 2003.

94. Eide AH et al. *Living conditions among people with activity limitations in Zimbabwe: a representative regional survey*. Oslo, SINTEF, 2003.

95. Eide AH, Loeb ME, eds. *Living conditions among people with activity limitations in Zambia: a national representative study*. Oslo, SINTEF, 2006.

96. Scheer J et al. Access barriers for persons with disabilities. *Journal of Disability Policy Studies*, 2003,13:221-230. doi:10.1177/104420730301300404

97. de Savigny D, Adam T, eds. *Systems thinking for health systems strengthening*. Geneva, World Health Organization, 2009 (http://www.who.int/alliance-hpsr/resources/9789241563895/en/index.html, accessed 25 March 2010).

98. Kickbusch I. The development of international health policies–accountability intact? *Social Science & Medicine (1982)*, 2000,51:979-989. doi:10.1016/S0277-9536(00)00076-9 PMID:10972440

99. Marks BA, Heller T. Bridging the equity gap: health promotion for adults with intellectual and developmental disabilities. *The Nursing Clinics of North America*, 2003,38:205-228. doi:10.1016/S0029-6465(02)00049-X PMID:12914305

100. Nilsen ES et al. Methods of consumer involvement in developing healthcare policy and research, clinical practice guidelines and patient information material. *Cochrane Database of Systematic Reviews (Online)*, 2006,3:CD004563- PMID:16856050

101. Walmsley J. Inclusive learning disability research: the (nondisabled) researcher's role. *British Journal of Learning Disabilities*, 2004,32:65-71. doi:10.1111/j.1468-3156.2004.00281.x

102. Truman C, Raine P. Experience and meaning of user involvement: some explorations from a community mental health project. *Health & Social Care in the Community*, 2002,10:136-143. doi:10.1046/j.1365-2524.2002.00351.x PMID:12121249

103. Hayward R, Cutler P. What contribution can ordinary people make to national mental health policies? *Community Mental Health Journal*, 2007,43:517-526. doi:10.1007/s10597-007-9086-7 PMID:17514505

104. Tomes N. The patient as a policy factor: a historical case study of the consumer/survivor movement in mental health. *Health Affairs (Project Hope)*, 2006,25:720-729. doi:10.1377/hlthaff.25.3.720 PMID:16684736

105. Sloper P, Lightfoot J. Involving disabled and chronically ill children and young people in health service development. *Child: Care, Health and Development*, 2003,29:15-20. doi:10.1046/j.1365-2214.2003.00315.x PMID:12534563

106. . Bedfordshire Community Health ServicesNothing about us without us: involving families in early support. *Community Practitioner: the journal of the Community Practitioners' & Health Visitors' Association*, 2009,82:26-29. PMID:19552112

107. Roulstone A, Hudson V. Carer participation in England, Wales and Northern Ireland: a challenge for interprofessional working. *Journal of Interprofessional Care*, 2007,21:303-317. doi:10.1080/13561820701327822 PMID:17487708

108. Ali M, Miyoshi C, Ushijima H. Emergency medical services in Islamabad, Pakistan: a public-private partnership. *Public Health*, 2006,120:50-57. doi:10.1016/j.puhe.2005.03.009 PMID:16198384

109. Gottret P, Schieber G. *Health financing revisited: a practitioners guide*. Washington, World Bank, 2006.

110. *The World Health Report 2010 – Health systems financing: the path to universal coverage*. Geneva, World Health Organization, 2010.

111. Lagarde M, Palmer N. The impact of health financing strategies on access to health service in low and middle income countries (protocol). *Cochrane Database of Systematic Reviews*, 2006,3CD006092-

112. Saxena S, Sharan P, Saraceno B. Budget and financing of mental health services: baseline information on 89 countries from WHO's project atlas. *The Journal of Mental Health Policy and Economics*, 2003,6:135-143. PMID:14646006

113. Dixon A et al. Financing mental health services in low- and middle-income countries. *Health Policy and Planning*, 2006,21:171-182. doi:10.1093/heapol/czl004 PMID:16533860

114. White PH. Access to health care: health insurance considerations for young adults with special health care needs/disabilities. *Pediatrics*, 2002,110:1328-1335. PMID:12456953

115. Pre-Existing Condition Insurance Plan (PCIP). Washington, United States Department of Health and Human Services, 2010 (http://www.healthcare.gov/law/provisions/preexisting/index.html, accessed 6 December 2010).

116. Kruk ME, Freedman LP. Assessing health system performance in developing countries: a review of the literature. *Health Policy (Amsterdam, Netherlands)*, 2008,85:263-276. PMID:17931736

117. Salti N, Chaaban J, Raad F. Health equity in Lebanon: a microeconomic analysis. *International Journal for Equity in Health*, 2010,9:11- doi:10.1186/1475-9276-9-11 PMID:20398278

118. Jeffrey AE, Newacheck PW. Role of insurance for children with special health care needs: a synthesis of the evidence. *Pediatrics*, 2006,118:e1027-e1038. doi:10.1542/peds.2005-2527 PMID:16966391

119. Newacheck PW et al. The future of health insurance for children with special health care needs. *Pediatrics*, 2009,123:e940-e947. doi:10.1542/peds.2008-2921 PMID:19403486

120. Ayanian JZ et al. Unmet health needs of uninsured adults in the United States. *JAMA: Journal of the American Medical Association*, 2000,284:2061-2069. doi:10.1001/jama.284.16.2061 PMID:11042754

121. Lin JD et al. Primary health care for people with an intellectual disability: a mission impossible? *Journal of Medical Science*, 2005,25:109-118.

122. Gwatkin DR, Bhuiya A, Victora CG. Making health systems more equitable. *Lancet*, 2004,364:1273-1280. doi:10.1016/S0140-6736(04)17145-6 PMID:15464189

123. McAvoy BR, Coster GD. General practice and the New Zealand health reforms – lessons for Australia? *Australia and New Zealand Health Policy*, 2005,2:1-11. doi:10.1186/1743-8462-2-26 PMID:15679895

124. *Primary health care: care plus*. Wellington, New Zealand Ministry of Health, 2007 (http://www.moh.govt.nz/moh.nsf/indexmh/phcs-projects-careplusservice, accessed 6 December 2010).

125. Meng H et al. Impact of a health promotion nurse intervention on disability and health care costs among elderly adults with heart conditions. *The Journal of Rural Health: official journal of the American Rural Health Association and the National Rural Health Care Association*, 2007,23:322-331. doi:10.1111/j.1748-0361.2007.00110.x PMID:17868239

126. Al Ahmadi A. Cash transfers and persons with disabilities in practice: The case of Yemen. *Disability Monitor Initiative-Middle East Journal*, 2009, 1:27–29. (http://www.disabilitymonitor-me.org/, accessed 14 April 2011).

127. South-North Centre for Dialogue and Development. *Global survey on government action on the implementation of the standard rules of the equalization of opportunities for persons with disabilities*. Amman, Office of the UN Special Rapporteur on Disabilities. 2006.

128. Lagarde M, Haines A, Palmer N. The impact of conditional cash transfers on health outcomes and use of health services in low and middle income countries. *Cochrane Database of Systematic Reviews (Online)*, 2009,4CD008137- PMID:19821444

129. Barber SL, Gertler PJ. Empowering women to obtain high quality care: evidence from an evaluation of Mexico's conditional cash transfer programme. *Health Policy and Planning*, 2009,24:18-25. doi:10.1093/heapol/czn039 PMID:19022854

130. Morris SS et al. Monetary incentives in primary health care and effects on use and coverage of preventive health care interventions in rural Honduras: cluster randomised trial. *Lancet*, 2004,364:2030-2037. doi:10.1016/S0140-6736(04)17515-6 PMID:15582060

131. Fiszbein A, Schady N. *Conditional cash transfers: reducing present and future poverty*. Washington, World Bank, 2009.

132. Kaplan C. Special issues in contraception: caring for women with disabilities. *Journal of Midwifery & Women's Health*, 2006,51:450-456. doi:10.1016/j.jmwh.2006.07.009 PMID:17081935

133. *The World Health Report 2001 – Mental health: New understanding, new hope*. Geneva, World Health Organization, 2001.

134. Saxena S et al. Resources for mental health: scarcity, inequity, and inefficiency. *Lancet*, 2007,370:878-889. doi:10.1016/S0140-6736(07)61239-2 PMID:17804062

135. Dollars, DALYs and decisions. Geneva, World Health Organization, 2006.

136. *Mental health systems in selected low- and middle-income countries: a WHO-AIMS cross national analysis*. Geneva, World Health Organization, 2009.

137. Siqueira FC et al. [Architectonic barriers for elderly and physically disabled people: an epidemiological study of the physical structure of health service units in seven Brazilian states] *Ciência & Saúde Coletiva*, 2009,14:39-44. PMID:19142307

138. Trösken T, Geraedts M. [Accessibility of doctors' surgeries in Essen, Germany] *Gesundheitswesen (Bundesverband der Arzte des Offentlichen Gesundheitsdienstes (Germany))*, 2005,67:613-619. PMID:16217715

139. Huber M et al. *Quality in and equality of access to healthcare services*. Brussels, European Commission, 2008.

140. Park JH et al. Disparities between persons with and without disabilities in their participation rates in mass screening. *European Journal of Public Health*, 2009,19:85-90. doi:10.1093/eurpub/ckn108 PMID:19158103

141. Ubido J, Huntington J, Warburton D. Inequalities in access to healthcare faced by women who are deaf. *Health & Social Care in the Community*, 2002,10:247-253. doi:10.1046/j.1365-2524.2002.00365.x PMID:12193168

142. Smith DL. Disparities in patient-physician communication for persons with a disability from the 2006 Medical Expenditure Panel Survey (MEPS). *Disability and Health Journal*, 2009,2:206-215. doi:10.1016/j.dhjo.2009.06.002 PMID:21122761

143. Phillips A, Morrison J, Davis RW. General practitioners' educational needs in intellectual disability health. *Journal of Intellectual Disability Research: JIDR*, 2004,48:142-149. doi:10.1111/j.1365-2788.2004.00503.x PMID:14723656

144. Iezzoni LI, Ramanan RA, Lee S. Teaching medical students about communicating with patients with major mental illness. *Journal of General Internal Medicine*, 2006,b21:1112-1115. doi:10.1111/j.1525-1497.2006.00521.x PMID:16970561

145. Shakespeare T, Iezzoni LI, Groce NE. Disability and the training of health professionals. *Lancet*, 2009,374:1815-1816. doi:10.1016/S0140-6736(09)62050-X PMID:19957403

146. Banda I. Disability, poverty and HIV/AIDS. *Newsletter of Disabled Persons*, 2006, South Africa.

147. Antonelli RC, McAllister JW, Popp J. *Making care coordination a critical component of the pediatric health system: a multidisciplinary framework*. New York, The Commonwealth Fund, 2009.

148. David TJ. Transition from the paediatric clinic to the adult service. *Journal of the Royal Society of Medicine*, 2001,94:373-374. PMID:11461978

149. Honey A et al. Approaching adulthood with a chronic health condition: professionals' and young people's perspectives. In: Bennett D et al., eds. *Challenges in adolescent health: an Australian perspective*. Hauppauge, Nova Science Publishers, 2009:177–188.

150. Shaw KL, Southwood TR, McDonagh JE. British Paediatric Rheumatology GroupUser perspectives of transitional care for adolescents with juvenile idiopathic arthritis. *Rheumatology (Oxford, England)*, 2004,43:770-778. doi:10.1093/rheumatology/keh175 PMID:15039498

151. Stewart D. Transition to adult services for young people with disabilities: current evidence to guide future research. *Developmental Medicine and Child Neurology*, 2009,51:Suppl 4169-173. doi:10.1111/j.1469-8749.2009.03419.x PMID:19740226

152. Binks JA et al. What do we really know about the transition to adult-centered health care? A focus on cerebral palsy and spina bifida. *Archives of Physical Medicine and Rehabilitation*, 2007,88:1064-1073. doi:10.1016/j.apmr.2007.04.018 PMID:17678671

153. Davis M, Sondheimer DL. State child mental health efforts to support youth in transition to adulthood. *The Journal of Behavioral Health Services & Research*, 2005,32:27-42. doi:10.1007/BF02287326 PMID:15632796

154. Kroll T, Neri MT. Experiences with care co-ordination among people with cerebral palsy, multiple sclerosis, or spinal cord injury. *Disability and Rehabilitation*, 2003,25:1106-1114. doi:10.1080/0963828031000152002 PMID:12944150

155. Bodenheimer T. Coordinating care–a perilous journey through the health care system. *The New England Journal of Medicine*, 2008,358:1064-1071. doi:10.1056/NEJMhpr0706165 PMID:18322289

156. Smith RD. Promoting the health of people with physical disabilities: a discussion of the financing and organization of public health services in Australia. *Health Promotion International*, 2000,15:79-86. doi:10.1093/heapro/15.1.79

157. Aulagnier M et al. General practitioners' attitudes towards patients with disabilities: the need for training and support. *Disability and Rehabilitation*, 2005,27:1343-1352. doi:10.1080/09638280500164107 PMID:16321918

158. Coleman R, Loppy L, Walraven G. The treatment gap and primary health care for people with epilepsy in rural Gambia. *Bulletin of the World Health Organization*, 2002,80:378-383. PMID:12077613

159. Summers SJ, Jones J. Cross-cultural working in community learning disabilities services: clinical issues, dilemmas and tensions. *Journal of Intellectual Disability Research: JIDR*, 2004,48:687-694. doi:10.1111/j.1365-2788.2004.00601.x PMID:15357689

160. Ory MG, DeFriese GH. *Self-care in later life: research, program and policy issues*. New York, Springer Publishing Company, 1998.

161. *Integrating mental health into primary care: a global perspective*. Singapore, World Health Organization and World Organization of Family Doctors, 2008.

162. *Mental health and development: targeting people with mental health conditions as a vulnerable group*. Geneva, World Health Organization, 2010.

163. Krahn GL, Ritacco B. Public health as a change agent for disability. In: Drum C, Krahn G, Bersani H, eds. *Disability and public health*. Washington, American Public Health Association, 2009:183–204.

164. Tomlinson M et al. Research priorities for health of people with disabilities: an expert opinion exercise. *Lancet*, 2009,374:1857-1862. doi:10.1016/S0140-6736(09)61910-3 PMID:19944866

165. Patel V et al. Treatment and prevention of mental disorders in low-income and middle-income countries. *Lancet*, 2007,370:991-1005. doi:10.1016/S0140-6736(07)61240-9 PMID:17804058

166. World Health Organization, United Nations Educational, Scientific and Cultural Organization, International Labour Organization, International Disability and Development Consortium. *Community-based rehabilitation: CBR guidelines*. Geneva, World Health Organization, 2010.

167. Final technical report: Raising the voice of the African Decade of Disabled Persons: Phase II: Training emerging leaders in the disability community, promoting disability rights and developing HIV/AIDS awareness and prevention programs for adolescents and young adults with disabilities in Africa. *New York, Rehabilitation International, 2007.*

168. Drum CE et al. Guidelines and criteria for the implementation of community-based health promotion programs for individuals with disabilities. *American Journal of Health Promotion: AJHP*, 2009,b24:93-101, ii. doi:10.4278/ajhp.090303-CIT-94 PMID:19928482

169. Durvasula S, Beange H. Health inequalities in people with intellectual disability: strategies for improvement. *Health Promotion Journal of Australia*, 2001,11:27-31.

170. *The World Health Report 2008: Primary health care, now more than ever*. Geneva, World Health Organization, 2008 (http://www.who.int/whr/2008/en/index.html, accessed 11 April 2010).

171. van Loon J, Knibbe J, Van Hove G. From institutional to community support: consequences for medical care. *Journal of Applied Research in Intellectual Disabilities*, 2005,18:175-180. doi:10.1111/j.1468-3148.2005.00246.x

172. Balogh R et al. Organising health care services for persons with an intellectual disability. *Cochrane Database of Systematic Reviews (Online)*, 2008,4CD007492- PMID:18843752

173. *Strengthening care for the injured: Success stories and lessons learned from around the world.* Geneva, World Health Organization, 2010.

174. Lennox N et al. Effects of a comprehensive health assessment programme for Australian adults with intellectual disability: a cluster randomized trial. *International Journal of Epidemiology*, 2007,36:139-146. doi:10.1093/ije/dyl254 PMID:17218326

175. Lorig KR et al. Internet-based chronic disease self-management: a randomized trial. *Medical Care*, 2006,44:964-971. doi:10.1097/01.mlr.0000233678.80203.c1 PMID:17063127

176. Wagner EH et al. Finding common ground: patient-centeredness and evidence-based chronic illness care. *Journal of Alternative and Complementary Medicine (New York, NY)*, 2005,11:Suppl 1S7-S15. PMID:16332190

177. *Innovative care for chronic conditions: building blocks for actions: global report.* Geneva, World Health Organization, 2002.

178. *New paradigm of medical care for persons with disability: a multi-country action research joint initiative of WHO/DAR & AIFO/Italy.* Piedecuesta, ASODISPIE, 2007 (http://www.aifo.it/english/proj/aifo-who/romemeeting_dec07/Colombia_piedecuesta-descriptive.pdf, accessed 6 January 2011).

179. Allen M et al. Improving patient-clinician communication about chronic conditions: description of an internet-based nurse E-coach intervention. *Nursing Research*, 2008,57:107-112. doi:10.1097/01.NNR.0000313478.47379.98 PMID:18347482

180. Leveille SG et al. Health coaching via an internet portal for primary care patients with chronic conditions: a randomized controlled trial. *Medical Care*, 2009,47:41-47. doi:10.1097/MLR.0b013e3181844dd0 PMID:19106729

181. Beran D et al. Diabetes care in Nicaragua: results of the RAPIA study. *Diabetes Voice*, 2007,52:38-40.

182. Lindsey M. Comprehensive health care services for people with learning disabilities. *Advances in Psychiatric Treatment*, 2002,8:138-147. doi:10.1192/apt.8.2.138

183. Jamoom EW et al. The effect of caregiving on preventive care for people with disabilities. *Disability and Health Journal*, 2008,1:51-57. doi:10.1016/j.dhjo.2007.11.005 PMID:21122711

184. Kendall E, Clapton J. Time for a shift in Australian rehabilitation? *Disability and Rehabilitation*, 2006,28:1097-1101. doi:10.1080/09638280500531784 PMID:16950740

185. Schillinger D et al. Effects of primary care coordination on public hospital patients. *Journal of General Internal Medicine*, 2000,15:329-336. doi:10.1046/j.1525-1497.2000.07010.x PMID:10840268

186. Boling PA. Care transitions and home health care. *Clinics in Geriatric Medicine*, 2009,25:135-148, viii. doi:10.1016/j.cger.2008.11.005 PMID:19217498

187. Zwarenstein M, Reeves S, Perrier L. Effectiveness of pre-licensure interprofessional education and post-licensure collaborative interventions. *Journal of Interprofessional Care*, 2005,19:Suppl 1148-165. doi:10.1080/13561820500082800 PMID:16096152

188. Nielsen PR et al. Costs and quality of life for prehabilitation and early rehabilitation after surgery of the lumbar spine. *BMC Health Services Research*, 2008,8:209- doi:10.1186/1472-6963-8-209 PMID:18842157

189. Battersby MW. SA HealthPlus TeamHealth reform through coordinated care: SA HealthPlus. *BMJ (Clinical research ed.)*, 2005,330:662-665. doi:10.1136/bmj.330.7492.662 PMID:15775001

190. Engle PL et al. International Child Development Steering GroupStrategies to avoid the loss of developmental potential in more than 200 million children in the developing world. *Lancet*, 2007,369:229-242. doi:10.1016/S0140-6736(07)60112-3 PMID:17240290

191. Elliott J, Hatton C, Emerson E. The health of people with intellectual disabilities in the UK: evidence and implications for the NHS. *Journal of Integrated Care*, 2003,11:9-17.

192. Stewart D et al. A critical appraisal of literature reviews about the transition to adulthood for youth with disabilities. *Physical & Occupational Therapy in Pediatrics*, 2006,26:5-24. PMID:17135067

193. Gething L, Fethney J. The need for disability awareness training among rurally based Australian general medical practitioners. *Disability and Rehabilitation*, 1997,19:249-259. doi:10.3109/09638289709166535 PMID:9195143

194. Haggerty JL et al. Continuity of care: a multidisciplinary review. *BMJ (Clinical research ed.)*, 2003,327:1219-1221. doi:10.1136/bmj.327.7425.1219 PMID:14630762

195. Elrod CS, DeJong G. Determinants of utilization of physical rehabilitation services for persons with chronic and disabling conditions: an exploratory study. *Archives of Physical Medicine and Rehabilitation*, 2008,89:114-120. doi:10.1016/j.apmr.2007.08.122 PMID:18164340

196. Darrah J, Magil-Evans J, Adkins R. How well are we doing? Families of adolescents or young adults with cerebral palsy share their perceptions of service delivery. *Disability and Rehabilitation*, 2002,24:542-549. doi:10.1080/09638280210121359 PMID:12171644

197. Stille CJ, Antonelli RC. Coordination of care for children with special health care needs. *Current Opinion in Pediatrics*, 2004,16:700-705. doi:10.1097/01.mop.0000144442.68016.92 PMID:15548935

198. Bordé A et al. *Information and communication technologies for development: health.* New York, Global Alliance for ICT and Development, 2010.

199. Gagnon MP et al. Interventions for promoting information and communication technologies adoption in healthcare professionals. [review]*Cochrane Database of Systematic Reviews (Online)*, 2009,1CD006093- PMID:19160265

200. Crosson JC et al. Implementing an electronic medical record in a family medicine practice: communication, decision making, and conflict. *Annals of Family Medicine*, 2005,3:307-311. doi:10.1370/afm.326 PMID:16046562

201. Rowe N et al. Ten-year experience of a private nonprofit telepsychiatry service. *Telemedicine and e-Health: the official journal of the American Telemedicine Association*, 2008,14:1078-1086. doi:10.1089/tmj.2008.0037 PMID:19119830

202. Taylor DM et al. Exploring the feasibility of videoconference delivery of a self-management program to rural participants with stroke. *Telemedicine and e-Health: the official journal of the American Telemedicine Association*, 2009,15:646-654. doi:10.1089/tmj.2008.0165 PMID:19694589

203. Murray E et al. Interactive health and communication applications for people with chronic disease. *Cochrane Database of Systematic Reviews*, 2005,4CD004274-

204. Seren E. Web-based hearing screening test. *Telemedicine and e-Health: the official journal of the American Telemedicine Association*, 2009,15:678-681. doi:10.1089/tmj.2009.0013 PMID:19694590

205. Maulik PK, Darmstadt GL. Childhood disability in low- and middle-income countries: overview of screening, prevention, services, legislation, and epidemiology. *Pediatrics*, 2007,120:Suppl 1S1-S55. doi:10.1542/peds.2007-0043B PMID:17603094

206. Loon J, Knibbe J, Van Hove G. From institutional to community support: consequences for medical care. *Journal of Applied Research in Intellectual Disabilities*, 2005,18:175-180. doi:10.1111/j.1468-3148.2005.00246.x

207. Hewitt-Taylor J. Children with complex, continuing health needs and access to facilities. *Nursing Standard (Royal College of Nursing (Great Britain): 1987)*, 2009,23:35-41. PMID:19413072

208. Liu SY, Clark MA. Breast and cervical cancer screening practices among disabled women aged 40–75: does quality of the experience matter? *Journal of Women's Health (2002)*, 2008,17:1321-1329. doi:10.1089/jwh.2007.0591 PMID:18788985

209. Morrison EH, George V, Mosqueda L. Primary care for adults with physical disabilities: perceptions from consumer and provider focus groups. *Family Medicine*, 2008,40:645-651. PMID:18830840

210. Sabharwal S, Sebastian JL, Lanouette M. An educational intervention to teach medical students about examining disabled patients. *JAMA: Journal of the American Medical Association*, 2000,284:1080-1081. doi:10.1001/jama.284.9.1080-a PMID:10974684

211. Wong JG, Scully P. A practical guide to capacity assessment and patient consent in Hong Kong. *Hong Kong Medical Journal = Xianggang yi xue za zhi/Hong Kong Academy of Medicine*, 2003,9:284-289. PMID:12904617

212. Maart S, Jelsma J. The sexual behaviour of physically disabled adolescents. *Disability and Rehabilitation*, 2010,32:438-443. doi:10.3109/09638280902846368 PMID:20113191

213. Dyer O. Gynaecologist is struck off for sterilising women without their consent. *British Medical Journal*, 2002,325:1260- doi:10.1136/bmj.325.7375.1260

214. Grover SR. Menstrual and contraceptive management in women with an intellectual disability. *The Medical Journal of Australia*, 2002,176:108-110. PMID:11936305

215. Servais L. Sexual health care in persons with intellectual disabilities. *Mental Retardation and Developmental Disabilities Research Reviews*, 2006,12:48-56. doi:10.1002/mrdd.20093 PMID:16435330

216. Stansfield AJ, Holland AJ, Clare ICH. The sterilisation of people with intellectual disabilities in England and Wales during the period 1988 to 1999. *Journal of Intellectual Disability Research: JIDR*, 2007,51:569-579. doi:10.1111/j.1365-2788.2006.00920.x PMID:17598870

217. Nieuwenhuijsen C et al. Unmet needs and health care utilization in young adults with cerebral palsy. *Disability and Rehabilitation*, 2008,30:1254-1262. doi:10.1080/09638280701622929 PMID:18821192

218. Tracy J, Iacono T. People with developmental disabilities teaching medical students–does it make a difference? *Journal of Intellectual & Developmental Disability*, 2008,33:345-348. doi:10.1080/13668250802478633 PMID:19039695

219. Graham CL et al. Teaching medical students about disability in family medicine. *Family Medicine*, 2009,41:542-544. PMID:19724936

220. Duggan A et al. What can I learn from this interaction? A qualitative analysis of medical student self-reflection and learning in a standardized patient exercise about disability. *Journal of Health Communication*, 2009,14:797-811. doi:10.1080/10810730903295526 PMID:20029712

221. Saketkoo L et al. Effects of a disability awareness and skills training workshop on senior medical students as assessed with self ratings and performance on a standardized patient case. *Teaching and Learning in Medicine*, 2004,16:345-354. doi:10.1207/s15328015tlm1604_7 PMID:15582871

222. Packer TL et al. Attitudes to disability of Russian occupational therapy and nursing students. *International Journal of Rehabilitation Research. Internationale Zeitschrift fur Rehabilitationsforschung. Revue Internationale de Recherches de Réadaptation*, 2000,23:39-47. PMID:10826124

223. Thompson TL, Emrich K, Moore G. The effect of curriculum on the attitudes of nursing students toward disability. *Rehabilitation Nursing: the official journal of the Association of Rehabilitation Nurses*, 2003,28:27-30. PMID:12567819

224. Melville CA et al. Enhancing primary health care services for adults with intellectual disabilities. *Journal of Intellectual Disability Research: JIDR*, 2005,49:190-198. doi:10.1111/j.1365-2788.2005.00640.x PMID:15713194

225. *National programme on orientation of medical officers working in primary health centres to disability management.* New Dehli, Rehabilitation Council of India, 2009 (http://www.rehabcouncil.nic.in/projects/phc.htm, accessed 30 September 2010).

226. *Clinical guidelines and integrated care pathways for the oral health care of people with learning disabilities.* London, British Society for Disability and Oral Health and The Royal College of Surgeons of England, 2001.

227. Kerac M. The Malawi directory of disability organizations. In: Hartley S, ed. *CBR as part of community development: a poverty eradication strategy.* London, University College London, Centre for International Child Health, 2006.

228. Pappaioanou M et al. Strengthening capacity in developing countries for evidence-based public health: the data for decision-making project. *Social Science & Medicine (1982)*, 2003,57:1925-1937. doi:10.1016/S0277-9536(03)00058-3 PMID:14499516

229. Oxman AD et al. SUPPORT Tools for evidence-informed health policymaking (STP) 1: What is evidence-informed policymaking? *Health Research Policy and Systems/BioMed Central*, 2009,7:Suppl 1S1- doi:10.1186/1478-4505-7-S1-S1 PMID:20018099

230. Armour BS, Thierry JM, Wolf LA. State-level differences in breast and cervical cancer screening by disability status: United States, 2008. *Women's Health Issues: official publication of the Jacobs Institute of Women's Health*, 2009,19:406-414. doi:10.1016/j.whi.2009.08.006 PMID:19879454

231. Jamison DT et al., eds. *Priorities in health.* Washington, World Bank, 2006.

232. Tercero F et al. The epidemiology of moderate and severe injuries in a Nicaraguan community: a household-based survey. *Public Health*, 2006,120:106-114. doi:10.1016/j.puhe.2005.07.005 PMID:16260010

233. Adams E et al. Fundamentals of disability epidemiology. In: Drum CE, Krahn GL, Bersani H, eds. *Disability and public health.* Washington, American Public Health Association, 2009:105–124.

234. Baquet CR et al. Recruitment and participation in clinical trials: socio-demographic, rural/urban, and health care access predictors. *Cancer Detection and Prevention*, 2006,30:24-33. doi:10.1016/j.cdp.2005.12.001 PMID:16495020

235. Mactavish JB, Lutfiyya ZM, Mahon MJ. "I can speak for myself": involving individuals with intellectual disabilities as research participants. *Mental Retardation*, 2000,38:216-227. doi:10.1352/0047-6765(2000)038<0216:ICSFMI>2.0.CO;2 PMID:10900929

236. Rimmer JH et al. Exercise intervention research on persons with disabilities: what we know and where we need to go. *American Journal of Physical Medicine & Rehabilitation/Association of Academic Physiatrists*, 2010,89:249-263. doi:10.1097/PHM.0b013e3181c9fa9d PMID:20068432

237. Lollar DJ. Public health and disability: emerging opportunities. *Public Health Reports (Washington, DC: 1974)*, 2002,117:131-136. doi:10.1016/S0033-3549(04)50119-X PMID:12356997

238. Seekins T, Kimpton T. *Evidence-based health promotion interventions for people with disabilities: results of a systematic review of literature.* Portland, Rehabilitation Research and Training Center, 2008 (http://www.ohsu.edu/oidd/rrtc/archive/SOS2008/briefs/promotion_seekins_review.cfm, accessed 30 September 2010)

239. Heald A. Physical health in schizophrenia: a challenge for antipsychotic therapy. *European Psychiatry: the journal of the Association of European Psychiatrists*, 2010,25:Suppl 2S6-S11. doi:10.1016/S0924-9338(10)71700-4 PMID:20620888

240. Gilbert T. Involving people with learning disabilities in research: issues and possibilities. *Health & Social Care in the Community*, 2004,12:298-308. doi:10.1111/j.1365-2524.2004.00499.x PMID:15272885

241. Lin PI, Shuldiner AR. Rethinking the genetic basis for comorbidity of schizophrenia and type 2 diabetes. *Schizophrenia Research*, 2010,123:234-243. doi:10.1016/j.schres.2010.08.022 PMID:20832248

242. Alzheimer's Society [web site]. (http://alzheimers.org.uk, accessed 30 September 2010).

243. Jette AM, Keysor JJ. Uses of evidence in disability outcomes and effectiveness research. *The Milbank Quarterly*, 2002,80:325-345. doi:10.1111/1468-0009.t01-1-00006 PMID:12101875

Chapter 4

Rehabilitation

"Being an amputee myself with functional lower limb prosthetics, I can say that the device enable me to function normally. My prosthetics brought back my confidence and self esteem to participate in mainstream activities of the society, thus changing my outlook in life to positive to more positive. Definitely, my prosthetics had an impact on my present status or the quality of life I am enjoying now because I basically perform all the task that is assigned to me which at the end the day results to quality output and good pay."

Johnny

"Coming from a country where there is not much awareness and resources for dealing with post-spinal cord injured victims, my return home was indeed an enormous challenge. Living in a house that was inaccessible, members of my family have had to persevere with daily lifting me up and down the house. Physiotherapy had become a crucial necessity and as a result of the continuous costs incurred, my mother took up the task to administer physiotherapy as well as stand in as my caretaker. During my rehabilitation process, getting admitted for treatment during times of illness or to use physiotherapy facilities was close to impossible as a result of the overwhelming numbers on the waiting list. My rehabilitation period despite challenging was a humbling moment of my life and a continuous process that I face until today. I have learned disability is not inability and a strong mentality and great attitude have been very important!"

Casey

"Families find themselves in difficulty after a member of the family has a stroke. I consider myself a stroke survivor but my family are stroke victims. I have been fortunate and have been able to return to work, but I have had to battle all the way. We do not get the help we need, services are so variable and there is not enough speech and language therapy and physiotherapy. After my stroke I had to learn to do everything again, including swallowing and to learn to talk. The first thing that came back to me with my speech was swearing, my first sentence had four expletives in it, but I am told that was normal."

Linda

"If you don't have a proper wheelchair, that is when you really feel that you are disabled. But if you have a proper wheelchair, which meets your needs and suits you, you can forget about your disability."

Faustina

4

Rehabilitation

Rehabilitation has long lacked a unifying conceptual framework (*1*). Historically, the term has described a range of responses to disability, from interventions to improve body function to more comprehensive measures designed to promote inclusion (see **Box 4.1**). The *International Classification of Functioning, Disability and Health* (ICF) provides a framework that can be used for all aspects of rehabilitation (*11–14*).

For some people with disabilities, rehabilitation is essential to being able to participate in education, the labour market, and civic life. Rehabilitation is always voluntary, and some individuals may require support with decision-making about rehabilitation choices. In all cases rehabilitation should help to empower a person with a disability and his or her family.

Article 26, Habilitation and Rehabilitation, of the United Nations *Convention on the Rights of Persons with Disabilities* (CRPD) calls for:

"… appropriate measures, including through peer support, to enable persons with disabilities to attain and maintain their maximum independence, full physical, mental, social and vocational ability, and full inclusion and participation in all aspects of life".

The Article further calls on countries to organize, strengthen, and extend comprehensive rehabilitation services and programmes, which should begin as early as possible, based on multidisciplinary assessment of individual needs and strengths, and including the provision of assistive devices and technologies.

This chapter examines some typical rehabilitation measures, the need and unmet need for rehabilitation, barriers to accessing rehabilitation, and ways in which these barriers can be addressed.

Understanding rehabilitation

Rehabilitation measures and outcomes

Rehabilitation measures target body functions and structures, activities and participation, environmental factors, and personal factors. They contribute

Box 4.1. What is rehabilitation?

This Report defines **rehabilitation** as "a set of measures that assist individuals who experience, or are likely to experience, disability to achieve and maintain optimal functioning in interaction with their environments". A distinction is sometimes made between habilitation, which aims to help those who acquire disabilities congenitally or early in life to develop maximal functioning; and rehabilitation, where those who have experienced a loss in function are assisted to regain maximal functioning (2). In this chapter the term "rehabilitation" covers both types of intervention. Although the concept of rehabilitation is broad, not everything to do with disability can be included in the term. Rehabilitation targets improvements in individual functioning – say, by improving a person's ability to eat and drink independently. Rehabilitation also includes making changes to the individual's environment – for example, by installing a toilet handrail. But barrier removal initiatives at societal level, such as fitting a ramp to a public building, are not considered rehabilitation in this Report.

Rehabilitation reduces the impact of a broad range of health conditions. Typically rehabilitation occurs for a specific period of time, but can involve single or multiple interventions delivered by an individual or a team of rehabilitation workers, and can be needed from the acute or initial phase immediately following recognition of a health condition through to post-acute and maintenance phases.

Rehabilitation involves identification of a person's problems and needs, relating the problems to relevant factors of the person and the environment, defining rehabilitation goals, planning and implementing the measures, and assessing the effects (see figure below). Educating people with disabilities is essential for developing knowledge and skills for self-help, care, management, and decision-making. People with disabilities and their families experience better health and functioning when they are partners in rehabilitation (3–9).

The rehabilitation process

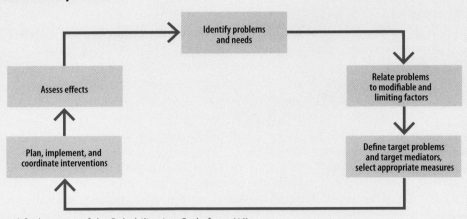

Source: A modified version of the Rehabilitation Cycle from (10).

Rehabilitation – provided along a continuum of care ranging from hospital care to rehabilitation in the community (12) – can improve health outcomes, reduce costs by shortening hospital stays (15–17), reduce disability, and improve quality of life (18–21). Rehabilitation need not be expensive.

Rehabilitation is cross-sectoral and may be carried out by health professionals in conjunction with specialists in education, employment, social welfare, and other fields. In resource-poor contexts it may involve non-specialist workers – for example, community-based rehabilitation workers in addition to family, friends, and community groups.

Rehabilitation that begins early produces better functional outcomes for almost all health conditions associated with disability (18–30). The effectiveness of early intervention is particularly marked for children with, or at risk of, developmental delays (27, 28, 31, 32), and has been proven to increase educational and developmental gains (4, 27).

to a person achieving and maintaining optimal functioning in interaction with their environment, using the following broad outcomes:

- prevention of the loss of function
- slowing the rate of loss of function
- improvement or restoration of function
- compensation for lost function
- maintenance of current function.

Rehabilitation outcomes are the benefits and changes in the functioning of an individual over time that are attributable to a single measure or set of measures (33). Traditionally, rehabilitation outcome measures have focused on the individual's impairment level. More recently, outcomes measurement has been extended to include individual activity and participation outcomes (34, 35). Measurements of activity and participation outcomes assess the individual's performance across a range of areas – including communication, mobility, self-care, education, work and employment, and quality of life. Activity and participation outcomes may also be measured for programmes. Examples include the number of people who remain in or return to their home or community, independent living rates, return-to-work rates, and hours spent in leisure and recreational pursuits. Rehabilitation outcomes may also be measured through changes in resource use – for example, reducing the hours needed each week for support and assistance services (36).

The following examples illustrate different rehabilitation measures:

- **A middle-aged woman with advanced diabetes**. Rehabilitation might include assistance to regain strength following her hospitalization for diabetic coma, the provision of a prosthesis and gait training after a limb amputation, and the provision of screen-reader software to enable her to continue her job as an accountant after sustaining loss of vision.
- **A young man with schizophrenia.** The man may have trouble with routine daily tasks, such as working, living independently, and

maintaining relationships. Rehabilitation might mean drug treatment, education of patients and families, and psychological support via outpatient care, community-based rehabilitation, or participation in a support group.

- **A child who is deafblind.** Parents, teachers, physical and occupational therapists, and other orientation and mobility specialists need to work together to plan accessible and stimulating spaces to encourage development. Caregivers will need to work with the child to develop appropriate touch and sign communication methods. Individualized education with careful assessment will help learning and reduce the child's isolation.

Limitations and restrictions for a child with cerebral palsy, and possible rehabilitation measures, outcomes, and barriers are described in Table 4.1.

Rehabilitation teams and specific disciplines may work across categories. Rehabilitation measures in this chapter are broadly divided into three categories:

- rehabilitation medicine
- therapy
- assistive technologies.

Rehabilitation medicine

Rehabilitation medicine is concerned with improving functioning through the diagnosis and treatment of health conditions, reducing impairments, and preventing or treating complications (12, 37). Doctors with specific expertise in medical rehabilitation are referred to as physiatrists, rehabilitation doctors, or physical and rehabilitation specialists (37). Medical specialists such as psychiatrists, paediatricians, geriatricians, ophthalmologists, neurosurgeons, and orthopaedic surgeons can be involved in rehabilitation medicine, as can a broad range of therapists. In many parts of the world where specialists in rehabilitation medicine are not available, services may be provided by doctors and therapists (see Box 4.2).

Table 4.1. Child with cerebral palsy and rehabilitation

Difficulties faced by the child	Rehabilitation measures	Possible outcomes	Potential barriers	People involved in the measures
Unable to care for self	▶ Therapy – Training for the child on different ways to complete the task. – Assessment and provision of equipment, training parents to lift, carry, move, feed and otherwise care for the child with cerebral palsy. – Teaching parents and family members to use and maintain equipment. – Provision of information and support for parents and family. – Counselling the family. ▶ Assistive technology – Provision of equipment for maintaining postures and self-care, playing and interaction, such as sitting or standing (when age-appropriate)	– Parents better able to care for their child and be proactive. – Reduced likelihood of compromised development, deformities, and contractures. – Reduced likelihood of respiratory infections. – Access to support groups or peer support. – Coping with stress and other psychological demands. – Better posture, respiration, feeding, speech, and physical activity performance.	– Timeliness of interventions. – Availability of family and support. – Financial capacity to pay for services and equipment. – Availability of well trained staff. – Attitudes and understanding of others involved in the rehabilitation measure. – Physical access to home environment, community, equipment, assistive devices and services.	– The child, parents, siblings, and extended family. – Depending on the setting and resources available: physiotherapists, occupational therapists, speech and language therapists, orthotists and technicians, doctors, psychologists, social workers, community-based rehabilitation workers, schoolteachers, teaching assistants.
Difficulty walking	▶ Rehabilitation medicine – Botulinum toxin injections. – Surgical treatment of contractures and deformities (therapy interventions usually complement these medical interventions). ▶ Therapy – Therapy, exercises and targeted play activities to train effective movements. ▶ Assistive technology – Orthotics, wheelchair or other equipment.	– Decreased muscle tone, better biomechanics of walking. – Decrease in self-reported limitations. – Increased participation in education and social life.	– Access to post-acute rehabilitation.	– Doctor, parents, therapist, orthotist.
Communication difficulties	▶ Therapy – Audiology. – Activities for language development. – Conversation skills. – Training conversation partners. ▶ Assistive technology – Training to use and maintain aids and equipment, which may include hearing aids and augmentative and alternative communication devices.	– Better communication skills. – Participation in social, educational and occupational life opportunities. – Improved relationships with family, friends, and the wider community. – Reduced risk of distress, educational failure, and antisocial behaviour.	– Availability of speech language therapists. – Social and economic status of the family. – Costs of purchasing and maintaining devices.	– Parents, speech and language pathologist/therapist, communication disorders assistant, community-based rehabilitation worker, teachers, and assistants.

Note: The table shows some potential rehabilitation measures for a child with cerebral palsy, possible outcomes, potential barriers, and the various people involved in care.

Box 4.2. Clubfoot treatment in Uganda

Clubfoot, a congenital deformity involving one or both feet, is commonly neglected in low and middle-income countries. If left untreated, clubfoot can result in physical deformity, pain in the feet, and impaired mobility, all of which can limit community participation, including access to education.

In Uganda the incidence of clubfoot is 1.2 per 1000 live births. The condition is usually not diagnosed, or if diagnosed it is neglected because conventional invasive surgery treatment is not possible with the resources available (*38*).

The Ponseti clubfoot treatment involving manipulation, casting, Achilles tenotomy, and fitting of foot braces has proven to result in a high rate of painless, functional feet (Ponseti, 1996). The benefits of this approach for developing countries are low cost, high effectiveness, and the possibility to train service providers other than medical doctors to perform the treatment. The results of a clubfoot project in Malawi, where the treatment was conducted by trained orthopaedic clinical officers, showed that initial good correction was achieved in 98% of cases (*39*).

The Ugandan Sustainable Clubfoot Care Project – a collaborative partnership between the Ugandan Ministry of Health, CBM International, and Ugandan and Canadian universities – is funded by the Canadian International Development Agency. Its purpose is to make sustainable, universal, effective, and safe treatment of clubfoot in Uganda using the Ponseti method. It built on the existing health care and education sectors and has incorporated research to inform the project's activities and evaluate outcomes.

The project has resulted in many positive achievements in two years including:

- The Ugandan Ministry of Health has approved the Ponseti method as the preferred treatment for clubfoot in all its hospitals.
- 36% of the country's public hospitals have built the capacity to do the Ponseti procedure and are using the method.
- 798 health-care professionals received training to identify and treat clubfoot.
- Teaching modules on clubfoot and the Ponseti method are being used in two medical and three paramedical schools.
- 1152 students in various health disciplines received training in the Ponseti method.
- 872 children with clubfoot received treatment, an estimated 31% of infants born with clubfoot during the sample period – very high, given that only 41% of all births occur in a health care centre.
- Public awareness campaigns were implemented – including radio messages and distribution of posters and pamphlets to village health teams – to inform the general public that clubfoot is correctable.

The project shows that clubfoot detection and treatment can quickly be incorporated into settings with few resources. The approach requires:

- Screening infants at birth for foot deformity to detect the impairment.
- Building the capacity of health-care professionals across the continuum of care, from community midwives screening for deformity, to NGO technicians making braces, and orthopaedic officers performing tenotomies.
- Decentralizing clubfoot care services, including screening in the community, for example through community-based rehabilitation workers, and treatment in local clinics, to address treatment adherence barriers.
- Incorporating Ponseti method training into the education curricula of medical, nursing, paramedical, and infant health-care students.
- Establishing mechanisms to address treatment adherence barriers including travel distance and costs.

Rehabilitation medicine has shown positive outcomes, for example, in improving joint and limb function, pain management, wound healing, and psychosocial well-being (40–47).

Therapy

Therapy is concerned with restoring and compensating for the loss of functioning, and preventing or slowing deterioration in functioning in every area of a person's life. Therapists and rehabilitation workers include occupational therapists, orthotists, physiotherapists, prosthetists, psychologists, rehabilitation and technical assistants, social workers, and speech and language therapists.

Therapy measures include:
- training, exercises, and compensatory strategies
- education
- support and counselling
- modifications to the environment
- provision of resources and assistive technology.

Convincing evidence shows that some therapy measures improve rehabilitation outcomes (see Box 4.3). For example, exercise therapy in a broad range of health conditions – including cystic fibrosis, frailness in elderly people, Parkinson disease, stroke, osteoarthritis in the knee and hip, heart disease, and low back pain – has contributed to increased strength, endurance, and flexibility of joints. It can improve balance, posture, and range of motion or functional mobility, and reduce the risk of falls (49–51). Therapy interventions have also been found to be suitable for the long-term care of older persons to reduce disability (18). Some studies show that training in activities of daily living have positive outcomes for people with stroke (52).

Box 4.3. Money well spent: The effectiveness and value of housing adaptations

Public spending on housing adaptations for people with difficulties in functioning in the United Kingdom of Great Britain and Northern Ireland amounted to more than £220 million in 1995, and both the number of demands and unit costs are growing. A 2000 research study examined the effectiveness of adaptations in England and Wales, using interviews with recipients of major adaptations, postal questionnaires returned by recipients of minor adaptations, administrative records, and the views of visiting professionals. The main measure of "effectiveness" was the degree to which the problems experienced by the respondent before adaptation were overcome by the adaptation, without causing new problems. The study found that:

- Minor adaptations (rails, ramps, over-bath showers, and door entry systems, for example) – most costing less than £500 – produced a range of lasting, positive consequences for virtually all recipients: 62% of respondents suggested they felt safer from the risk of accident, and 77% perceived a positive effect on their health.
- Major adaptations (bathroom conversions, extensions, lifts, for example) in most cases had transformed people's lives. Before adaptations, people used words like "prisoner", "degraded", and "afraid' to describe their situations; following adaptations, they spoke of themselves as "independent", "useful", and "confident".
- Where major adaptations failed, it was typically because of weaknesses in the original specification. Adaptations for children sometimes failed to allow for the child's growth, for example. In other cases, policies intended to save money resulted in major waste. Examples included extensions that were too small or too cold to use, and cheap but ineffective substitutes for proper bathing facilities.
- The evidence from recipients suggests that successful adaptations keep people out of hospitals, reduce strain on carers, and promote social inclusion.
- Benefits were most pronounced where careful consultation with users took place, where the needs of the whole family had been considered, and where the integrity of the home had been respected.

Adaptations appear to be a highly effective use of public resources, justifying investment in health and rehabilitation resources. Further research is needed in diverse contexts and settings.

Source (48).

Distance training was used in Bangladesh for mothers of children with cerebral palsy in an 18-month therapy programme: it promoted the development of physical and cognitive skills and improved motor skills in the children (53). Counselling, information, and training on adaptive methods, aids, and equipment have been effective for individuals with spinal cord injury and younger people with disabilities (54–56). Many rehabilitation measures help people with disabilities to return or continue to work, including adjusting the content or schedule of work, and making changes to equipment and the work environment (57, 58).

Assistive technologies

An assistive technology device can be defined as "any item, piece of equipment, or product, whether it is acquired commercially, modified, or customized, that is used to increase, maintain, or improve the functional capabilities of individuals with disabilities" (59).

Common examples of assistive devices are:
- crutches, prostheses, orthoses, wheelchairs, and tricycles for people with mobility impairments;
- hearing aids and cochlear implants for those with hearing impairments;
- white canes, magnifiers, ocular devices, talking books, and software for screen magnification and reading for people with visual impairments;
- communication boards and speech synthesizers for people with speech impairments;
- devices such as day calendars with symbol pictures for people with cognitive impairment.

Assistive technologies, when appropriate to the user and the user's environment, have been shown to be powerful tools to increase independence and improve participation. A study of people with limited mobility in Uganda found that assistive technologies for mobility created greater possibilities for community participation, especially in education and employment

(60). For people in the United Kingdom with disabilities resulting from brain injuries, technologies such as personal digital assistants, and simpler technologies such as wall charts, were closely associated with independence (61). In a study of Nigerians with hearing impairments, provision of a hearing aid was associated with improved function, participation and user satisfaction (62).

Assistive devices have also been reported to reduce disability and may substitute or supplement support services – possibly reducing care costs (63). In the United States of America, data over 15 years from the National Long-Term Care Survey found that increasing use of technology was associated with decreasing reported disability among people aged 65 years and older (64). Another study from the United States showed that users of assistive technologies such as mobility aids and equipment for personal care reported less need for support services (65).

In some countries, assistive devices are an integral part of health care and are provided through the national health care system. Elsewhere, assistive technology is provided by governments through rehabilitation services, vocational rehabilitation, or special education agencies (66), insurance companies, and charitable and nongovernmental organizations.

Rehabilitation settings

The availability of rehabilitation services in different settings varies within and across nations and regions (67–70). Medical rehabilitation and therapy are typically provided in acute care hospitals for conditions with acute onset. Follow-up medical rehabilitation, therapy, and assistive devices could be provided in a wide range of settings, including specialized rehabilitation wards or hospitals; rehabilitation centres; institutions such as residential mental and nursing homes, respite care centres, hospices, prisons, residential educational institutions, and military residential settings; or single or multiprofessional practices (office or clinic). Longer-term rehabilitation may be provided within community settings and facilities such as primary health care centres, schools, workplaces, or home-care therapy services (67–70).

Needs and unmet needs

Global data on the need for rehabilitation services, the type and quality of measures provided, and estimates of unmet need do not exist. Data on rehabilitation services are often incomplete and fragmented. When data are available, comparability is hampered by differences in definitions, classifications of measures and personnel, populations under study, measurement methods, indicators, and data sources – for example, individuals with disabilities, service providers, or programme managers may experience needs and demands differently (71, 72).

Unmet rehabilitation needs can delay discharge, limit activities, restrict participation, cause deterioration in health, increase dependency on others for assistance, and decrease quality of life (37, 73–77). These negative outcomes can have broad social and financial implications for individuals, families, and communities (78–80).

Despite acknowledged limitations such as the quality of data and cultural variations in perception of disabilities, the need for rehabilitation services can be estimated in several ways. These include data on the prevalence of disability; disability-specific surveys; and population and administrative data.

Prevalence data on health conditions associated with disability can provide information to assess rehabilitation needs (81). As Chapter 2 indicated, disability rates correlate with the increase in noncommunicable conditions and global ageing. The need for rehabilitation services is projected to increase (82, 83) due to these demographic and epidemiological factors. Strong evidence suggests that impairments related to ageing and many health conditions can be reduced and functioning improved with rehabilitation (84–86).

Higher rates of disability indicate a greater potential need for rehabilitation. Epidemiological evidence together with an examination of the number, type, and severity of impairments, and the activity limitations and participation restrictions that may benefit from various rehabilitation measures, can help measure the need for services and may be useful for setting appropriate priorities for rehabilitation (87).

- The number of people needing hearing aids worldwide is based on 2005 World Health Organization estimates that about 278 million people have moderate to profound hearing impairments (88). In developed countries, industry experts estimate that about 20% of people with hearing impairments need hearing aids (89), suggesting 56 million potential hearing-aid users worldwide. Hearing aid producers and distributors estimate that hearing aid production currently meets less than 10% of global need (88), and less than 3% of the hearing aid needs in developing countries are met annually (90).

- The International Society for Prosthetics and Orthotics and the World Health Organization have estimated that people needing prostheses or orthotics and related services represent 0.5% of the population in developing countries; and 30 million people in Africa, Asia, and Latin America (91) require an estimated 180 000 rehabilitation professionals. In 2005 there were 24 prosthetic and orthotic schools in developing countries, graduating 400 trainees annually. Worldwide existing training facilities for prosthetic and orthotic professionals and other providers of essential rehabilitation services are deeply inadequate in relation to the need (92).

- A national survey of musculoskeletal impairment in Rwanda concluded that 2.6% of children are impaired and that about 80 000 need physical therapy, 50 000 need orthopaedic surgery, and 10 000 need assistive devices (93).

Most of the available data on national supply and unmet need are derived from disability-specific surveys on specific populations such as:

- National studies on living conditions of people with disabilities conducted in Malawi, Mozambique, Namibia, Zambia, and Zimbabwe (94–98) revealed large gaps in the provision of medical rehabilitation and assistive devices (see Table 2.5 in Chapter 2). Gender inequalities in access to assistive devices were evident in Malawi (men 25.3% and women 14.1%) and Zambia (men 15.7% and women 11.9%) (99).

- A survey of physical rehabilitation medicine in Croatia, the Czech Republic, Hungary, Slovakia, and Slovenia found a general lack of access to rehabilitation in primary, secondary, tertiary, and community health care settings, as well as regional and socioeconomic inequalities in access (100).

- In a study of people identified as disabled from three districts in Beijing, China, 75% of those interviewed expressed a need for a range of rehabilitation services, of which only 27% had received such services (101). A national Chinese study of the need for rehabilitation in 2007 found that unmet need was particularly high for assistive devices and therapy (102).

- United States surveys report considerable unmet needs – often caused by funding problems – for assistive technologies (103).

Unmet need for rehabilitation services can also be estimated from administrative and population survey data. The supply of rehabilitation services can be estimated from administrative data on the provision of services, and measures such as waiting times for rehabilitation services can proxy the extent to which demand for services is being met.

A recent global survey (2006–2008) of vision services in 195 countries found that waiting times in urban areas averaged less than one month, while waiting times in rural areas ranged from six months to a year (104). Proxy measures may not always be reliable. In the case of waiting times, for instance, lack of awareness of services and beliefs about disability influence treatment-seeking, while restrictions on who is legitimately waiting for services can complicate data interpretation (105–107).

Indicators on the number of people demanding but not receiving services, or receiving inadequate or inappropriate services, can provide useful planning information (108). Data on rehabilitation often are not disaggregated from other health care services, however, and rehabilitation measures are not included in existing classification systems, which could provide a framework for describing and measuring rehabilitation. Administrative data on supply are often fragmented because rehabilitation can take place in a variety of settings and be performed by different personnel.

Comparing multiple data sources can provide more robust interpretations, if a common framework like the ICF is used. As an example, the Arthritis Community Research and Evaluation Unit in Toronto merged administrative data sources to profile rehabilitation demand and supply across all regions of the province of Ontario (109). The researchers triangulated population data with the number of health-care workers per region to estimate the number of workers per person: they found that the higher concentration of workers in the southern region did not coincide with the highest areas of demand, causing unmet demand for rehabilitation.

Addressing barriers to rehabilitation

The barriers to rehabilitation service provision can be overcome through a series of actions, including:

- reforming policies, laws, and delivery systems, including development or revision of national rehabilitation plans;
- developing funding mechanisms to address barriers related to financing of rehabilitation;

- increasing human resources for rehabilitation, including training and retention of rehabilitation personnel;
- expanding and decentralizing service delivery;
- increasing the use and affordability of technology and assistive devices;
- expanding research programmes, including improving information and access to good practice guidelines.

Reforming policies, laws, and delivery systems

A 2005 global survey (*110*) of the implementation of the nonbinding, United Nations *Standard Rules on the Equalization of Opportunities for Persons with Disabilities* found that:

- in 48 of 114 (42%) countries that responded to the survey, rehabilitation policies were not adopted;
- in 57 (50%) countries legislation on rehabilitation for people with disabilities was not passed;
- in 46 (40%) countries rehabilitation programmes were not established.

Many countries have good legislation and related policies on rehabilitation, but the implementation of these policies, and the development and delivery of regional and local rehabilitation services, have lagged. Systemic barriers include:

- **Lack of strategic planning**. A study of rehabilitation medicine related to physical impairments – excluding assistive technology, sensory impairments, and specialized disciplines – in five central and eastern European countries suggested that the lack of strategic planning for services had resulted in an uneven distribution of service capacity and infrastructure (*100*).
- **Lack of resources and health infrastructure**. Limited resources and health infrastructure in developing countries, and in rural and remote communities in developed

countries, can reduce access to rehabilitation and quality of services (*111*). In a survey on the reasons for not using needed health facilities in two Indian states, 52.3% of respondents indicated that no healthcare facility in the area was available (*112*). Other countries lack rehabilitation services that have proven effective at reducing long-term costs, such as early intervention for children under the age of 5 (*5, 113–115*). A study of users of community-based rehabilitation (CBR) in Ghana, Guyana, and Nepal showed limited impact on physical well-being because CBR workers had difficulties providing physical rehabilitation, assistive devices, and referral services (*116*). In Haiti, before the 2010 earthquake, an estimated three quarters of amputees received prosthetic management due to the lack of availability of services (*117*).

- **Lack of agency responsible to administer, coordinate, and monitor services**. In some countries all rehabilitation is integrated in health care and financed under the national health system (*118, 119*). In other countries responsibilities are divided between different ministries, and rehabilitation services are often poorly integrated into the overall system and not well coordinated (*120*). A report of 29 African countries found that many lack coordination and collaboration among the different sectors and ministries involved in disability and rehabilitation, and 4 of the 29 countries did not have a lead ministry (*119*).
- **Inadequate health information systems and communication strategies** can contribute to low rates of participation in rehabilitation. Aboriginal Australians have high rates of cardiovascular disease but low rates of participation in cardiac rehabilitation, for example. Barriers to rehabilitation include poor communication across the health care sector and between providers (notably between primary and secondary care), inconsistent and insufficient data collection processes, multiple clinical information systems,

and incompatible technologies (*121*). Poor communication results in ineffective coordination of responsibilities among providers (*75*).

- **Complex referral systems can limit access**. Where access to rehabilitation services is controlled by doctors (*77*), medical rules or attitudes of primary physicians can obstruct individuals with disabilities from obtaining services (*122*). People are sometimes not referred, or inappropriately referred, or unnecessary medical consultations may increase their costs (*123–126*). This is particularly relevant to people with complex needs requiring multiple rehabilitation measures.
- **Absence of engagement with people with disabilities**. The study of 114 countries mentioned above did not consult with disabled people's organizations in 51 countries, and did not consult with families of persons with disabilities about design, implementation, and evaluation of rehabilitation programmes in 57 of the study countries (*110*).

Countries that lack policies and legislation on rehabilitation should consider introducing them, especially countries that are signatories to the CRPD, as they are required to align national law with Articles 25 and 26 of the Convention. Rehabilitation can be incorporated into general legislation on health, and into relevant employment, education, and social services legislation, as well as into specific legislation for persons with disabilities.

Policy responses should emphasize early intervention and use of rehabilitation to enable people with a broad range of health conditions to improve or maintain their level of functioning, with a specific focus on ensuring participation and inclusion, such as continuing to work (*127*). Services should be provided as close as possible to communities where people live, including in rural areas (*128*).

Development, implementation, and monitoring of policy and laws should include users (see Box 4.4) (*132*). Rehabilitation professionals must be aware of the policies and programmes given the role of rehabilitation in keeping people with disabilities participating in society (*133, 134*).

National rehabilitation plans and improved collaboration

Creating or amending national plans on rehabilitation, and establishing infrastructure and capacity to implement the plan are critical to improving access to rehabilitation. Plans should be based on analysis of the current situation, consider the main aspects of rehabilitation provision – leadership, financing, information, service delivery, products and technologies, and the rehabilitation workforce (*135*) – and define priorities based on local need. Even if it is not immediately possible to provide rehabilitation services for all who need them, a plan involving smaller, annual investments may progressively strengthen and expand the rehabilitation system.

Successful implementation of the plan depends on establishing or strengthening mechanisms for intersectoral collaboration. An interministerial committee or agency for rehabilitation can coordinate across organizations. For example, a Disability Action Council with representatives from the government, NGOs, and training programmes was established in Cambodia in 1997, to support coordination and cooperation across rehabilitation providers, decrease duplication and improve distribution of services and referral systems, and promote joint ventures in training (*136*). The Council has been very successful in developing physical rehabilitation and supporting professional training (physical therapy, prosthetics, orthotics, wheelchairs, and CBR) (*137*). Further benefits include (*136*):

- joint negotiation for equipment and supplies;
- sharing knowledge and expertise;
- continuing education through sharing specialist educators, establishing clinical education sites, reviewing and revising curricula, and disseminating information;

Box 4.4. Reform of mental health law in Italy – closing psychiatric institutions is not enough

In 1978 Italy introduced Law No. 180 gradually phasing out psychiatric hospitals and introducing a community-based system of psychiatric care. Social psychiatrist Franco Basaglia was a leading figure behind the new law that rejected the assumption that people with mental illness were a danger to society. Basaglia had become appalled by the inhuman conditions he witnessed as the director of a psychiatric hospital in northern Italy. He viewed social factors as the main determinants in mental illness, and became a champion of community mental health services and beds in general hospitals instead of psychiatric hospitals (129).

Thirty years later, Italy is the only country where traditional mental hospitals are prohibited by law. The law comprised framework legislation, with individual regions tasked with implementing detailed norms, methods, and timetables for action. As a result of the law, no new patients were admitted to psychiatric hospitals, and a process of deinstitutionalization of psychiatric inpatients was actively promoted. The inpatient population dropped by 53% between 1978 and 1987, and the final dismantling of psychiatric hospitals was completed by 2000 (130).

Treatment for acute problems is delivered in general hospital psychiatric units, each with a maximum of 15 beds. A network of community mental health and rehabilitation centres support mentally ill people, based on a holistic perspective. The organization of services uses a departmental model to coordinate a range of treatments, phases, and professionals. Campaigns against stigma, for social inclusion of people with mental health problems, and empowerment of patients and families have been promoted and supported centrally and regionally.

As a consequence of these policies, Italy has fewer psychiatric beds than other countries – 1.72 per 10 000 people in 2001. While Italy has a comparable number of psychiatrists per head of population to the United Kingdom, it has one third the psychiatric nurses and psychologists, and one tenth of the social workers. Italy also has lower rates of compulsory admissions (2.5 per 10 000 people in 2001, compared with 5.5 per 10 000 in England) (131), and lower use of psychotropic drugs than other European countries. "Revolving door" readmissions are evident only in regions with poor resources.

Yet Italian mental health care is far from perfect (130). In place of public sector mental hospitals, the government operates small, protected communities or apartments for long-term patients, and private facilities provide long-term care in some regions. But support for mental health varies significantly by region, and the burden of care still falls on families in some areas. Community mental health and rehabilitation services have in some areas failed to innovate, and optimal treatments are not always available. Italy is preparing a new national strategy to reinforce the community care system, face emerging priorities, and standardize regional mental health care performance.

Italy's experience shows that closing psychiatric institutions must be accompanied by alternative structures. Reform laws should provide minimum standards, not just guidelines. Political commitment is necessary, as well as investment in buildings, staff, and training. Research and evaluation is vital, together with central mechanisms for verification, control, and comparison of services.

- support for the transition from expatriate professional services to local management.

Developing funding mechanisms for rehabilitation

The cost of rehabilitation can be a barrier for people with disabilities in high-income as well as low-income countries. Even where funding from governments, insurers, or NGOs is available, it may not cover enough of the costs to make rehabilitation affordable (117). People with disabilities have lower incomes and are often unemployed, so are less likely to be covered by employer-sponsored health plans or private voluntary health insurance (see Chapter 8). If they have limited finances and inadequate public health coverage, access to rehabilitation may also be limited, compromising activity and participation in society (138).

Lack of financial resources for assistive technologies is a significant barrier for many (101). People with disabilities and their families purchase more than half of all assistive devices directly (139). In a national survey in India, two thirds of the assistive technology users reported having paid for their devices themselves (*112*). In Haiti, poor access to prosthetic services was attributed partially to users being unable to pay (*117*).

Spending on rehabilitation services is difficult to determine because it generally is not disaggregated from other health care expenditure. Limited information is available on expenditure for the full range of rehabilitation measures (*68, 74, 138*). Governments in 41 of 114 countries did not provide funding for assistive devices in 2005 (*110*). Even in the 79 countries where insurance schemes fully or partially covered assistive devices, 16 did not cover poor people with disabilities, and 28 did not cover all geographical locations (*110*). In some cases existing programmes did not cover maintenance and repairs for assistive devices, which can leave individuals with defective equipment and limit its use (*76, 112, 140*). One third of the 114 countries providing data to the 2005 global study did not allocate specific budgets for rehabilitation services (*110*). OECD countries appear to be investing more in rehabilitation than in the past, but the spending is still low (*120*). For example, unweighted averages for all OECD countries between 2006 and 2008 indicate that public spending on rehabilitation as part of labour market programmes was 0.02% of GDP with no increase over time (*127*).

Health care funding often provides selective coverage for rehabilitation services – for example, by restricting the number or type of assistive devices, the number of therapy visits over a specific time, or the maximum cost (*77*) – in order to control cost. While cost controls are needed, they should be balanced with the need to provide services to those who can benefit. In the United States, government and private insurance plans limit coverage of assistive technologies and may not replace ageing devices until they are broken, sometimes requiring a substantial waiting period (*77*). A study of assistive device use by people with rheumatic disease in Germany and the Netherlands found significant differences between the two countries, thought to result from differences in country-related health care systems with respect to prescription and reimbursement rules (*141*).

Policy actions require a budget matching the scope and priorities of the plan. The budget for rehabilitation services should be part of the regular budgets of relevant ministries – notably health – and should consider ongoing needs. Ideally, the budget line for rehabilitation services would be separated to identify and monitor spending.

Many countries – particularly low-income and middle-income countries – struggle to finance rehabilitation, but rehabilitation is a good investment because it builds human capital (*36, 142*). Financing strategies can improve the provision, access, and coverage of rehabilitation services, particularly in low-income and middle-income countries. Any new strategy should be carefully evaluated for its applicability and cost–effectiveness before being implemented. Financing strategies may include the following:

- **Reallocate or redistribute resources**. Public rehabilitation services should be reviewed and evaluated, with resources reallocated effectively. Possible modifications include:
  - changing from hospital or clinic-based rehabilitation to community-based interventions (*74, 83*);
  - reorganizing and integrating services to make them more efficient (*26, 74, 143*);
  - relocating equipment to where it is most needed (*144*).
- **Cooperate internationally**. Developed countries, through their development aid, could provide long-term technical and financial assistance to developing countries to strengthen rehabilitation services, including rehabilitation personnel development. Aid agencies from Australia, Germany, Italy, Japan, New Zealand, Norway, Sweden, the United Kingdom, and the United States have supported such activities (*145–147*).

- **Include rehabilitation services in foreign aid for humanitarian crises**. Conflict and natural disaster cause injuries and disabilities and make people with existing disabilities even more vulnerable – for example, after an earthquake there are increased difficulties in moving around due to the rubble from collapsed buildings and the loss of mobility devices. Foreign aid should also include trauma care and rehabilitation services (*135, 142, 148*).
- **Combine public and private financing**. Clear demarcation of responsibilities and good coordination among sectors is needed for this strategy to be effective. Some services could be publicly funded but privately provided – as in Australia, Cambodia, Canada, and India.
- **Target poor people with disabilities**. The essential elements of rehabilitation need to be identified, publicly funded, and made available for free to people with low incomes, as in South Africa (*149*) and India (*8*).
- **Evaluate coverage of health insurance, including criteria for equitable access**. A study in the United States on access to physical therapy found that health care funding sources provided different coverage for physical therapy services depending on whether people had cerebral palsy, multiple sclerosis, or spinal cord injury (*74*).

Increasing human resources for rehabilitation

Global information about the rehabilitation workforce is inadequate. In many countries national planning and review of human resources for health do not refer to rehabilitation (*135*). Many lack the technical capacity to accurately monitor their rehabilitation workforce, so data are often unreliable and out-of-date. Furthermore, the terms to describe the workers vary, proven analytical tools are absent, and skills and experience for assessing crucial policy issues are lacking (*150, 151*).

Many countries, developing and developed, report inadequate, unstable, or nonexistent supplies, (*83, 152, 153*) and unequal geographic distribution of, rehabilitation professionals (*82, 140*). Developed countries such as Australia, Canada, and the United States report shortages of rehabilitation personnel in rural and remote areas (*154–156*).

The low quality and productivity of the rehabilitation workforce in low-income countries are disconcerting. The training for rehabilitation and other health personnel in developing countries, can be more complex than in developed countries. Training needs to consider the absence of other practitioners for consultation and advice and the lack of medical services, surgical treatment, and follow-up care through primary health care facilities. Rehabilitation personnel working in low-resource settings require extensive knowledge on pathology, and good diagnostic, problem-solving, clinical decision-making, and communication skills (*136*).

Physiotherapy services are the ones most often available, often in small hospitals (*144*). A recent comprehensive survey of rehabilitation in Ghana identified no rehabilitation doctor or occupational therapist in the country, and only a few prosthetists, orthotists, and physical therapists, resulting in very limited access to therapy and assistive technologies (*68*). Services such as speech pathology are nearly absent in many countries (*144*). In India people with speech impairments were much less likely to receive assistive devices than people with visual impairments (*112*).

An extensive survey of rehabilitation doctors in sub-Saharan Africa identified only six, all in South Africa, for more than 780 million people, while Europe has more than 10 000 and the United States more than 7000 (*142*). Discrepancies are also large for other rehabilitation professions: 0.04–0.6 psychologists per 100 000 population in low-income and lower middle-income countries, compared with 1.8 in upper middle-income countries and 14 in high-income countries; and 0.04 social workers per 100 000 population in low-income countries compared with 15.7 in high-income countries (*157*). Data from official statistical sources showing the large disparities in supply of physiotherapists are shown in Fig. 4.1, and data from a survey by the World Federation of Occupational Therapists showing the disparities in occupational therapists are shown in Fig. 4.2.

The lack of women in rehabilitation professions, and the cultural attitudes towards gender, affect rehabilitation services in some contexts. The low number of women technicians in India, for example, may partly explain why women with disabilities were less likely than men to receive assistive devices (*112*). Female patients in Afghanistan can be treated only by female therapists, and men only by men. Restrictions on travel for women

Fig. 4.1.   Physiotherapists per 10 000 population in selected countries

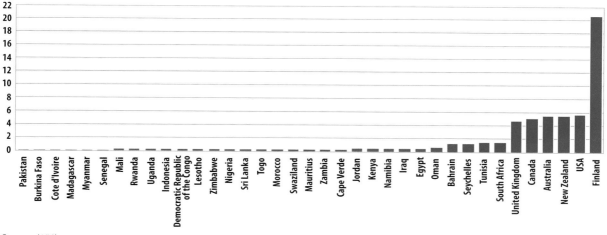

Source (*158*).

Fig. 4.2.   Occupational therapists per 10 000 population in selected countries

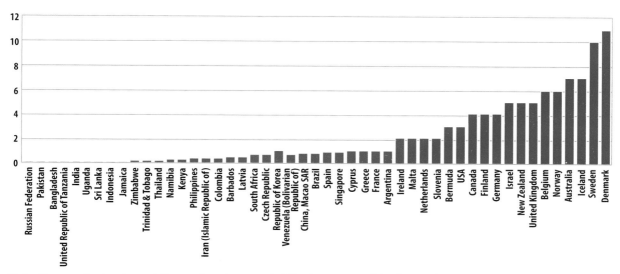

Note: Many professional associations collect data on rehabilitation personnel. Professionals are not obliged, however, to be members or to respond to the survey questionnaires. This data was collated from 65 member organizations with a 93% response rate.
Source (*159*).

prevent female physiotherapists from participating in professional development and training workshops and limit their ability to make home visits (*160*).

Expanding education and training

Many developing countries do not have educational programmes for rehabilitation professionals. According to the 2005 global survey of 114 countries, 37 had not taken action to train rehabilitation personnel and 56 had not updated medical knowledge of health-care providers on disability (*110*).

Differences across countries in the type of training and the competency standards required influence the quality of services (*92, 136, 161*). University training for rehabilitation personnel may not be feasible in all developing countries because of the academic expertise required, the time and expense, and the ability of national governments and NGOs to sustain the training (*162–165*). Long-term funding commitment from Governments and donors is required (*136, 166*).

Education for rehabilitation personnel – commonly institutional and urban-based – is not always relevant to the needs of the population, especially in rural communities (*167*). In Afghanistan one study found that physical therapists with two years of training had difficulty with clinical reasoning and that clinical competencies varied, especially for managing complex disabilities and identifying their own training needs (*168*).

Given the global lack of rehabilitation professionals, mixed or graded levels of training may be required to increase the provision of essential rehabilitation services. Where graded training is used, consideration should be given to career development and continuing education opportunities between levels.

University professional education – advocated by developed countries and professional associations – builds discipline-specific qualifications in physical and occupational therapy, prosthetics and orthotics, and speech and language, among others (*162–165*). Professional associations support minimum standards for training (*162–164, 169*). The complexity of working in resource-poor contexts suggests the importance of either university or strong technical diploma education (*136*). The feasibility of establishing and sustaining tertiary training needs is determined by several factors including political stability, availability of trained educators, availability of financial support, educational standards within the country, and the cost and time for training.

Low- and middle-income countries such as China, India, Lebanon, Myanmar, Thailand, Viet Nam, and Zimbabwe have responded to the lack of professional resources by establishing mid-level training programmes (*92, 170*). Rehabilitation training times have been shortened after wars and conflicts when the number of people with impairments has increased sharply – for example, in the United States after World War I, and in Cambodia after its civil war (*126, 136, 171*). Mid-level therapists are also relevant in developed countries: a collaborative project in north-eastern England compensated for difficulties in recruiting qualified professionals by training rehabilitation assistants to work alongside rehabilitation therapists (*152*).

Mid-level workers, therapists and technicians can be trained as multipurpose rehabilitation workers with basic training in a range of disciplines (occupational therapy, physical therapy, speech therapy, for example), or as profession-specific assistants that provide rehabilitation services under supervision (*152, 170*). Prosthetics and orthotics courses meet the WHO/ISPO standards in several developing countries including Afghanistan, Cambodia, Ethiopia, El Salvador, India, Indonesia, United Republic of Tanzania, Thailand, Togo, Sri Lanka, Pakistan, Sudan, and Viet Nam (see Box 4.5) (*92, 172*). A positive side-effect of mid-level training is that trained professionals are limited in their ability to emigrate to developed countries

Box 4.5. Education in prosthetics and orthotics through the University Don Bosco

In 1996 the University Don Bosco in San Salvador, El Salvador, started the first formal training programme for prosthetics and orthotics in Central America, with support from the German Technical Cooperation organization.

The University Don Bosco, now the leading institution for prosthetics and orthotics education in Latin America, has graduated about 230 prosthetists and orthotists from 20 countries. Programmes continued to expand even after external funding ended. The university now employs nine full-time prosthetics and orthotics teachers, and cooperates with the International Society for Prosthetics and Orthotics and other international organizations such as the World Health Organization (WHO), other universities, and private companies.

Several approaches were instrumental in the success of this training initiative:

- **Strong partnership**. An established education institution with strong pedagogical expertise, University Don Bosco was identified to assume overall responsibility for the training. The German Technical Cooperation agency, experienced in developing prosthetics and orthotics training programmes in Asia and Africa, provided the technical and financial support.
- **Long-term vision for sustainable training provision**. A six-month orientation phase enabled the different partners to agree on details of project implementation, including objectives, activities, indicators, responsibilities, and resources. A 7–10 year strategy enabled the programme to become self-sustaining.
- **Internationally recognized guidelines**. All University Don Bosco training programmes have been developed with support from the International Society for Prosthetics and Orthotics, accredited based on the international guidelines for training developed by the Society and by WHO.
- **Capacity building**. Technical content was developed and delivered by two advisors from the German Technical Cooperation for the initial three-year training programme (ISPO/WHO Category II). From the first intake of 25 students, two outstanding graduates were selected for postgraduate studies in Germany. Following their return in 2000, responsibilities were gradually transferred from the advisors to the graduates. In 2000 the programme expanded to accept up to 25 students from all over Latin America, and in 2002 additional support from WHO helped establish a distance-learning programme for prosthetist and orthotist personnel with a minimum of five years of experience. The distance-learning programme, available in Spanish, Portuguese, English, and French, is now also offered in Angola and Bosnia and Herzegovina. In 2006 a five-year degree programme in prosthetics and orthotics (ISPO /WHO Category I) was started.
- **Ensuring recruitment**. Prosthetic and orthotic technicians and engineers were integrated into the general health system in El Salvador, and support was provided to other countries to establish similar programmes.
- **Choosing appropriate technologies**. Identifying and developing appropriate technologies ensured sustainable provision.

(*136*). Mid-level training is also less expensive, and although insufficient by itself, it may be an option for extending services in the absence of full professional training (*136*).

Community-based workers – a third level of training – shows promise in addressing geographical access (*173*, *174*). They can work across traditional health and social services boundaries to provide basic rehabilitation in the community while referring patients to more specialized services as needed (*152*, *175*). CBR workers generally have minimal training, and rely on established medical and rehabilitation services for specialist treatment and referral.

Providing opportunities for people with disabilities to train as rehabilitation personnel would broaden the pool of qualified people and could benefit patients through improved empathy, understanding, and communication (*176*).

Training existing health-care personnel in rehabilitation

The duration of specialist training for doctors in Physical and Rehabilitation Medicine varies across the world: three years in China (Chinese Standards), at least four years in Europe (*37*), and five years in the United States (*177*). Some countries have used shorter courses to meet the urgent need for rehabilitation doctors: in China, for example, a one-year certificate course in applied rehabilitation, run between 1990 and 1997, was developed at Tongji Medical University, Wuhan, graduating 315 doctors now working across 30 provinces (Nan, personal communication 2010).

Primary health-care workers can benefit from broad rehabilitation training (using the biopsychosocial framework proposed by the ICF) (*178*). In the absence of rehabilitation specialists, health staff with appropriate training can help meet service shortages or supplement services. For example, nurses and health-care assistants can follow up on therapy services (*179*). Training programmes for health-care professionals should be user-driven, need-based, and relevant to the roles of the professionals (*180*).

Building training capacity

Academic institutions and universities in developed countries and international NGOs – with support from international donors and in partnership with governments or a local NGO – can build training capacity by helping train educators and supporting the upgrade of training courses in developing countries (*136, 142, 181*). The Cambodian School of Prosthetics and Orthotics, with La Trobe University in Australia, recently upgraded a programme from Category II (orthopaedic technologist) to a bachelor's degree in Prosthetics and Orthotics using distance education (*182*). This approach has enabled students to remain in their home country, and is more cost-effective than full-time study in Australia (*182*).

Where training capacity does not exist in one country, regional training centres may provide a transitional solution (see Box 4.5). Mobility India trains rehabilitation therapy assistants, and provides specific training in prosthetics and orthotics, to students from India, Bangladesh, Nepal, and Sri Lanka. But this approach generates only a limited number of graduates, and travel and subsistence increase costs – so it cannot meet the vast personnel needs of other developing countries.

Curricula content

Training for rehabilitation personnel should include an overview of relevant national and international legislation, including the CRPD, that promotes client-centred approaches and shared decision-making between people with disabilities and professionals (*167*).

The ICF can create a common understanding among health-care staff, and facilitate communication, the use of assessment tools, and standardized outcome measures to better manage rehabilitation interventions (*17, 178*).

Tertiary and mid-level education can be made more relevant to the needs of people in rural communities by including content on community needs, using appropriate technologies, and using progressive education methods including active learning and problem-based orientation (*167, 175, 183, 184*). Including content on the social, political, cultural, and economic factors that affect the health and quality of life of persons with disabilities can make the curriculum more relevant to the context in which rehabilitation personnel will work (*167, 185–187*). Studies have also shown that interdisciplinary team training develops collaboration, reduces staff burnout, improves rehabilitation implementation, and increases client participation and satisfaction (*188*).

Recruiting and retaining rehabilitation personnel

Mechanisms to ensure employment for rehabilitation graduates are vital to the future of graduates and the sustainability of training. The WHO code of practice on the recruitment of health-care workers (*189*) reflects a commitment to strengthen health systems globally, and to address the unequal distribution of health-care workers both within countries and throughout the world, particularly in sub-Saharan Africa and developing countries. The code stresses the need for awareness of local health care needs in low-income countries, and for promotion of worker exchanges and training between countries.

Several countries have training programmes that target potential rehabilitation and health students from the local community, especially in rural or remote areas (*190*). In Nepal the Institute of Medicine accepts local, mid-level health workers with a minimum of three years' experience for medical training. The rationale is that locally recruited and trained personnel may be better equipped and prepared for living in the local community (*183*). Thailand has used this strategy for rural recruitment and training, adapting it so that workers are assigned public sector positions in their home towns (*190*).

Even where training programmes exist, staff are often difficult to retain, particularly in rural and remote areas. Despite a huge need for rehabilitation services in both urban and rural Cambodia, for example, hospitals cannot afford to hire rehabilitation professionals (*136*). Like other health staff, retaining rehabilitation professionals is affected by poor working conditions, safety concerns, poor management, conflict, inadequate training, and lack of career development and continuing education opportunities (*68, 175, 190–192*).

International demand for skills also influence where rehabilitation workers seek work (*190, 193*). Health-care workers often relocate from low-income countries to high-income countries, in search of better living standards, political stability, and professional opportunities (*82, 144, 194, 195*). While most attention has been given to medical and nursing professionals, a wave of physical therapists have also emigrated from developing countries such as Brazil, Egypt, India, Nigeria, and the Philippines (*196, 197*).

Long-term retention of personnel, using various incentives and mechanisms, is fundamental to continuing services (see Table 4.2).

Table 4.2. Incentives and mechanisms for retaining personnel

Mechanisms	Examples
Financial rewards	Financial bonuses for working in areas of need, or incentives such as subsidized housing, contributions to school fees, housing loans, and the provision of vehicles. In some countries governments subsidize training costs in return for a guaranteed period of service in rural or remote areas. Approaches should be evaluated and compared with the costs of alternative schemes such as the use of temporaries or overseas recruitment (*190, 191, 194, 198*).
Financial incentives for return to service	Expatriate rehabilitation professionals from developing countries can contribute significantly to the development of the rehabilitation infrastructure in their home countries. Providing financial incentives requires careful long-term evaluation (*198*).
Career development	Opportunities for promotion, recognition of skills and responsibilities, good supervision and support, practical training of resident medical and therapy workers (*68, 181*). Several countries are encouraging international undergraduate and graduate experience, with employers providing support – such as unpaid leave and subsidized travel costs.
Continuing education and professional development	Opportunities to attend in-service training, seminars and conferences, receive online and postgraduate training courses, and benefit from professional associations that promote quality in-service training (*188, 195*).
A good work environment	Improvements to building design, ensuring the safety and comfort of the workplace, and providing adequate equipment and resources for the work. Supportive and efficient management practices, including good management of workloads and the recognition of service (*175, 190, 191, 194*).

Expanding and decentralizing service delivery

Rehabilitation services are often located too far from where a person with a disability lives (*199–201*). Major rehabilitation centres are usually located in urban areas; even basic therapeutic services often are not available in rural areas (*202, 203*). Travelling to secondary or tertiary rehabilitation services can be costly and time-consuming, and public transport is often not adapted for people with mobility difficulties (*77, 174*). In Uganda two studies on clubfoot treatment protocols found a significant association between treatment adherence and the distance patients had to travel to the clinic (*38, 204*).

Some people with disabilities have complex rehabilitation needs requiring intensive or expert management in tertiary care settings (see Box 4.6) (*77, 207, 208*). However the majority of people require fairly low-cost, modest rehabilitation services in primary and secondary health care settings (*119, 207*). Integrating rehabilitation into primary and secondary health care settings can:

- Help coordinate the delivery of rehabilitation services (*126*), and having an interdisciplinary health care team under one roof can provide essential health care at an affordable cost (*209*).
- Improve availability, accessibility, and affordability (*200*) which can overcome barriers to referral, such as inaccessible locations, inadequate services, and the high costs of private rehabilitation (*100, 126, 210*).
- Improve patient experience by ensuring services are available early and that waiting time and travelling time are reduced. Together with patient involvement in service development, this can produce better outcomes, improve compliance with treatment, and increase satisfaction among patients and rehabilitation personnel (*211*).

Referral systems are required between different modes of service delivery (inpatient, outpatient, home-based care) and levels of health service provision (primary, secondary, and tertiary care facilities and community settings) (*100, 136, 212*).

Integration and decentralization are therefore beneficial for people with conditions requiring regular or protracted interventions, and for elderly people (*213*). Evaluation of a primary care-based, low-vision service in Wales, showed that low-vision assessments increased by 51%; waiting time fell from more than six months to less than two months; travel time to the nearest provider was reduced for 80% of people; visual disability scores improved significantly; and 97% of patients said that they found the service helpful (*214*).

Coordinated multidisciplinary rehabilitation

Coordination is required to ensure the continuity of care when more than one provider is involved in rehabilitation (*216*). The aim of coordinated rehabilitation is to improve functional outcomes and reduce costs. Evidence has shown that the provision of coordinated, multidisciplinary rehabilitation services can be effective and efficient (*208*).

Multidisciplinary teams can convey many rehabilitation benefits to patients. For example, multidisciplinary rehabilitation for persons with disabilities associated with obstructive pulmonary disease has been found to reduce the use of health services (*217*). Multidisciplinary therapy services for elderly people showed that patients' ability to engage in activities of daily living improved, and the loss of functioning decreased (*6, 218*). Using a team approach to improve participation in society for young people with physical disabilities has proven cost-effective (*219*).

Community-delivered services

Community-delivered rehabilitation interventions are an important part of the continuum of rehabilitation services, and can help improve efficiency and effectiveness of inpatient rehabilitation services (*220*). A systematic review of the

Box 4.6. Brazil – Simplified rehabilitation programs in a hospital in São Paulo

São Paulo has seen a great increase in the number of people with injury-related disabilities. The Orthopaedic and Traumatology Institute at the Clinical Hospital of the Faculty of Medicine, University of São Paulo – a public referral hospital with 162 beds – receives the most severe cases of traumatic injury. Of the 1400 emergency patients admitted each month, about 50 have significant impairments that need extensive long-term rehabilitation services, including spinal cord injuries, hip fractures in the elderly, limb amputations, and patients with multiple injuries. In the 1980s and 1990s patients with injury-related disability could wait for a year or more before receiving placement at a rehabilitation centre. This delay increased the number of secondary complications – contractures, pressure sores, and infections – which reduced the effectiveness of rehabilitation services when they eventually became available.

In response, the Institute at the hospital created the Simplified Rehabilitation Program initially for people with spinal cord injuries, which was later extended to elderly persons with hip fractures and individuals with severe musculoskeletal injuries. The Program aims to prevent joint deformities and pressure sores, promote mobility and wheelchair transfers, manage bladder and bowel issues, control pain, improve self-care independence, and train caregivers (especially for quadriplegics and elderly patients).

The rehabilitation team also provides advice about assistive devices and home modifications. It comprises a physiatrist, physiotherapist, and rehabilitation nurse for the orientation work with patients and caregivers. In addition, a psychologist, social assistant, and occupational therapist may be involved for persons with multiple or complex impairments, such as those with quadriplegia. The team does not have its own specific unit in the hospital, but cares for patients on the general wards.

The Program is primarily educational and needs no special equipment. It usually starts in the second or third week after injury when the patient has become clinically stable, and continues for the two months that most patients remain in the hospital. Patients return for their first follow-up evaluation 30–60 days after discharge and periodically thereafter as needed. These visits focus on general medical care, prevention of complications, and basic rehabilitative care to maximize function. The Program has had a profound effect on the prevention of secondary complications (see table below).

Complications in patients with traumatic spinal cord injuries: comparative data between 1981–1991 and 1999–2008

Complications	1981–1991 (*n* = 186)	1999–2008 (*n* = 424)	Percentage point reduction
Urinary infection	85%	57%	28
Pressure sore	65%	42%	23
Pain[a]	86%	63%	23
Spasticity	30%	10%	20
Joint deformity	31%	8%	23

[a] Pain is chronic pain that interfered with functional recovery.

Note: Patients in the two time periods were fairly comparable in terms of age (mean 29 years before, 35 years after) and gender (70% male before, 84% male after). Etiology differed between the before and after groups, with 54% of patients in the before group having sustained gunshot wounds, compared with only 19% after. Level of injury in the before group was 65% paraplegic and 35% quadriplegic, while the after group was 59% paraplegic and 41% quadriplegic.

Sources (*205, 206*).

This example suggests that developing countries with limited resources and large numbers of injuries can benefit from basic rehabilitation strategies, to reduce secondary conditions. This requires:

- acute care doctors recognizing patients with disabling injuries, and involving the rehabilitation team in their care as early as possible;
- a small and well trained team in the general hospital;
- basic rehabilitative care directed towards health promotion and prevention of complications, initiated soon after the acute phase of trauma care;
- provision of basic equipment and supplies.

Source (*215*).

Box 4.7. Physical assistance to earthquake victims and rehabilitation service strengthening in Gujarat, India

On 26 January 2001 an earthquake measuring 6.9 on the Richter scale struck Gujarat State, India. An estimated 18 000 people were killed and 130 000 people were injured in the Kutchch District of Gujarat, creating a heavy burden on an already fragmented health care system. The response shows that overall care – particularly rehabilitation services for people with disabilities – can be considerably strengthened affordably and sustainably even in low-income and post-disaster settings.

In the wake of the disaster, a partnership between the state government of Gujarat, Handicap International (an international nongovernment organization) and the Blind People's Association (a local cross-disability NGO) was established to build the capacity of existing services.

Tertiary level

- The project improved equipment and infrastructure for physiotherapy and other aspects of facility-based rehabilitation at the Civil Paraplegic Hospital and in Kutchch.
- It improved discharge planning for people with disabilities admitted to the Civil Paraplegic Hospital Centre through the training of social workers.
- Prior to the earthquake no referral system existed. Referral rates improved for people with disabilities from the Civil Hospital to a new community network of 39 disability and development organizations supporting community-based rehabilitation services.

District, secondary level

- The project improved rehabilitation service delivery by providing technical assistance to the Blind People's Association to establish one secondary-level rehabilitation centre – providing prosthetics and orthotics, and physical therapy (by eight visually impaired physiotherapists) near the new Kutchch District Hospital. Nearly 3000 people received orthopaedic devices, an additional 598 received free assistive devices through the Government assistance scheme, and 208 people were fitted with devices in their homes by physical therapists. The referral centre supported satellite centres for six months after the earthquake.
- Coordination improved between different levels of government health providers, and between government health providers and nongovernmental organizations, with mechanisms for referral, treatment, and follow-up, which helped ensure access and continuity of service. An individual case record system and a directory of all rehabilitation facilities in and around Kutchch were developed and managed by the primary health care centres.

Community level

- The project strengthened primary health care, training 275 health-care workers to identify people with disabilities and provide appropriate interventions and referral. An evaluation eight months after the training showed high knowledge retention, with many workers able to identify children with disabilities under 10 months old.
- It improved the provision of rehabilitation services at a community health centre through the establishment of a physiotherapy programme.
- It included the people with disabilities in development initiatives by training 24 community development workers, in 84 of 128 villages, to identify people with disabilities, deliver basic care and refer.
- It increased the proportion of persons with paraplegia having access to both hospital and community-based rehabilitation services.
- It increased awareness among community and family members, disabled persons, and professionals about disability prevention and disability management, through publishing eight new awareness materials in the local language.

Initial activities in 2001–2002 focused on people with spinal cord injury, and mortality within five years of being discharged from the hospital came down from 60% before the programme to 4% afterwards. As the project became successful, it expanded both geographically and to cover all types of disabilities. It now encompasses the entire state of Gujarat, where disability-related activities have been integrated into all levels of the government-run health care system.

Source Handicap International, internal reports.

effectiveness of community-based interventions to maintain physical function and independence in elderly people found that the interventions reduced the number of falls and admissions to nursing homes and hospitals, and improved physical function (*6*). Community-delivered services also respond to workforce shortages, geographical population dispersion, changing demographics, and technological innovations (*175, 221*). Efforts to provide rehabilitation more flexibly are increasing, including through home-based services and schools (*222*). Rehabilitation services should be provided as close as possible to people's homes and communities (*223, 224*).

In low-resource, capacity-constrained settings, efforts should focus on accelerating the supply of services in communities through CBR (*112, 175*), complemented with referral to secondary services (see Box 4.7) (*175*). Examples of measures in community-based rehabilitation include:

- Identifying people with impairments and facilitating referrals. CBR workers in Bangladesh were trained as "key informants" to identify and refer children with visual impairments to specialist eye camps; referrals by the informants accounted for 64% of all referrals to the eye camps. Children were identified earlier and were more representative of the overall incidence of blindness across the community (*225*). A subsequent review of 11 similar studies that used Participatory Rural Appraisal and informants to identify disabled children concluded that community-based methods were consistently less expensive than other methods, and that children benefited from longer engagement with subsequent community interventions (*226*).
- Delivering simple therapeutic strategies through rehabilitation workers, or taught to individuals with disabilities or a family member. Examples include adopting a better posture to prevent contractures, and training in daily living skills (*227*).

- Providing individual or group-based educational, psychological, and emotional support services for persons with disabilities and their families. A study of a CBR model for people with chronic schizophrenia in rural India found that while the community-based rehabilitation model was more time- and resource-intensive than outpatient services, it was more efficient, better at overcoming economic, cultural, and geographic barriers, better for programme compliance, and appropriate for resource-poor settings (*211*). Another study on CBR in Italy found that people with mental illness experienced improved interpersonal relationships and social inclusion. Very isolated people also benefited from the close relationship developed between the patient and the CBR worker (*228*).
- Involving the community. In Thailand a study in two rural districts building capacity for CBR used group meetings for people with disabilities, their families, and community members to manage rehabilitation problems collaboratively (*167*).

Increasing the use and affordability of technology

Assistive devices

Many people around the world acquire assistive technology on the open market. Access to assistive technology can be improved by improving economies of scale in purchasing and production to reduce cost. Centralized, large-scale collective purchasing, or consortium buying, nationally or regionally, can reduce costs. For example, the General Eye and Low Vision Centre in China, in the Hong Kong Special Administrative Region, has a centralized system that purchases bulk supplies of high-quality but affordable low-vision devices. The centre also undertakes quality control and distributes low-vision devices to more than 70 non-commercial organizations in all regions (*229*).

Mass production can lower costs if the device uses universal design principles, and is marketed widely (see Chapter 6 for further details). Expanding markets beyond regional or national boundaries may generate the volume necessary to achieve economies of scale and to produce assistive devices at competitive prices (*230, 231*).

Manufacturing or assembling products locally, using local materials, can reduce cost and ensure that devices are suitable for the context. Locally-made products may be complex items such as wheelchairs, or simpler items such as seating. Other production options include importing the components and assembling the final product locally. Some governments offer low-interest loans to enterprises producing aids for people with disabilities, while others – Viet Nam, for example – offer tax exemptions and other subsidies to such manufacturers (*232*).

Reducing duty and import taxes can help where countries need to import assistive devices – for instance, because the local market is too small to sustain local production. Viet Nam does not impose import taxes on assistive devices for persons with disabilities (*232*), and Nepal has reduced duties for institutions importing assistive devices (*233*).

Even where free or subsidized schemes for provision of assistive devices are available, unless professionals and people with disabilities are aware of their existence, they will not benefit from them, so information sharing and awareness is vital (*112, 234*).

To ensure that assistive devices are appropriate, suitable and of high quality (*89, 235–237*), the devices need to:

- **Suit the environment**. A large number of wheelchairs in low-income and middle-income countries, donated by the international community without related services, are rejected because they are not appropriate for the user in their environment (*238, 239*).

- **Be suitable for the user**. Poor selection and fit of assistive devices, or lack of training in their use, may cause further problems and secondary conditions. Devices should be selected carefully and fitted properly. Users should be engaged in assessment and selection to minimize abandonment because of a mismatch between need and device.

- **Include adequate follow-up to ensure safe and efficient use**. A study in rural Finland on why prescribed hearing aids remain unused found that follow-up care, including counselling, resulted in increased and more consistent use of the devices. Availability and affordability of local maintenance is also important. Access to batteries affects ongoing hearing-aid use, for instance. Improved hearing-aid battery technologies are needed for resource-poor settings. A project in Botswana discovered that rechargeable batteries using solar power offered a promising option (*240*).

Telerehabilitation

The use of information, communication, and related technologies for rehabilitation is an emerging resource that can enhance the capacity and accessibility of rehabilitation measures by providing interventions remotely (*241–243*).

Telerehabilitation technologies include:
- video and teleconferencing technologies in accessible formats;
- mobile phones;
- remote data-collection equipment and telemonitoring – for example, cardiac monitors.

Technology may be used by people with disabilities, rehabilitation workers, peers, trainers, supervisors, and community workers and families.

Where the Internet is available, e-health (telehealth or telemedicine) and telerehabilitation techniques have enabled people in remote areas to receive expert treatment from specialists located elsewhere. Examples of telerehabilitation include:

- telepsychiatry services (*244*), cardiac rehabilitation (*245–247*), speech and language therapy (*248, 249*), and cognitive rehabilitation for people with traumatic brain injury (*250, 251*);
- remote assessments to provide home modification services to underserved elderly people (*252*);
- training and support of health-care personnel (*210*);
- computerized guidelines to help clinicians use appropriate interventions (*253*);
- consultation between tertiary hospital and community hospitals for problems related to prosthetics, orthotics, and wheelchair prescription (*254*);
- sharing professional expertise between countries, as well as at critical times such as in the aftermath of a disaster (*181*).

Growing evidence on the efficacy and effectiveness of telerehabilitation shows that telerehabilitation leads to similar or better clinical outcomes when compared to conventional interventions (*255*). Further information on resource allocation and costs is needed to support policy and practice (*255*).

Expanding research and evidence-based practice

Some aspects of rehabilitation have benefited from significant research, but others have received little attention. Validated research on specific rehabilitation interventions and programmes for people with disabilities – including medical, therapeutic, assistive, and community-based rehabilitation – is limited (*256–258*). Rehabilitation lacks randomized controlled trials – widely recognized as the most rigorous method of testing interventions efficacy (*259, 260*).

Lack of reliable research hinders the development and implementation of effective rehabilitation policies and programmes. More research on rehabilitation in different contexts is needed, particularly on (*261, 262*):

- the link between rehabilitation needs, receipt of services, health outcomes (functioning and quality of life), and costs;
- access barriers and facilitators for rehabilitation, models of service provision, approaches to human resource development, financing modalities, among others;
- cost–effectiveness and sustainability of rehabilitation measures, including community-based rehabilitation programmes.

Obstacles to strengthening research capacity include insufficient rehabilitation researchers, inadequate infrastructure to train and mentor researchers, and the absence of partnerships between relevant disciplines and organizations representing persons with disabilities.

Research on rehabilitation has several characteristics that differ fundamentally from biomedical research, and which can make the research difficult:

1. There is no common taxonomy of rehabilitation measures (*12, 257*).
2. Rehabilitation outcomes can be difficult to characterize and study (*257*) given the breadth and complexity of measures. Rehabilitation often employs several measures simultaneously, and involves workers from different disciplines. This can often make it difficult to measure changes resulting from interventions, such as the specific outcomes from therapy compared to an assistive device where the two are used concurrently.
3. Few valid outcome measures for activity limitations and participation restrictions can be reliably scored by different health professionals within a multidisciplinary team (*263, 264*).
4. Sample sizes are often too small. The range of disabilities is extremely large, and conditions diverse. Rehabilitation measures are

highly individualized and based on health condition, impairments, and contextual factors, and often the numbers of people within homogeneous groups that can be included in research studies are small. This may preclude the use of controlled trials (*37*).

5. The need to allow for participation of people with disabilities – in decision-making through the process of rehabilitation – requires research designs and methods that may not be considered rigorous under current grading systems.

6. Research-controlled trials, which require blinding and placebo controls, may not be feasible or ethical if services are denied for control groups (*260, 265*).

Information and good practice guidelines

Information to guide good practice is essential for building capacity, strengthening rehabilitation systems, and producing cost-effective services and better outcomes.

Good rehabilitation practice uses research evidence. It is derived not from single studies, but from an interpretation of one or more studies, or systematic reviews of studies (*265–267*), and provides the best available research on techniques, effectiveness, cost–benefits, and consumer perspectives. Rehabilitation professionals can obtain information on good practices through:

- Guidelines that apply research knowledge, usually on a specific health condition, to actual practice for clinicians.
- An independent search for specific interventions.
- Continuing professional education.
- Clinical guidance notes on good practice from employers and health organizations.
- Discipline-specific Internet databases that appraise the research for clinicians. A wide variety of sources, including general bibliographic databases and databases specializing in rehabilitation research, are available on the Internet. Most of these databases

have already evaluated the research for quality, provided ratings of research studies, and summarized the evidence.

Evidence-based practice attempts to apply the most recent, appropriate, and effective rehabilitation interventions drawn from research (*259*). Barriers to the development of guidelines and to the integration of evidence into practice include: lack of professional time and skills, limited access to evidence (including language barriers), difficulty in arriving at a consensus, and adapting existing guidelines to local contexts. These issues are particularly relevant to developing countries (*195, 268*). A study from Botswana, for example, highlights the lack of policy implementation and use of research findings (*269*).

Where evidence is lacking, the expertise of clinicians and consumers could be used to develop consensus-based practice guidance. For instance, a "consensus conference" laid the foundation for WHO guidelines on the provision of manual wheelchairs in less-resourced settings. The guidelines were developed in partnership with the International Society for Prosthetics and Orthotics and the US Agency for International Development (*270*).

New Zealand's pioneering *Autistic Spectrum Disorder Guidelines*, developed in response to gaps in service, provide a good example of the evidence-based approach. The guidelines cover identification and diagnosis of conditions, and discuss access to interventions and services (*271*). A wide range of stakeholders were involved in developing the guidelines, including people with autism, parents of children with autism, medical, educational, and community providers, and researchers from New Zealand and elsewhere, with particular attention to the perspectives and experiences of Māori and Pacific people. As a result of these guidelines, proven programmes have been scaled-up, increasing numbers of people trained in assessment and diagnosis of autism, and increasing numbers of people enquiring about and receiving information on the condition. A range of programmes to help support families of people with disabilities have also been started (*272*). Guidelines developed for one setting may need adaptation for implementation in another setting.

Research, data, and information

Better data are needed on service provision, service outcomes, and the economic benefits of rehabilitation (*273*). Evidence for the effectiveness of interventions and programmes is extremely beneficial to:
- guide policy-makers in developing appropriate services
- allow rehabilitation workers to employ appropriate interventions
- support people with disabilities in decision-making.

Long-term longitudinal studies are needed to ascertain if expenditure for health and health-related services decreases if rehabilitation services are provided. Research is also needed on the effect rehabilitation has on families and communities, for example, the benefits accrued when caregivers return to paid work, when support services or ongoing long-term care costs are reduced, and when persons with disabilities and their families feel less isolated. A broad approach is required as benefits of rehabilitation often accrue to a different government budget line from that funding rehabilitation (*207*).

Relevant strategies for addressing barriers in research include the following:
- Involve end-users in planning and research, including people with disabilities and rehabilitation workers, to increase the probability that the research will be useful (*269, 274*).
- Use the ICF framework to help develop a global common language and assist with global comparisons (*12, 17*).
- Use a range of methodologies. More research such as that by the Cochrane

Collaboration (Rehabilitation and Related Therapies) (*208*) is needed when feasible. Alternative, rigorous research methodologies are indicated, including qualitative research, prospective observational cohort design (*259*), or high-quality, quasi-experimental designs that suit the research questions (*265*), including research studies on CBR (*173*).
- Systematically disseminate results so that: policy across government reflects research findings, clinical practice can be evidence-based, and people with disabilities and their families can influence the use of research (*269*).
- Enhance the clinical and research environment. Providing international learning and research opportunities will often involve linking universities in developing countries with those in high-income and middle-income countries (*68*). Countries in a particular region, such as South-East Asia, can also collaborate on research projects (*275*).

Conclusion and recommendations

The priority is to ensure access to appropriate, timely, affordable, and high-quality rehabilitation interventions, consistent with the CRPD, for all those who need them.

In middle-income and high-income countries with established rehabilitation services, the focus should be on improving efficiency and effectiveness, by expanding the coverage and improving the relevance, quality, and affordability of services.

In lower-income countries the focus should be on introducing and gradually expanding rehabilitation services, prioritizing cost-effective approaches.

A broad range of stakeholders have roles to play:
- Governments should develop, implement, and monitor policies, regulatory

mechanisms, and standards for rehabilitation services, as well as promoting equal access to those services.

- Service providers should provide the highest quality of rehabilitation services.
- Other stakeholders (users, professional organizations etc.) should increase awareness, participate in policy development, and monitor implementation.
- International cooperation can help share good and promising practices and provide technical assistance to countries that are introducing and expanding rehabilitation services.

Policies and regulatory mechanisms

- Assess existing policies, systems, services, and regulatory mechanisms, identifying gaps and priorities to improve provision.
- Develop or revise national rehabilitation plans, in accord with situation analysis, to maximize functioning within the population in a financially sustainable manner.
- Where policies exist, make the necessary changes to ensure consistency with the CRPD.
- Where policies do not exist, develop policies, legislation and regulatory mechanisms coherent with the country context and with the CRPD. Prioritize setting of minimum standards and monitoring.

Financing

Develop funding mechanisms to increase coverage and access to affordable rehabilitation services. Depending on each country's specific circumstances, these could include a mix of:

- Public funding targeted at persons with disabilities, with priority given to essential elements of rehabilitation including assistive devices and people with disability who cannot afford to pay.

- Promoting equitable access to rehabilitation through health insurance.
- Expanding social insurance coverage.
- Public-private partnership for service provision.
- Reallocation and redistribution of existing resources.
- Support through international cooperation including in humanitarian crises.

Human resources

Increase the numbers and capacity of human resources for rehabilitation. Relevant strategies include:

- Where specialist rehabilitation personnel are in short supply, develop standards in training for different types and levels of rehabilitation personnel that can enable career development and continuing education across levels.
- Establish strategies to build training capacity in accord with national rehabilitation plans.
- Identify incentives and mechanisms for retaining personnel especially in rural and remote areas.
- Train non-specialist health professionals (doctors, nurses, primary care workers) on disability and rehabilitation relevant to their roles and responsibilities.

Service delivery

Where there are none, or only limited, services introduce minimum services within existing health and social service provision. Relevant strategies include:

- Developing basic rehabilitation services within the existing health infrastructure.
- Strengthening rehabilitation service provision through community-based rehabilitation.

- Prioritizing early identification and intervention strategies using community workers and health personnel.

Where services exist, expand service coverage and improve service quality. Relevant strategies include:
- Developing models of service provision that encourage multidisciplinary and client-centred approaches.
- Ensuring availability of high quality services in the community.
- Improving efficiency by improved coordination between levels and across sectors.

In all settings, three principles are relevant:
- Include service-users in decision-making.
- Base interventions on sound research evidence.
- Monitor and evaluate outcomes.

Technology

Increase access to assistive technology that is appropriate, sustainable, affordable, and accessible. Relevant strategies include:
- Establishing service provision for assistive devices.

- Training users and following up.
- Promoting local production.
- Reducing duty and import tax.
- Improving economies of scale based on established need.

To further enhance capacity, accessibility and coordination of rehabilitation measures the use of information and communication technologies - telerehabilitation - can be explored.

Research and evidence-based practice

- Increase research and data on needs, type and quality of services provided, and unmet need (disaggregated by sex, age, and associated health condition).
- Improve access to evidence-based guidelines on cost-effective rehabilitation measures.
- Disaggregate expenditure data on rehabilitation services from other health care services.
- Assess the service outcomes and economic benefits of rehabilitation.

References

1. Stucki G, Cieza A, Melvin J. The International Classification of Functioning, Disability and Health (ICF): a unifying model for the conceptual description of the rehabilitation strategy. *Journal of Rehabilitation Medicine: official journal of the UEMS European Board of Physical and Rehabilitation Medicine*, 2007,39:279-285. doi:10.2340/16501977-0041 PMID:17468799
2. *Swedish disability policy: services and care for people with functional impairments: habilitation, rehabilitation, and technical aids* [Article No. 2006–114–24]. Stockholm, Socialstyrelsen, The National Board of Health and Welfare, 2006 (http://www.socialstyrelsen.se/Lists/Artikelkatalog/Attachments/9548/2006-114-24_200611424.pdf, accessed 11 May 2010).
3. Llewellyn G et al. Development and psychometric properties of the Family Life Interview. *Journal of Applied Research in Intellectual Disabilities*, 2010,23:52-62. doi:10.1111/j.1468-3148.2009.00545.x
4. *Learning disabilities and young children: identification and intervention* [Fact sheet]. New York, National Joint Committee on Learning Disabilities, 2006 (http://www.ldonline.org/article/Learning_Disabilities_and_Young_Children%3A_Identification_and_Intervention?theme=print, accessed 2 May 2010).
5. Storbeck C, Pittman P. Early intervention in South Africa: moving beyond hearing screening. *International Journal of Audiology*, 2008,47:Suppl 1S36-S43. doi:10.1080/14992020802294040 PMID:18781512
6. Beswick AD et al. Complex interventions to improve physical function and maintain independent living in elderly people: a systematic review and meta-analysis. *Lancet*, 2008,371:725-735. doi:10.1016/S0140-6736(08)60342-6 PMID:18313501
7. Velema JP, Ebenso B, Fuzikawa PL. Evidence for the effectiveness of rehabilitation-in-the-community programmes. *Leprosy Review*, 2008,79:65-82. PMID:18540238
8. Norris G et al. Addressing Aboriginal mental health issues on the Tiwi Islands. *Australasian Psychiatry: bulletin of Royal Australian and New Zealand College of Psychiatrists*, 2007,15:310-314. doi:10.1080/10398560701441687 PMID:17612884

9. Mola E, De Bonis JA, Giancane R. Integrating patient empowerment as an essential characteristic of the discipline of general practice/family medicine. *The European Journal of General Practice*, 2008,14:89-94. doi:10.1080/13814780802423463 PMID:18821139

10. Steiner WA et al. Use of the ICF model as a clinical problem-solving tool in physical therapy and rehabilitation medicine. *Physical Therapy*, 2002,82:1098-1107. PMID:12405874

11. Bickenbach JE et al. Models of disablement, universalism and the international classification of impairments, disabilities and handicaps. *Social Science & Medicine (1982)*, 1999,48:1173-1187. doi:10.1016/S0277-9536(98)00441-9 PMID:10220018

12. Stucki G, Reinhardt JD, Grimby G. Organizing human functioning and rehabilitation research into distinct scientific fields. Part II: Conceptual descriptions and domains for research. *Journal of Rehabilitative Medicine: official journal of the UEMS European Board of Physical and Rehabilitation Medicine*, 2007,39:299-307. doi:10.2340/16501977-0051 PMID:17468802

13. Rimmer JH. Use of the ICF in identifying factors that impact participation in physical activity/rehabilitation among people with disabilities. *Disability and Rehabilitation*, 2006,28:1087-1095. doi:10.1080/09638280500493860 PMID:16950739

14. *World Health Organization International classification of functioning, disability, and health*. Geneva, World Health Organization, 2001.

15. Stucki G, Ustün TB, Melvin J. Applying the ICF for the acute hospital and early post-acute rehabilitation facilities. *Disability and Rehabilitation*, 2005,27:349-352. doi:10.1080/09638280400013941 PMID:16040535

16. Stucki G et al. Rationale and principles of early rehabilitation care after an acute injury or illness. *Disability and Rehabilitation*, 2005,27:353-359. doi:10.1080/09638280400014105 PMID:16040536

17. Rauch A, Cieza A, Stucki G. How to apply the International Classification of Functioning Disability and health (ICF) for rehabilitation management in clinical practice. *European Journal of Physical Rehabilitation Medicine*, 2008,44:439-442.

18. Forster A et al. Rehabilitation for older people in long-term care. *Cochrane Database of Systematic Reviews (Online)*, 2009,1CD004294- PMID:19160233

19. Khan F et al. Multidisciplinary rehabilitation for adults with multiple sclerosis. *Cochrane Database of Systematic Reviews (Online)*, 2007,2CD006036- PMID:17443610

20. Lacasse Y et al. Pulmonary rehabilitation for chronic obstructive pulmonary disease. *Cochrane Database of Systematic Reviews (Online)*, 2006,4CD003793- PMID:17054186

21. Davies EJ et al. Exercise based rehabilitation for heart failure. *Cochrane Database of Systematic Reviews (Online)*, 2010,4CD003331- PMID:20393935

22. Iyengar KP et al. Targeted early rehabilitation at home after total hip and knee joint replacement: Does it work? *Disability and Rehabilitation*, 2007,29:495-502. doi:10.1080/09638280600841471 PMID:17364804

23. Choi JH et al. Multimodal early rehabilitation and predictors of outcome in survivors of severe traumatic brain injury. *The Journal of Trauma*, 2008,65:1028-1035. doi:10.1097/TA.0b013e31815eba9b PMID:19001970

24. Petruševičienė D, Krisciūnas A. Evaluation of activity and effectiveness of occupational therapy in stroke patients at the early stage of rehabilitation. [Kaunas]*Medicina (Kaunas, Lithuania)*, 2008,44:216-224. PMID:18413989

25. Scivoletto G, Morganti B, Molinari M. Early versus delayed inpatient spinal cord injury rehabilitation: an Italian study. *Archives of Physical Medicine and Rehabilitation*, 2005,86:512-516. doi:10.1016/j.apmr.2004.05.021 PMID:15759237

26. Nielsen PR et al. Costs and quality of life for prehabilitation and early rehabilitation after surgery of the lumbar spine. *BMC Health Services Research*, 2008,8:209- doi:10.1186/1472-6963-8-209 PMID:18842157

27. Global Early Intervention Network [website]. (http://www.atsweb.neu.edu/cp/ei/, accessed 11 May 2010).

28. Roberts G et al. Rates of early intervention services in very preterm children with developmental disabilities at age 2 years. *Journal of Paediatrics and Child Health*, 2008,44:276-280. doi:10.1111/j.1440-1754.2007.01251.x PMID:17999667

29. Clini EM et al. Effects of early inpatient rehabilitation after acute exacerbation of COPD. *Respiratory Medicine*, 2009,103:1526-1531. doi:10.1016/j.rmed.2009.04.011 PMID:19447015

30. Rahman A et al. Cluster randomized trial of a parent-based intervention to support early development of children in a low-income country. *Child: Care, Health and Development*, 2009,35:56-62. doi:10.1111/j.1365-2214.2008.00897.x PMID:18991970

31. Hadders-Algra M. General movements: a window for early identification of children at high risk for developmental disorders. *The Journal of Pediatrics*, 2004,145:Supp112-18. doi:10.1016/j.jpeds.2004.05.017 PMID:15238899

32. Overview of Early Intervention. Washington, National Dissemination Center for Children with Disabilities, 2009 (http://www.nichcy.org/babies/overview/Pages/default.aspx, accessed 2 May 2010).

33. Finch E et al. *Physical rehabilitation outcome measures: a guide to enhanced clinical decision-making*, 2nd editon. Hamilton, Ontario, Canadian Physiotherapy Association, 2002.

34. Scherer MJ. Assessing the benefits of using assistive technologies and other supports for thinking, remembering and learning. *Disability and Rehabilitation*, 2005,27:731-739. doi:10.1080/09638280400014816 PMID:16096225

35. Scherer MJ et al. Predictors of assistive technology use: the importance of personal and psychosocial factors. *Disability and Rehabilitation*, 2005,27:1321-1331. doi:10.1080/09638280500164800 PMID:16298935

36. Turner-Stokes L et al. *Evidence-based guidelines for clinical management of traumatic brain injury: British national guidelines*. London, British Society of Rehabilitation Medicine Publications Unit, Royal College of Physicians, 2005.

37. Gutenbrunner C, Ward AB, Chamberlain MA. White book on Physical and Rehabilitation Medicine in Europe. *Journal of Rehabilitation Medicine: official journal of the UEMS European Board of Physical and Rehabilitation Medicine*, 2007,45:Suppl6-47. PMID:17206318

38. Pirani S et al. Towards effective Ponseti clubfoot care: the Uganda sustainable clubfoot care project. *Clinical Orthopaedics and Related Research*, 2009,467:1154-1163. doi:10.1007/s11999-009-0759-0 PMID:19308648

39. Tindall AJ et al. Results of manipulation of idiopathic clubfoot deformity in Malawi by orthopaedic clinical officers using the Ponseti method: a realistic alternative for the developing world? *Journal of Pediatric Orthopedics*, 2005,25:627-629. doi:10.1097/01.bpo.0000164876.97949.6b PMID:16199944

40. Wallen M, Gillies D. Intra-articular steroids and splints/rest for children with juvenile idiopathic arthritis and adults with rheumatoid arthritis. *Cochrane Database of Systematic Reviews (Online)*, 2006,1CD002824- PMID:16437446

41. Shah N, Lewis M. Shoulder adhesive capsulitis: systematic review of randomised trials using multiple corticosteroid injections. *The British Journal of General Practice: the journal of the Royal College of General Practitioners*, 2007,57:662-667. PMID:17688763

42. Bellamy N et al. Intraarticular corticosteroid for treatment of osteoarthritis of the knee. *Cochrane Database of Systematic Reviews (Online)*, 2006,2CD005328- PMID:16625636

43. Lambert RG et al. Steroid injection for osteoarthritis of the hip: a randomized, double-blind, placebo-controlled trial. *Arthritis and Rheumatism*, 2007,56:2278-2287. doi:10.1002/art.22739 PMID:17599747

44. Manheimer E et al. Meta-analysis: acupuncture for osteoarthritis of the knee. *Annals of Internal Medicine*, 2007,146:868-877. PMID:17577006

45. Tomassini V et al. Comparison of the effects of acetyl L-carnitine and amantadine for the treatment of fatigue in multiple sclerosis: results of a pilot, randomised, double-blind, crossover trial. *Journal of the Neurological Sciences*, 2004,218:103-108. doi:10.1016/j.jns.2003.11.005 PMID:14759641

46. Kranke P et al. Hyperbaric oxygen therapy for chronic wounds. *Cochrane Database of Systematic Reviews (Online)*, 2004,2CD004123- PMID:15106239

47. Quinn TJ et al. European Stroke Organisation (ESO) Executive CommitteeESO Writing CommitteeEvidence-based stroke rehabilitation: an expanded guidance document from the European Stroke Organisation (ESO) guidelines for management of ischaemic stroke and transient ischaemic attack 2008. *Journal of Rehabilitation Medicine: official journal of the UEMS European Board of Physical and Rehabilitation Medicine*, 2009,41:99-111. doi:10.2340/16501977-0301 PMID:19225703

48. Heywood F. *Money well spent: the effectiveness and value of housing adaptations*. Bristol, The Policy Press, 2001.

49. Fransen M, McConnell S, Bell M. Exercise for osteoarthritis of the hip or knee. *Cochrane Database of Systematic Reviews (Online)*, 2003,3CD004286- PMID:12918008

50. Jolliffe J et al. Exercise-based rehabilitation for coronary heart disease. *Cochrane Database of Systematic Reviews (Online)*, 2009,1CD001800-

51. Rees K et al. Exercise based rehabilitation for heart failure. *Cochrane Database of Systematic Reviews (Online)*, 2004,3CD003331- PMID:15266480

52. Legg L et al. Occupational therapy for patients with problems in personal activities of daily living after stroke: systematic review of randomised trials. *BMJ (Clinical research ed.)*, 2007,335:922- doi:10.1136/bmj.39343.466863.55 PMID:17901469

53. McConachie H et al. Difficulties for mothers in using an early intervention service for children with cerebral palsy in Bangladesh. *Child: Care, Health and Development*, 2001,27:1-12. doi:10.1046/j.1365-2214.2001.00207.x PMID:11136337

54. Heiman JR. Psychologic treatments for female sexual dysfunction: are they effective and do we need them? *Archives of Sexual Behavior*, 2002,31:445-450. doi:10.1023/A:1019848310142 PMID:12238613

55. Alexander MS, Alexander CJ. Recommendations for discussing sexuality after spinal cord injury/dysfunction in children, adolescents, and adults. *The Journal of Spinal Cord Medicine*, 2007,30:Suppl 1S65-S70. PMID:17874689

56. Sipski ML et al. Effects of vibratory stimulation on sexual response in women with spinal cord injury. *Journal of Rehabilitation Research and Development*, 2005,42:609-616. doi:10.1682/JRRD.2005.01.0030 PMID:16586186

57. Waddell G, Burton AK, Kendall NAS. *Vocational rehabilitation: what works, for whom and when?* London, The Stationery Office, 2008.

58. *Employment assistance for people with mental illness. Literature review.* Commonwealth of Australia, 2008 (http://workplace.gov.au/NR/rdonlyres/39A1C4CE-0DE3-4049-A410-8B61D5509C#(/0/MentalHealthEmplomentAssistanceLiteratureReview_web.doc, accessed 7 November 2008).

59. Assistive Technology Act. United States Congress 2004 (Public Law 108–364) (http://www.ataporg.org/atap/atact_law.pdf, accessed 12 December 2010)

60. Hunt PC et al. Demographic and socioeconomic factors associated with disparity in wheelchair customizability among people with traumatic spinal cord injury. *Archives of Physical Medicine and Rehabilitation*, 2004,85:1859-1864. doi:10.1016/j.apmr.2004.07.347 PMID:15520982

61. Evans JJ et al. Who makes good use of memory aids? Results of a survey of people with acquired brain injury. *Journal of the International Neuropsychological Society: JINS*, 2003,9:925-935. doi:10.1017/S1355617703960127 PMID:14632251

62. Olusanya BO. Classification of childhood hearing impairment: implications for rehabilitation in developing countries. *Disability and Rehabilitation*, 2004,26:1221-1228. doi:10.1080/09638280410001724852 PMID:15371023

63. Persson J et al. *Costs and effects of prescribing walkers.* Sweden, Center for Technology Assessment, 2007 (CMT rapport 2007:3).

64. Spillman BC. Changes in elderly disability rates and the implications for health care utilization and cost. *The Milbank Quarterly*, 2004,82:157-194. doi:10.1111/j.0887-378X.2004.00305.x PMID:15016247

65. Agree EM, Freedman VA. A comparison of assistive technology and personal care in alleviating disability and unmet need. *The Gerontologist*, 2003,43:335-344. PMID:12810897

66. Basavaraj V. Hearing aid provision in developing countries: an Indian case study. In: McPherson B, Brouillette R, eds. *Audiology in developing countries.* Boston, MA, Nova Science Publishers, 2008a.

67. Haig AJ. Developing world rehabilitation strategy II: flex the muscles, train the brain, and adapt to the impairment. *Disability and Rehabilitation*, 2007,29:977-979. doi:10.1080/09638280701480369 PMID:17577733

68. Tinney MJ et al. Medical rehabilitation in Ghana. *Disability and Rehabilitation*, 2007,29:921-927. doi:10.1080/09638280701240482 PMID:17577726

69. Buntin MB. Access to postacute rehabilitation. *Archives of Physical Medicine and Rehabilitation*, 2007,88:1488-1493. doi:10.1016/j.apmr.2007.07.023 PMID:17964894

70. Ottenbacher KJ, Graham JE. The state-of-the-science: access to postacute care rehabilitation services. A review. *Archives of Physical Medicine and Rehabilitation*, 2007,88:1513-1521. doi:10.1016/j.apmr.2007.06.761 PMID:17964898

71. Kephart G, Asada Y. Need-based resource allocation: different need indicators, different results? *BMC Health Services Research*, 2009,9:122- doi:10.1186/1472-6963-9-122 PMID:19622159

72. K Graham S, Cameron ID. A survey of rehabilitation services in Australia. *Australian Health Review: a publication of the Australian Hospital Association*, 2008,32:392-399. doi:10.1071/AH080392 PMID:18666866

73. Darrah J, Magil-Evans J, Adkins R. How well are we doing? Families of adolescents or young adults with cerebral palsy share their perceptions of service delivery. *Disability and Rehabilitation*, 2002,24:542-549. doi:10.1080/09638280210121359 PMID:12171644

74. Elrod CS, DeJong G. Determinants of utilization of physical rehabilitation services for persons with chronic and disabling conditions: an exploratory study. *Archives of Physical Medicine and Rehabilitation*, 2008,89:114-120. doi:10.1016/j.apmr.2007.08.122 PMID:18164340

75. Kroll T, Neri MT. Experiences with care co-ordination among people with cerebral palsy, multiple sclerosis, or spinal cord injury. *Disability and Rehabilitation*, 2003,25:1106-1114. doi:10.1080/0963828031000152002 PMID:12944150

76. Neri MT, Kroll T. Understanding the consequences of access barriers to health care: experiences of adults with disabilities. *Disability and Rehabilitation*, 2003,25:85-96. PMID:12554383

77. Dejong G et al. The organization and financing of health services for persons with disabilities. *The Milbank Quarterly*, 2002,80:261-301. doi:10.1111/1468-0009.t01-1-00004 PMID:12101873

78. Chi MJ et al. Social determinants of emergency utilization associated with patterns of care. *Health Policy (Amsterdam, Netherlands)*, 2009,93:137-142. PMID:19665250

79. Hatano T et al. Unmet needs of patients with Parkinson's disease: interview survey of patients and caregivers. *The Journal of International Medical Research*, 2009,37:717-726. PMID:19589255

80. Fulda KG et al. Unmet mental health care needs for children with special health care needs stratified by socioeconomic status. *Child and Adolescent Mental Health*, 2009,14:190-199. doi:10.1111/j.1475-3588.2008.00521.x

81. The Global Burden of Disease. *2004 Update.* Geneva, World Health Organization, 2008a. (http://www.who.int/healthinfo/global_burden_disease/2004_report_update/en/index.htm, accessed 2 May 2010).

82. Landry MD, Ricketts TC, Verrier MC. The precarious supply of physical therapists across Canada: exploring national trends in health human resources (1991 to 2005). *Human Resources for Health*, 2007,5:23-http://www.human-resources-health.com/content/5/1/23 doi:10.1186/1478-4491-5-23 PMID:17894885

83. Bo W et al. The demand for rehabilitation therapists in Beijing health organizations over the next five years. *Disability and Rehabilitation*, 2008,30:375-380. doi:10.1080/09638280701336496 PMID:17852203

84. Lysack JT et al. Designing appropriate rehabilitation technology: a mobility device for women with ambulatory disabilities in India. *International Journal of Rehabilitation Research. Internationale Zeitschrift fur Rehabilitationsforschung. Revue Internationale de Recherches de Réadaptation*, 1999,22:1-9. PMID:10207746

85. Israsena P, Dubsok P, Pan-Ngum S. A study of low-cost, robust assistive listening system (ALS) based on digital wireless technology. *Disability and Rehabilitation. Assistive Technology*, 2008,3:295-301. doi:10.1080/17483100802323392 PMID:19117189

86. Lamoureux EL et al. The effectiveness of low-vision rehabilitation on participation in daily living and quality of life. *Investigative Ophthalmology & Visual Science*, 2007,48:1476-1482. doi:10.1167/iovs.06-0610 PMID:17389474

87. Durkin M. The epidemiology of developmental disabilities in low-income countries. *Mental Retardation and Developmental Disabilities Research Reviews*, 2002,8:206-211. doi:10.1002/mrdd.10039 PMID:12216065

88. *Deafness and hearing impairment*. Geneva, World Health Organization, 2010 (Fact sheet No. 300) (http://www.who.int/mediacentre/factsheets/fs300/en/print.html, accessed 7 June 2010)

89. McPherson B, Brouillette R. A fair hearing for all: providing appropriate amplification in developing countries. *Communication Disorders Quarterly*, 2004,25:219-223. doi:10.1177/15257401040250040601

90. *Guidelines for hearing aids and services for developing countries*. Geneva, World Health Organization, 2004.

91. Lindstrom A. Appropriate technologies for assistive devices in low-income countries. In: Hsu JD, Michael JW, Fisk JR, eds. *AAOS Atlas of orthoses and assistive devices*. Philadelphia, PA, Mosby/Eslevier, 2008.

92. World Health Organization, International Society for Prosthetics and Orthotics. *Guidelines for training personnel in developing countries for prosthetics and orthotics services*. Geneva, World Health Organization, 2005.

93. Atijosan O et al. The orthopaedic needs of children in Rwanda: results from a national survey and orthopaedic service implications. *Journal of Pediatric Orthopedics*, 2009,29:948-951. PMID:19934715

94. Loeb ME, Eide AH, eds. *Living conditions among people with activity limitations in Malawi: a national representative study*. Oslo, SINFEF, 2004.

95. Eide AH, Yusman K. *Living conditions among people with disabilities in Mozambique: a national representative study*. Oslo, SINTEF, 2009.

96. Eide AH et al. *Living conditions among people with activity limitations in Zimbabwe: a representative regional survey*. Oslo, SINTEF, 2003.

97. Eide AH, Loeb ME, eds. *Living conditions among people with activity limitations in Zambia: a national representative study*. Oslo, SINTEF, 2006.

98. Eide AH, van Rooy G, Loeb ME. *Living conditions among people with activity limitations in Namibia: a representative national survey*. Oslo, SINTEF, 2003.

99. Eide AH, Øderud T. Assistive technology in low income countries. In: Maclachlan M, Swartz L, eds. *Disability and international development*, Dordrecht, the Netherlands, Springer, 2009.

100. Eldar R et al. Rehabilitation medicine in countries of central/eastern Europe. *Disability and Rehabilitation*, 2008,30:134-141. doi:10.1080/09638280701191776 PMID:17852214

101. Zongjie Y, Hong D, Zhongxin X, Hui X. A research study into the requirements of disabled residents for rehabilitation services in Beijing. *Disability and Rehabilitation*, 2007,29:825-833. doi:10.1080/09638280600919657 PMID:17457741

102. Qiu ZY. *Rehabilitation need of people with disability in China: analysis and strategies* [in Chinese]. Beijing, Huaxia Press, 2007.

103. Carlson D, Ehrlich N. Assistive Technology and information technology use and need by persons with disabilities in the United States, 2001. Washington, DC, National Institute on Disability and Rehabilitation Research, U.S. Department of Education, 2005 (http://www.ed.gov/rschstat/research/pubs/at-use/at-use-2001.pdf, accessed 27 April 2007).

104. Chiang PPC. *The Global mapping of low vision services*. Melbourne, University of Melbourne, 2010.

105. Miller AR et al. Waiting for child developmental and rehabilitation services: an overview of issues and needs. *Developmental Medicine and Child Neurology*, 2008,50:815-821. doi:10.1111/j.1469-8749.2008.03113.x PMID:18811706

106. Passalent LA, Landry MD, Cott CA. Wait times for publicly funded outpatient and community physiotherapy and occupational therapy services: implications for the increasing number of persons with chronic conditions in Ontario, Canada. *Physiotherapy Canada. Physiothérapie Canada*, 2009,61:5-14. doi:10.3138/physio.61.1.5 PMID:20145747

107. El Sharkawy G, Newton C, Hartley S. Attitudes and practices of families and health care personnel toward children with epilepsy in Kilifi, Kenya. *Epilepsy & Behavior: E&B*, 2006,8:201-212. doi:10.1016/j.yebeh.2005.09.011 PMID:16275111

108. *Unmet need for disability services: effectiveness of funding and remaining shortfall*. Canberra, Australian Institute of Health and Welfare, 2002.

109. Cott C, Passalent LA, Borsey E. Ontario community rehabilitation: a profile of demand and provision. Toronto, Arthritis Community Research & Evaluation Unit, 2007 (Working Paper 07–1-A) (http://www.acreu.ca/pub/working-paper-07-01.html, accessed 30 April 2010).

110. South-North Centre for Dialogue and Development. *Global survey of government actions on the implementation of the standard rules of the equalisation of opportunities for persons with disabilities*. Amman, Office of the UN Special Rapporteur on Disabilities, 2006:141.

111. Middleton JW et al. Issues and challenges for development of a sustainable service model for people with spinal cord injury living in rural regions. *Archives of Physical Medicine and Rehabilitation*, 2008,89:1941-1947. doi:10.1016/j.apmr.2008.04.011 PMID:18929022

112. *People with disabilities in India: from commitments to outcomes*. Washington, World Bank, 2009. (http://imagebank.worldbank.org/servlet/WDSContentServer/IW3P/IB/2009/09/02/000334955_20090902041543/Rendered/PDF/502090WP0Peopl1Box0342042B01PUBLIC1.pdf, accessed 8 December 2010).

113. *Birth defects: revision of draft resolution considered by the Executive Board at its 125th session reflecting comments and proposals made by Bahamas, Canada, Chile, Mauritius, New Zealand, Oman and Paraguay.* Geneva, World Health Organization, 2009 (EB 126/10 Add. 1) (http://apps.who.int/gb/ebwha/pdf_files/EB126/B126_10Add1-en.pdf, accessed 2 May 2010).

114. de Souza N et al. The determination of compliance with an early intervention programme for high-risk babies in India. *Child: Care, Health and Development*, 2006,32:63-72. doi:10.1111/j.1365-2214.2006.00576.x PMID:16398792

115. Cooper SA et al. Improving the health of people with intellectual disabilities: outcomes of a health screening programme after 1 year. *Journal of Intellectual Disability Research: JIDR*, 2006,50:667-677. doi:10.1111/j.1365-2788.2006.00824.x PMID:16901294

116. World Health Organization, Swedish Organizations of Disabled Persons International Aid Association. *Part 1. Community-Based Rehabilitation as we experienced it ... voices of persons with disabilities.* Geneva, World Health Organization, 2002.

117. Bigelow J et al. A picture of amputees and the prosthetic situation in Haiti. *Disability and Rehabilitation*, 2004,26:246-252. doi:10.1080/09638280310001644915 PMID:15164958

118. Lilja M et al. Disability policy in Sweden: policies concerning assistive technology and home modification services. *Journal of Disability Policies Studies*, 2003,14:130-135. doi:10.1177/10442073030140030101

119. *Disability and rehabilitation status review of disability issues and rehabilitation services in 29 African Countries.* Geneva, World Health Organization, 2004.

120. *Modernizing sickness and disability policy: OECD thematic review on sickness, disability and work issues paper and progress report.* Paris, Organisation for Economic Co-operation and Development, 2008.

121. Digiacomo M et al. Health information system linkage and coordination are critical for increasing access to secondary prevention in Aboriginal health: a qualitative study. *Quality in Primary Care*, 2010,18:17-26. PMID:20359409

122. Hilberink SR et al. Health issues in young adults with cerebral palsy: towards a life-span perspective. *Journal of Rehabilitation Medicine: official journal of the UEMS European Board of Physical and Rehabilitation Medicine*, 2007,39:605-611. doi:10.2340/16501977-0103 PMID:17896051

123. Holdsworth LK, Webster V, McFadyen A. Self-referral to physiotherapy: deprivation and geographical setting – is there a relationship? Results of a national trial. *Physiotherapy*, 2006,92:16-25. doi:10.1016/j.physio.2005.11.003

124. Holdsworth LK, Webster V, McFadyen A. What are the costs to NHS Scotland of self-referral to physiotherapy? Results of a national trial. *Physiotherapy*, 2007,93:3-11. doi:10.1016/j.physio.2006.05.005

125. Holdsworth LK, Webster V, McFadyen A. Physiotherapists' and general practitioners' views of self-referral and physiotherapy scope of practice: results from a national trial. *Physiotherapy*, 2008,94:236-243. doi:10.1016/j.physio.2008.01.006

126. Eldar R. Integrated institution–community rehabilitation in developed countries: a proposal. *Disability and Rehabilitation*, 2000,22:266-274. doi:10.1080/096382800296728 PMID:10864129

127. Sickness, disability and work: keeping on track in the economic downturn. Paris, Organisation for Economic Co-operation and Development, 2009 (Background paper).

128. *Convention on the Rights of Persons with Disabilities.* Geneva, United Nations, 2006 (http://www2.ohchr.org/english/law/disabilities-convention.htm, accessed 16 May 2009).

129. Palermo GB. The 1978 Italian mental health law–a personal evaluation: a review. *Journal of the Royal Society of Medicine*, 1991,84:99-102. PMID:1999825

130. Barbui C, Tansella M. Thirtieth birthday of the Italian psychiatric reform: research for identifying its active ingredients is urgently needed. *Journal of Epidemiology and Community Health*, 2008,62:1021- doi:10.1136/jech.2008.077859 PMID:19008365

131. de Girolamo G et al. Compulsory admissions in Italy: results of a national survey. *International Journal of Mental Health*, 2008,37:46-60. doi:10.2753/IMH0020-7411370404

132. McColl MA, Boyce W. Disability advocacy organizations: a descriptive framework. *Disability and Rehabilitation*, 2003,25:380-392. doi:10.1080/0963828021000058521 PMID:12745947

133. Nunez G. Culture and disabilities. In: Drum CE, Krahn GL, Bersani H. *Disability and Public Health,* Washington, American Public Health Association, 2009:65–78.

134. *The Standard Rules on the Equalization of Opportunities for Persons with Disabilities.* New York, United Nations, 1993 (http://www.un.org/esa/socdev/enable/dissre00.htm, accessed 16 May 2009).

135. *Systems thinking for health systems strengthening. Alliance for Health Policy and Systems Research.* Geneva, World Health Organization, 2009b

136. Dunleavy K. Physical therapy education and provision in Cambodia: a framework for choice of systems for development projects. *Disability and Rehabilitation*, 2007,29:903-920. doi:10.1080/09638280701240433 PMID:17577725

137. *Annual Report 2009.* Phnom Penh, Disability Action Council, 2009. (http://www.dac.org.kh/cambodia_disability_resource_center/download/local-doc/DAC_Annual_Report_2009.pdf, accessed 12 July 2010).

138. Crowley JS, Elias R. *Medicaid's role for people with disabilities.* Washington, DC, Henry Kaiser Foundation, 2003.

139. Albrecht G, Seelman K, Bury M. *Handbook of Disability Studies.* London, Sage, 2003.

140. Sooful P, Van Dijk C, Avenant C. The maintenance and utilisation of government fitted hearing aids. *Central European Journal of Medicine*, 2009,4:110-118. doi:10.2478/s11536-009-0014-9

141. Veehof MM et al. What determines the possession of assistive devices among patients with rheumatic diseases? The influence of the country-related health care system. *Disability and Rehabilitation*, 2006,28:205-211. doi:10.1080/09638280500305064 PMID:16467055

142. Haig AJ et al. The practice of physical and rehabilitation medicine in sub-Saharan Africa and Antarctica: a white paper or a black mark? *Journal of Rehabilitation Medicine: official journal of the UEMS European Board of Physical and Rehabilitation Medicine*, 2009,41:401-405. doi:10.2340/16501977-0367 PMID:19479150

143. Woo J et al. In patient stroke rehabilitation efficiency: influence of organization of service delivery and staff numbers. *BMC Health Services Research*, 2008,8:86- doi:10.1186/1472-6963-8-86 PMID:18416858

144. Mock C et al., eds. *Strengthening care for the injured: Success stories and lessons learned from around the world*. Geneva, World Health Organization, 2010.

145. *Injuries, violence and disabilities biennial report 2008–2009*. Geneva, World Health Organization, 2010.

146. *Injuries, violence and disabilities biennial report 2006–2007*. Geneva, World Health Organization, 2008.

147. *Injuries, violence and disabilities biennial report 2004–2005*. Geneva, World Health Organization, 2006.

148. Massive need for rehabilitation and orthopedic equipment. Takoma Park, MD, Handicap International, 2010 (http://www.reliefweb.int/rw/rwb.nsf/db900SID/VVOS-7ZVSU6?OpenDocument, accessed 2 May 2010).

149. Goudge J et al. Affordability, availability and acceptability barriers to health care for the chronically ill: longitudinal case studies from South Africa. *BMC Health Services Research*, 2009,9:75- doi:10.1186/1472-6963-9-75 PMID:19426533

150. Brouillette R. The rehabilitation of hearing loss: challenges and opportunities in developing countries. In: McPherson B, Brouillette R, eds. *Audiology in developing countries*. Boston, MA, Nova Science Publishers, 2008b.

151. Dal Poz M et al., eds. *Handbook on monitoring and evaluation of human resources for health – with special applications for low- and middle-income countries*. Geneva, World Health Organization, 2009.

152. Stanmore E, Waterman H. Crossing professional and organizational boundaries: the implementation of generic rehabilitation assistants within three organizations in the northwest of England. *Disability and Rehabilitation*, 2007,29:751-759. doi:10.1080/09638280600902836 PMID:17453998

153. Al Mahdy H. Rehabilitation and community services in Iran. *Clinician in Management*, 2002,11:57-60.

154. Wilson RD, Lewis SA, Murray PK. Trends in the rehabilitation therapist workforce in underserved areas: 1980–2000. *The Journal of Rural Health: official journal of the American Rural Health Association and the National Rural Health Care Association*, 2009,25:26-32. doi:10.1111/j.1748-0361.2009.00195.x PMID:19166558

155. O'Toole K, Schoo AM. Retention policies for allied health professionals in rural areas: a survey of private practitioners. *Rural and Remote Health*, 2010,10:1331- PMID:20443649

156. MacDowell M et al. A national view of rural health workforce issues in the USA. *Rural and Remote Health*, 2010,10:1531- PMID:20658893

157. Saxena S et al. Resources for mental health: scarcity, inequity, and inefficiency. *Lancet*, 2007,370:878-889. doi:10.1016/S0140-6736(07)61239-2 PMID:17804062

158. *Global atlas of the health workforce*. Geneva, World Health Organization, 2008 (http://www.who.int/globalatlas/autologin/hrh_login.asp, accessed 1 June 2009).

159. *Occupational therapy human resources project 2010*. Melbourne, World Federation of Occupational Therapists, 2010.

160. Wickford J, Hultberg J, Rosberg S. Physiotherapy in Afghanistan–needs and challenges for development. *Disability and Rehabilitation*, 2008,30:305-313. doi:10.1080/09638280701257205 PMID:17852310

161. Higgs J, Refshauge K, Ellis E. Portrait of the physiotherapy profession. *Journal of Interprofessional Care*, 2001,15:79-89. doi:10.1080/13561820020022891 PMID:11705073

162. World Confederation for Physical Therapy [website]. (http://www.wcpt.org/, accessed 8 December 2010)

163. World Federation of Occupational Therapists [website]. (http://www.wfot.org/schoolLinks.asp, accessed 8 December 2010).

164. International Association of Logopedics and Phoniatrics [website]. (http://ialp.info/joomla/, accessed 8 December 2010).

165. International Society for Prosthetics and Orthotics [website]. (http://www.ispoint.org/, accessed 8 December 2010).

166. Leavitt R. The development of rehabilitation services and suggestions for public policy in developing nations. *Pediatric Physical Therapy*, 1995,7:112-117. doi:10.1097/00001577-199500730-00005

167. Nualnetre N. Physical therapy roles in community based rehabilitation: a case study in rural areas of north eastern Thailand. *Asia Pacific Disability Rehabilitation Journal*, 2009,20:1-12.

168. Armstrong J, Ager A. Physiotherapy in Afghanistan: an analysis of current challenges. *Disability and Rehabilitation*, 2006,28:315-322. doi:10.1080/09638280500160337 PMID:16492626

169. Smyth J. Occupational therapy training in Uganda: the birth of a profession. *World Federation of Occupational Therapists Bulletin*, 1996,34:26-31.

170. *The education of mid-level rehabilitation workers: Recommendations from country experiences*. Geneva, World Health Organization, 1992.

171. Gwyer J. Personnel resources in physical therapy: an analysis of supply, career patterns, and methods to enhance availability. *Physical Therapy*, 1995,75:56-65, discussion 65–67. PMID:7809199

172. Annual progress report to WHO. Brussels, International Society for Prosthetics and Orthotics, 2010.

173. Hartley S et al. Community-based rehabilitation: opportunity and challenge. *Lancet*, 2009,374:1803-1804. doi:10.1016/S0140-6736(09)62036-5 PMID:19944850

174. Penny N et al. Community-based rehabilitation and orthopaedic surgery for children with motor impairment in an African context. *Disability and Rehabilitation*, 2007,29:839-843. doi:10.1080/09638280701240052 PMID:17577718

175. *Increasing access to health workers in remote and rural areas through improved retention: Global policy recommendations.* Geneva, World Health Organization, 2010.

176. Shakespeare T, Iezzoni LI, Groce NE. Disability and the training of health professionals. *Lancet*, 2009,374:1815-1816. doi:10.1016/S0140-6736(09)62050-X PMID:19957403

177. Certification Booklet of Information 2010–2011 Examinations. Rochester, MN, ABPMR (American Board of Physical Medicine and Rehabilitation), 2010.

178. Reed GM et al. Three model curricula for teaching clinicians to use the ICF. *Disability and Rehabilitation*, 2008,30:927-941. doi:10.1080/09638280701800301 PMID:18484388

179. Atwal A et al. Multidisciplinary perceptions of the role of nurses and healthcare assistants in rehabilitation of older adults in acute health care. *Journal of Clinical Nursing*, 2006,15:1418-1425. doi:10.1111/j.1365-2702.2005.01451.x PMID:17038103

180. Fronek P et al. The effectiveness of a sexuality training program for the interdisciplinary spinal cord injury rehabilitation team. *Sexuality and Disability*, 2005,23:51-63. doi:10.1007/s11195-005-4669-0

181. Lee AC, Norton E. Use of telerehabilitation to address sustainability of international service learning in Mexico: pilot case study and lessons learned. *HPA Resource*, 2009,9:1-5.

182. Kheng S. The challenges of upgrading from ISPO Category II level to Bachelor Degree level by distance education. *Prosthetics and Orthotics International*, 2008,32:299-312. doi:10.1080/03093640802109764 PMID:18720252

183. Matock N, Abeykoon P. Innovative programmes of medical education in south-east Asia. New Delhi, World Health Organization, 1993.

184. *Increasing the relevance of education for health professionals*. Geneva, World Health Organization, 1993.

185. Watson R, Swartz L. *Transformation through occupation*. London, Whurr, 2004.

186. Chipps JA, Simpson B, Brysiewicz P. The effectiveness of cultural-competence training for health professionals in community-based rehabilitation: a systematic review of literature. *Worldviews on Evidence-Based Nursing/Sigma Theta Tau International, Honor Society of Nursing*, 2008,5:85-94. doi:10.1111/j.1741-6787.2008.00117.x PMID:18559021

187. Niemeier JP, Burnett DM, Whitaker DA. Cultural competence in the multidisciplinary rehabilitation setting: are we falling short of meeting needs? *Archives of Physical Medicine and Rehabilitation*, 2003,84:1240-1245. doi:10.1016/S0003-9993(03)00295-8 PMID:12917868

188. Corrigan PW, McCracken SG. Training teams to deliver better psychiatric rehabilitation programs. *Psychiatric Services (Washington, DC)*, 1999,50:43-45. PMID:9890577

189. *International recruitment of health personnel: draft global code of practice* [EB126/8]. Geneva, World Health Organization, 2009c.

190. Lehmann U, Dieleman M, Martineau T. Staffing remote rural areas in middle- and low-income countries: a literature review of attraction and retention. *BMC Health Services Research*, 2008,8:19- doi:10.1186/1472-6963-8-19 PMID:18215313

191. Tran D et al. Identification of recruitment and retention strategies for rehabilitation professionals in Ontario, Canada: results from expert panels. *BMC Health Services Research*, 2008,8:249- doi:10.1186/1472-6963-8-249 PMID:19068134

192. Crouch RB. SHORT REPORT Education and research in Africa: Identifying and meeting the needs. *Occupational Therapy International*, 2001,8:139-144. doi:10.1002/oti.141 PMID:11823878

193. Global Health Workforce Alliance [web site]. (http://www.ghwa.org/?74028ba8, accessed 30 April 2010).

194. Willis-Shattuck M et al. Motivation and retention of health workers in developing countries: a systematic review. *BMC Health Services Research*, 2008,8:247- doi:10.1186/1472-6963-8-247 PMID:19055827

195. Magnusson L, Ramstrand N. Prosthetist/orthotist educational experience & professional development in Pakistan. *Disability and Rehabilitation. Assistive Technology*, 2009,4:385-392. doi:10.3109/17483100903024634 PMID:19817652

196. Oyeyemi A. Nigerian physical therapists' job satisfaction: a Nigeria – USA comparison. *Journal of African Migration*, 2002,1:1-19.

197. Asis M. *Health worker migration: the case of the Philippines*. XVII general meeting of the Pacific Economic Cooperation Council. Sydney, 1–2 May 2007.

198. Bärnighausen T, Bloom DE. Financial incentives for return of service in underserved areas: a systematic review. *BMC Health Services Research*, 2009,9:86- doi:10.1186/1472-6963-9-86 PMID:19480656

199. Shaw A. Rehabilitation services in Papua New Guinea. *Papua and New Guinea Medical Journal*, 2004,47:215-227. PMID:16862945

200. De Angelis C, Bunker S, Schoo A. Exploring the barriers and enablers to attendance at rural cardiac rehabilitation programs. *The Australian Journal of Rural Health*, 2008,16:137-142. doi:10.1111/j.1440-1584.2008.00963.x PMID:18471183

201. Monk J, Wee J. Factors shaping attitudes towards physical disability and availability of rehabilitative support systems for disabled persons in rural Kenya. *Asia Pacific Disability and Rehabilitation Journal*, 2008,19:93-113.

202. *The United Nations Standard Rules on the equalization of opportunities for persons with disabilities: government responses to the implementation of the rules on medical care, rehabilitation, support services and personnel training* [Part 1. Summary]. Geneva, World Health Organization, 2001:20.

203. Siqueira FC et al. [Architectonic barriers for elderly and physically disabled people: an epidemiological study of the physical structure of health service units in seven Brazilian states] *Ciência & Saúde Coletiva*, 2009,14:39-44. PMID:19142307

204. Herman K. Barriers experienced by parents/caregivers of children with clubfoot deformity attending specific clinics in Uganda. Cape Town, Department of Physiotherapy in the Faculty of Community and Health Science, University of the Western Cape, 2006.

205. Greve JMD, Chiovato J, Batisttella LR. *Critical evaluation: 10 years SCI rehabilitation treatment in a developing country 1981–1991, Sao Pâulo, Brazil*. Free paper in the 3rd Annual Scientific Meeting of the International Medical Society of Paraplegia. Kobe, Japan, 30 May–2 June 1994.

206. Souza DR et al. *Characteristics of traumatic spinal cord injuries in a referral center: Institute of Orthopaedics and Traumatology, Clinical Hospital, Faculty of Medicine, University of São Paulo, IOT-HCFMUSP, São Paulo, Brazil*. Free paper in the International Society of Physical and Rehabilitation Medicine World Congress. Instanbul, Turkey, 13–17 June 2009.

207. Turner-Stokes L. Politics, policy and payment–facilitators or barriers to person-centred rehabilitation? *Disability and Rehabilitation*, 2007,29:1575-1582. doi:10.1080/09638280701618851 PMID:17922328

208. Wade DT, de Jong BA. Recent advances in rehabilitation. *BMJ (Clinical research ed.)*, 2000,320:1385-1388. doi:10.1136/bmj.320.7246.1385 PMID:10818031

209. *Declaration of Alma-Ata: International Conference on Primary Health Care, Alma-Ata, USSR, 6–12 September 1978*. Geneva, World Health Organization, 1978 (http://www.who.int/publications/almaata_declaration_en.pdf, accessed 2 May 2010).

210. Wakerman J et al. Primary health care delivery models in rural and remote Australia: a systematic review. *BMC Health Services Research*, 2008,8:276- doi:10.1186/1472-6963-8-276 PMID:19114003

211. Chatterjee S et al. Evaluation of a community-based rehabilitation model for chronic schizophrenia in rural India. *The British Journal of Psychiatry: the journal of mental science*, 2003,182:57-62. doi:10.1192/bjp.182.1.57 PMID:12509319

212. *The World Health Report 2008: Primary health care, now more than ever*. Geneva, World Health Organization, 2008 (http://www.who.int/whr/2008/en/index.html, accessed 11 April 2010).

213. Tyrell J, Burn A. Evaluating primary care occupational therapy: results from a London primary health care centre. *British Journal of Therapy and Rehabilitation*, 1996,3:380-385.

214. Ryan B et al. The newly established primary care based Welsh Low Vision Service is effective and has improved access to low vision services in Wales. *Ophthalmic & Physiological Optics: the journal of the British College of Ophthalmic Opticians (Optometrists)*, 2010,30:358-364. doi:10.1111/j.1475-1313.2010.00729.x PMID:20492541

215. Mock C et al. Evaluation of trauma care capabilities in four countries using the WHO-IATSIC Guidelines for Essential Trauma Care. *World Journal of Surgery*, 2006,30:946-956. doi:10.1007/s00268-005-0768-4 PMID:16736320

216. Boling PA. Care transitions and home health care. *Clinics in Geriatric Medicine*, 2009,25:135-148, viii. doi:10.1016/j.cger.2008.11.005 PMID:19217498

217. Griffiths TL et al. Results at 1 year of outpatient multidisciplinary pulmonary rehabilitation: a randomised controlled trial. *Lancet*, 2000,355:362-368. doi:10.1016/S0140-6736(99)07042-7 PMID:10665556

218. Legg L, Langhorne P. Outpatient Service TrialistsRehabilitation therapy services for stroke patients living at home: systematic review of randomised trials. *Lancet*, 2004,363:352-356. doi:10.1016/S0140-6736(04)15434-2 PMID:15070563

219. Bent N et al. Team approach versus ad hoc health services for young people with physical disabilities: a retrospective cohort study. *Lancet*, 2002,360:1280-1286. doi:10.1016/S0140-6736(02)11316-X PMID:12414202

220. Turner-Stokes L, Paul S, Williams H. Efficiency of specialist rehabilitation in reducing dependency and costs of continuing care for adults with complex acquired brain injuries. *Journal of Neurology, Neurosurgery, and Psychiatry*, 2006,77:634-639. doi:10.1136/jnnp.2005.073411 PMID:16614023

221. Kendall E, Marshall C. Factors that prevent equitable access to rehabilitation for Aboriginal Australians with disabilities: the need for culturally safe rehabilitation. *Rehabilitation Psychology*, 2004,49:5-13. doi:10.1037/0090-5550.49.1.5

222. Ameratunga S et al. Rehabilitation of the injured child. *Bulletin of the World Health Organization*, 2009,87:327-328. doi:10.2471/BLT.09.057067 PMID:19551242

223. Watermeyer BS et al., eds. *Disability and social change: South Africa agenda*. Pretoria, Human Sciences Research Council, 2006.

224. Higgins L, Dey-Ghatak P, Davey G. Mental health nurses' experiences of schizophrenia rehabilitation in China and India: a preliminary study. *International Journal of Mental Health Nursing*, 2007,16:22-27. doi:10.1111/j.1447-0349.2006.00440.x PMID:17229271

225. Muhit MA et al. The key informant method: a novel means of ascertaining blind children in Bangladesh. *The British Journal of Ophthalmology*, 2007,91:995-999. doi:10.1136/bjo.2006.108027 PMID:17431019

226. Gona JK et al. Identification of people with disabilities using participatory rural appraisal and key informants: a pragmatic approach with action potential promoting validity and low cost. *Disability and Rehabilitation*, 2010,32:79-85. doi:10.3109/09638280903023397 PMID:19925280

227. Hartley S, Okune J, eds. *CBR Policy development and implementation*. Norwich, University of East Anglia, 2008.

228. Barbato A et al. Outcome of community-based rehabilitation program for people with mental illness who are considered difficult to treat. *Journal of Rehabilitation Research and Development*, 2007,44:775-783. doi:10.1682/JRRD.2007.02.0041 PMID:18075936

229. General Eye and Low Vision Centre [web site]. (http://www.hksb.org.hk/en/index.php?option=com_content&view=article&id=39&Itemid=33, accessed 11 May 2010).

230. Bauer S, Lane J. Convergence of AT and mainstream products: keys to university participation in research, development and commercialization. *Technology and Disability*, 2006,18:67-78.

231. Lane J.. Delivering the D in R&D: recommendations for increasing transfer outcomes from development projects. *Assistive Technology Outcomes and Benefits*, 2008,(Fall special issue).

232. The Law on Persons with Disabilities. Hanoi, Socialist Republic of Viet Nam, 2010 (51/2010/QH12).

233. Production and distribution of assistive devices for people with disabilities [Part 1 chapter 5 and part 2 chapter 9]. Bangkok, United Nations Economic and Social Commission for Asia and the Pacific, 1997.

234. Field MJ, Jette AM, eds. *The future of disability in America*. Washington, The National Academies Press, 2007.

235. Borg J, Lindström A, Larsson S. Assistive technology in developing countries: national and international responsibilities to implement the Convention on the Rights of Persons with Disabilities. *Lancet*, 2009,374:1863-1865. doi:10.1016/S0140-6736(09)61872-9 PMID:19944867

236. Borg J, Larsson S. The right to assistive technology and its implementation. In: Bhanushali K, ed. *UN convention on rights of persons with disabilities*. Ahmedabad, India, ICFAI University Press, forthcoming.

237. Vuorialho A, Karinen P, Sorri M. Counselling of hearing aid users is highly cost-effective. *European Archives of Oto-Rhino-Laryngology: official journal of the European Federation of Oto-Rhino-Laryngological Societies (EUFOS): affiliated with the German Society for Oto-Rhino-Laryngology - Head and Neck Surgery*, 2006,263:988-995. doi:10.1007/s00405-006-0104-0 PMID:16799805

238. Mukherjee G, Samanta A. Wheelchair charity: a useless benevolence in community-based rehabilitation. *Disability and Rehabilitation*, 2005,27:591-596. doi:10.1080/09638280400018387 PMID:16019868

239. Oderud T et al. User satisfaction survey: an assessment study on wheelchairs in Tanzania. In: Sheldon S, Jacobs NA, eds. *Report of a consensus conference on wheelchairs for developing countries, Bengaluru, India, 6–11 November 2006*. Copenhagen, International Society for Prosthetics and Orthotics, 2007:112–117.

240. Godisa [website]. (http://www.godisa.org/, accessed 17 December 2010).

241. Seelman KD, Hartman LM. Telerehabilitation: policy issues and research tools. *International Journal of Telerehabilitation*, 2009,1:47-58. doi:10.5195/ijt.2009.6013

242. Taylor DM et al. Exploring the feasibility of video conference delivery of a self management program to rural participants with stroke. *Telemedicine and e-Health*, 2009,15:646-654. doi:10.1089/tmj.2008.0165 PMID:19694589

243. Vainoras A et al. Cardiological telemonitoring in rehabilitation and sports medicine. *Studies in Health Technology and Informatics*, 2004,105:121-130. PMID:15718601

244. Rowe N et al. Ten-year experience of a private nonprofit telepsychiatry service. *Telemedicine and e-Health: the official journal of the American Telemedicine Association*, 2008,14:1078-1086. doi:10.1089/tmj.2008.0037 PMID:19119830

245. Körtke H et al. New East-Westfalian Postoperative Therapy Concept: a telemedicine guide for the study of ambulatory rehabilitation of patients after cardiac surgery. *Telemedicine Journal and e-health: the official journal of the American Telemedicine Association*, 2006,12:475-483. doi:10.1089/tmj.2006.12.475 PMID:16942420

246. Giallauria F et al. Efficacy of telecardiology in improving the results of cardiac rehabilitation after acute myocardial infarction. *Monaldi Archives for Chest Disease = Archivio Monaldi per le malattie del torace / Fondazione clinica del lavoro, IRCCS [and] Istituto di clinica tisiologica e malattie apparato respiratorio, Università di Napoli, Secondo ateneo*, 2006,66:8-12. PMID:17125041

247. Ades PA et al. A controlled trial of cardiac rehabilitation in the home setting using electrocardiographic and voice transtelephonic monitoring. *American Heart Journal*, 2000,139:543-548. doi:10.1016/S0002-8703(00)90100-5 PMID:10689271

248. Sicotte C et al. Feasibility and outcome evaluation of a telemedicine application in speech-language pathology. *Journal of Telemedicine and Telecare*, 2003,9:253-258. doi:10.1258/135763303769211256 PMID:14599327

249. Theodoros DG. Telerehabilitation for service delivery in speech-language pathology. *Journal of Telemedicine and Telecare*, 2008,14:221-224. doi:10.1258/jtt.2007.007044 PMID:18632993

250. Tam SF et al. Evaluating the efficacy of tele-cognitive rehabilitation for functional performance in three case studies. *Occupational Therapy International*, 2003,10:20-38. doi:10.1002/oti.175 PMID:12830317

251. Man DW et al. A randomized clinical trial study on the effectiveness of a tele-analogy-based problem-solving programme for people with acquired brain injury (ABI). *NeuroRehabilitation*, 2006,21:205-217. PMID:17167189

252. Sanford JA, Butterfield T. Using remote assessment to provide home modification services to underserved elders. *The Gerontologist*, 2005,45:389-398. PMID:15933279

253. Damiani G et al. The effectiveness of computerized clinical guidelines in the process of care: a systematic review. *BMC Health Services Research*, 2010,10:2- doi:10.1186/1472-6963-10-2 PMID:20047686

254. Lemaire ED, Boudrias Y, Greene G. Low-bandwidth, Internet-based videoconferencing for physical rehabilitation consultations. *Journal of Telemedicine and Telecare*, 2001,7:82-89. doi:10.1258/1357633011936200 PMID:11331045

255. Kairy D et al. A systematic review of clinical outcomes, clinical process, healthcare utilization and costs associated with telerehabilitation. *Disability and Rehabilitation*, 2009,31:427-447. doi:10.1080/09638280802062553 PMID:18720118

256. Ebenbichler G et al. The future of physical & rehabilitation medicine as a medical specialty in the era of evidence-based medicine. *American Journal of Physical Medicine & Rehabilitation/Association of Academic Physiatrists*, 2008,87:1-3. doi:10.1097/PHM.0b013e31815e6a49 PMID:18158426

257. Dejong G et al. Toward a taxonomy of rehabilitation interventions: Using an inductive approach to examine the "black box" of rehabilitation. *Archives of Physical Medicine and Rehabilitation*, 2004,85:678-686. doi:10.1016/j.apmr.2003.06.033 PMID:15083447

258. Andrich R, Caracciolo A. Analysing the cost of individual assistive technology programmes. *Disability and Rehabilitation. Assistive Technology*, 2007,2:207-234. doi:10.1080/17483100701325035 PMID:19263539

259. Groah SL et al. Beyond the evidence-based practice paradigm to achieve best practice in rehabilitation medicine: a clinical review. *PM & R: the journal of injury, function, and rehabilitation*, 2009,1:941-950. PMID:19797005

260. Johnston MV et al. *The challenge of evidence in disability and rehabilitation research and practice: A position paper*. Austin, National Centre for the Dissemination of Disability Research, 2009.

261. Wee J. Creating a registry of needs for persons with disabilities in a Northern Canadian community: the disability registry project. *Asia Pacific Disability Rehabiliation Journal*, 2009,20:1-18.

262. Cornielje H, Velema JP, Finkenflügel H. Community based rehabilitation programmes: monitoring and evaluation in order to measure results. *Leprosy Review*, 2008,79:36-49. PMID:18540236

263. Greenhalgh J et al. "It's hard to tell": the challenges of scoring patients on standardised outcome measures by multidisciplinary teams: a case study of neurorehabilitation. *BMC Health Services Research*, 2008,8:217- doi:10.1186/1472-6963-8-217 PMID:18945357

264. Lamoureux EL et al. The Impact of Vision Impairment Questionnaire: an evaluation of its measurement properties using Rasch analysis. *Investigative Ophthalmology & Visual Science*, 2006,47:4732-4741. doi:10.1167/iovs.06-0220 PMID:17065481

265. Dijkers M. *When the best is the enemy of the good: the nature of research evidence used in systematic reviews and guidelines*. Austin, TX, National Center for the Dissemination of Disability Research, 2009.

266. Sudsawad P. *Knowledge translation: introduction to models, strategies, and measures*. Austin, TX, Southwest Educational Development Laboratory, National Center for the Dissemination of Disability Research, 2007 (http://www.ncddr.org/kt/products/ktintro/, accessed 2 May 2010).

267. Rogers J, Martin F. Knowledge translation in disability and rehabilitation research. *Journal of Disability Policy Studies*, 2009,20:110-126. doi:10.1177/1044207309332232

268. Turner TJ. Developing evidence-based clinical practice guidelines in hospitals in Australia, Indonesia, Malaysia, the Philippines and Thailand: values, requirements and barriers. *BMC Health Services Research*, 2009,9:235- doi:10.1186/1472-6963-9-235 PMID:20003536

269. Mmatli TO. Translating disability-related research into evidence-based advocacy: the role of people with disabilities. *Disability and Rehabilitation*, 2009,31:14-22. doi:10.1080/09638280802280387 PMID:18946807

270. World Health Organization, International Society for Prosthetics and Orthotics, United States Agency International Development. *Guidelines on the provision of manual wheelchairs in less-resourced settings*. Geneva, World Health Organization, 2008.

271. *New Zealand autism spectrum disorder guideline*. Wellington, New Zealand Ministries of Health and Education, 2008 (http://www.moh.govt.nz/moh.nsf/indexmh/nz-asd-guideline-apr08, accessed 15 March 2010).

272. *Disability support services*. Wellington, New Zealand Ministry of Health, 2009 (http://www.moh.govt.nz/moh.nsf/pagesmh/8594/$File/asd-newsletter-mar09.pdf, accessed 16 May 2009).

273. Tomlinson M et al. Research priorities for health of people with disabilities: an expert opinion exercise. *Lancet*, 2009,374:1857-1862. doi:10.1016/S0140-6736(09)61910-3 PMID:19944866

274. Stewart R, Bhagwanjee A. Promoting group empowerment and self-reliance through participatory research: a case study of people with physical disability. *Disability and Rehabilitation*, 1999,21:338-345. doi:10.1080/096382899297585 PMID:10471164

275. Chino N et al. Current status of rehabilitation medicine in Asia: a report from new millennium Asian symposium on rehabilitation medicine. *Journal of Rehabilitation Medicine: official journal of the UEMS European Board of Physical and Rehabilitation Medicine*, 2002,34:1-4. doi:10.1080/165019702317242631 PMID:11900256

Chapter 5

Assistance and support

"I don't know what to do for my mum. She is my earthly god. My family has been so supportive and helpful. They carry or feed me when I cannot. They have paid my bills. They have cared and loved me…I don't think [I will have children] unless when God does a miracle. I am very expensive to maintain, so how can I maintain my family?"

Irene

"In my town the programs work and the different social services talk to each other. The workers helped me get an apartment and gave me money for food when I didn't have anything to eat. I would have been kicked out of my apartment maybe two times if the worker didn't talk to my landlord because we were butting heads. I don't know if I would have made it without them. Those people really care about me and are committed to me. They are like my family and respect me. With the right support like that, people can grow into the right things and that needs to be thought of more. We don't need to be taken care of but to have someone to talk to and help us learn to solve our own problems."

Corey

"A revolution in life – and in my head! Personal Assistance [PA] means emancipation. PA means I am able to get up in the morning and to bed at night, that I can take care of my personal hygiene etc. but PA also means freedom to participate in society. I even have got a job! Now I can decide for myself how, when and by whom I shall be assisted. I get the housework and the gardening done, in addition to my personal things, and there are still hours left for recreational activities. I can also save hours, which makes it possible for me to go away on holiday."

Ellen

"At age 16 I was afraid to be 'weird'. As I saw no way out I conducted some suicide attempts. This led to an involuntary admission in a mental hospital with long-term seclusion, coercive medication, fixation, even body cavity searches to prevent me from self-harm or suicide. Caregivers confined me for months and months. As a result, I felt unwelcome and useless. Their treatment was not helping me at all. I got more depressed and suicidal, and refused to cooperate. I have been raised with a strong feeling of justice, and I believed this was not good care. There was no trust between the caregivers and me, only a fierce struggle. I felt like I was on a dead end and I saw no way out. I did not care for my life anymore and expected to die."

Jolijn

5

Assistance and support

For many people with disabilities, assistance and support are prerequisites for participating in society. The lack of necessary support services can make people with disabilities overly dependent on family members – and can prevent both the person with disability and the family members from becoming economically active and socially included. Throughout the world people with disabilities have significant unmet needs for support. Support services are not yet a core component of disability policies in many countries, and there are gaps in services everywhere.

No one model of support services will work in all contexts and meet all needs. A diversity of providers and models is required. But the overarching principle promoted by the United Nations *Convention on the Rights of Persons with Disabilities* (CRPD) (*1*) is that services should be provided in the community, not in segregated settings. Person-centred services are preferable, so that individuals are involved in decisions about the support they receive and have maximum control over their lives.

Many persons with disabilities need assistance and support to achieve a good quality of life and to be able to participate in social and economic life on an equal basis with others (*2*). A sign language interpreter, for instance, enables a Deaf person to work in a mainstream professional environment. A personal assistant helps a wheelchair user travel to meetings or work. An advocate supports a person with intellectual impairment to handle money or make choices (*2*). People with multiple impairments or older persons may require support to remain in their homes. These individuals are thus empowered to live in the community and participate in work and other activities, rather than be marginalized or left fully dependent on family support or social protection (*3, 4*).

Most assistance and support comes from family members or social networks. State supply of formal services is generally underdeveloped, not-for-profit organizations have limited coverage, and private markets rarely offer enough affordable support to meet the needs of people with disabilities (*5–7*). State funding of responsive formal support services is an important element of policies to enable the full participation of persons with disabilities in social and economic life. States also have an important role in setting standards, regulating, and providing services (*8*). Also by reducing the need for informal assistance, these services can enable family members to participate in paid or income-generating activity.

Box 5.1. Personal ombudsmen for supported decision-making in Sweden

Article 12 of the United Nations *Convention on the Rights of Persons with Disabilities* (CRPD) ensures that people cannot lose legal capacity simply because of disability. People may require support to exercise that capacity, and safeguards will be needed to prevent the abuse of such support. The CRPD obliges governments to take appropriate and effective measures so that people have the support they need to exercise their legal capacity.

Supported decision-making can take many forms. It involves people with disabilities having supporters, or advocates, who know them, can understand and interpret their choices and desires, and can communicate these choices and desires to others. Forms of supported decision-making may include support networks, personal "ombudspeople", community services, peer support, personal assistants and good advanced planning (9).

Satisfying these requirements is not always straightforward. People in institutions may be denied this support. There may be no relevant agencies. An individual may not be able to identify a trusted person. Also considerable effort and financial investment may be needed. However existing models of substitute decision-making or guardianship are also costly and complicated. Supported decision-making should thus be seen as a redistribution of existing resources, not as an additional expense (10). Examples of decision-making support models can be found in Canada and Sweden. The Personal Ombud (PO) programme in Skåne, the southernmost province of Sweden, supports people with psychosocial disabilities, helping them assert their legal rights and make major decisions about their lives (11).

PO-Skåne employs individuals with a professional degree – such as law or social work – who have the ability and interest to interact well with people with psychosocial disabilities. They do not work from an office but go out to meet the people they work with, wherever they are based. Only a verbal agreement is required to set up the service, which is confidential. This allows a relationship of trust to be established, even with individuals who have had experience of abuse by authorities claiming to help.

Once the PO relationship has been set up by agreement, the PO can act only on specific requests – for instance, to help the person obtain government benefits. Often, the greatest need is to talk about life. The PO may also be asked to help resolve long-standing problems, such as creating a better relationship with the family.

The PO programme has helped many people to manage their lives. The initial costs can be high, as people assert their rights and make full use of the services. But the costs fall as situations are resolved and the need for support declines.

Sources (12–14).

The CRPD sees support and assistance not as ends in themselves but as means to preserving dignity and enabling individual autonomy and social inclusion. Equal rights and participation are thus to be achieved, in part, through the provision of support services for people with disabilities and their families. Article 12 restores the capacity of decision-making to people with disabilities. Respecting individual wishes and preferences – whether through supported decision-making or otherwise—is a legal imperative (see Box 5.1). Articles 19 and 28 are concerned with "the right to live independently and be included in the community" with an "adequate standard of living and social protection". Article 21 upholds rights to freedom of expression and opinion and access to information through sign language and other forms of communication.

Evidence on the demand for and supply of support services and assistance is scarce, even in developed countries. This chapter presents evidence on the need and unmet need for support services, the barriers to formal provision, and what works in overcoming these barriers.

Understanding assistance and support

This chapter uses the phrase "assistance and support" to cover a range of interventions labelled elsewhere as "informal care", "support services", or "personal assistance", but as part of a broad category which also includes advocacy, communication support, and other non-therapeutic interventions.

Some of the more common types of assistance and support services include:

- **community support and independent living** – assistance with self-care, household care, mobility, leisure, and community participation;
- **residential support services** – independent housing and congregate living in group homes and institutional settings;
- **respite services** – short-term breaks for caregivers and people with disabilities;
- **support in education or employment** – such as a classroom assistant for a child with a disability, or personal support in the workplace;
- **communication support** – such as sign-language interpreters;
- **community access** – including day care centres;
- **information and advice services** – including professional, peer support, advocacy, and supported decision-making;
- **assistance animals** – such as dogs trained to guide people with a visual impairment.

This chapter deals mainly with assistance and support in the activities of daily life and community participation. Support services in education and employment, as well as environmental adaptations, are discussed elsewhere in the report.

When are assistance and support required?

The need for assistance and support can fluctuate, depending on environmental factors, the stage of life, the underlying health conditions, and the level of individual functioning.

Key factors determining the need for support services are the availability of appropriate assistive devices, the presence and willingness of family members to provide assistance, and the degree to which the environment facilitates participation of people with disabilities,

including older persons. When individuals with disabilities can independently get to a bathroom, for instance, they may not require another person to help them. When they have a suitable wheelchair, they may be able to negotiate their local environment without assistance. And if mainstream services are accessible, there will be less requirement for specialized support.

The need for assistance and support changes through stages of the lifecycle. Formal support may include:

- **in childhood** – respite care, special needs assistance in education;
- **in adulthood** – advocacy services, residential support, or personal assistance in the workplace;
- **in old age** – day centres, home-help services, assisted living arrangements, nursing homes, and palliative care.

Often, problems in service provision occur between these stages – such as between childhood and adulthood (*15*).

Needs and unmet needs

Data are sparse on the needs for national formal support services. Chapter 2 discussed evidence on support services. Most of the evidence about support services and assistance in this chapter comes from developed countries. This does not imply that formal assistance and support are not equally relevant in low-income settings; it suggests instead that they are rarely provided formally or that data about them are not collected.

Population surveys in Australia, Canada, New Zealand, and the United States of America have shown that between 60% and 80% of people with disabilities generally have their needs met for assistance with everyday activities (*16–19*). Most of the support in these countries is from informal sources, such as families and friends. For example, a survey of 1505 non-elderly adults in the United States with disability found that:

- 70% relied on family and friends for assistance with daily activities, and only 8% used home-health aides and personal assistants;

- 42% reported having failed to move in or out of a bed or a chair because no one was available to help;
- 16% of home-care users reported problems paying for home care in the previous 12 months;
- 45% of participants in the study worried that caring for them would become too much of a burden on the family;
- 23% feared having to go into a nursing home or other type of facility (20).

For most countries, including developed ones (21), and for many disability groups, there are large gaps in meeting needs for support:

- **Community support and independent living**. In China there is a shortage of community support services for people with disabilities who need personal care and lack family support (6, 22). In New Zealand a household disability survey of 14 500 children with physical disabilities reported that 10% of families reported unmet need for household care, and 7% for funding for respite care (23).
- **Communication support**. Deaf people frequently have difficulties in recruiting and training interpreters, particularly in rural or isolated communities (24, 25) (see Box 5.2). A survey on the human rights situation of Deaf people found that 62 of the 93 countries that responded have sign language interpreting services, 43 have some kind of sign language interpreters training, and 30 countries had 20 or fewer qualified sign language interpreters, including Iraq, Madagascar, Mexico, Sudan, Thailand, and the United Republic of Tanzania (27).
- **Respite services**. In the United Kingdom a large study of family caregivers of adults with intellectual disability found that 33% had a high but unmet need for respite services and 30% a high but unmet need for home-based services (28). A 2001 United States cross-sectional survey of children with special health care needs found that of the 38 831 respondents, 3178 (8.8%)

reported a need for respite care in the prior 12 months, especially among younger children, mothers with low education, low-income households, and minority race or ethnicity (29).

Social and demographic factors affecting demand and supply

Population growth affects the supply of care. Growth in older age cohorts and their rates of disability influence both supply and demand, and changes in family structure impact on the availability and willingness to provide care.

- The ageing of consumers and ageing of family members who provide support point to a greatly increased demand for support services. The number of people aged 60 years or over worldwide has roughly tripled – from 205 million in 1950 to 606 million in 2000 – and is projected to triple again by 2050 (30). The likelihood of acquiring a health condition increases as people age – something relevant to prospective users of support services and to family members who provide support.
- Despite high proportions of young people in many countries – for example in Kenya 50% of the population is under 15 years of age (31) – there has been a decrease in the number of children per family (32). Over 1980–2001 fertility rates declined in developed countries (from 1.5 to 1.2) and in developing countries (from 3.6 to 2.6). Even though infant and child mortality rates have been steadily falling in most countries, the counteracting impact of falling fertility rates is greater, with the net effect that smaller family sizes are projected (33), indicating less family care.
- In most countries there has been an increase in geographical mobility. With young people moving more readily from rural areas to urban centres or abroad, and with changing attitudes, shared living arrangements within families are becoming less common (33).

Box 5.2. **Signs of progress with community-based rehabilitation**

The Ugandan government piloted a community-based rehabilitation (CBR) programme in Tororo district of Eastern Uganda in the 1990s, with support from partners, notably the Norwegian Association of the Disabled. During the initial phases Deaf people realized that they were missing out on rehabilitation services. They responded through their national umbrella organization – Uganda National Association of the Deaf (UNAD) – alerting the CBR managers and other development partners to the fact that Deaf people were being excluded because the CBR workers could not use sign language, and so could not communicate with them, and therefore could not help them to access services, information, and support.

Uganda Sign Language (USL), developed informally by UNAD in the 1970s, came to be formally recognized and approved by the Ugandan government in 1995. UNAD devised a pilot project for teaching CBR workers sign language in Tororo in 2003. The main objective was to enable Deaf people's inclusion and participation in communities and realize their full physical and mental potential. Twelve Deaf volunteers run USL training for the CBR workers, the Deaf people and their families. So far, more than 45 CBR workers have been taught sign language: although only about 10 are fluent, the rest have a basic USL, which allows them to greet Deaf people and to provide the key information about education and employment and health among other things.

Although the project has been largely successful, some major problems encountered include the high expectations from target groups, the inadequate funds to expand to a wider area, the persistence of negative attitudes, and the high illiteracy and poverty among Deaf people and their families. These obstacles have been tackled through sensitization and awareness campaigns, intensive fundraising activities, and collaboration with the government to mainstream Deaf people's issues in their programmes and budgets.

The story of Okongo Joseph, a Deaf beneficiary, gives an idea of how such an initiative can change lives, by enabling the CBR programmes to offer services that include the Deaf community. Okongo lives in a remote location, was born deaf, and never went to school, but has now learned sign language from UNAD volunteers who visited him at his home. Okongo writes:

"I would like to send my sincere vote of thanks to UNAD for the development you have brought to me as a Deaf person and to my family members at large. I have achieved a lot since this programme started. I really thank UNAD for the sign language programme they have taught me, my family and my new friends who work in CBR. I am now not a primitive person like before. The goat I was given is in good condition. I request for more from you. I wish you good luck."

Source (*26*).

It is uncertain whether informal care and existing provisions for supporting older people with a disability will cope with these demographic shifts (*34*). Modelling from Australia suggests that fears about future lack of caregivers may be misplaced (*35*).

Consequences for caregivers of unmet need for formal support services

Informal care can be an efficient and cost-effective way of supporting people with disabilities. But exclusive reliance on informal support can have adverse consequences for caregivers.

- **Stress**. The demands of caring often result in stress for families, particularly for women, who tend to be responsible for domestic labour, with care for family members with disability representing a significant share (*36*). In older age, men may also care for spouses (*37*). Factors contributing to stress – and possibly affecting the caregiver's personal health – include increased time spent on care for the person with a disability, increased housework, disruptions to sleep, and the emotional impact of care (*38*). Caregivers also report isolation and loneliness (*39*).

- **Fewer opportunities for employment**. Where employment would otherwise be an option, caring for a family member with a disability is likely to result in lost economic opportunities, as caregivers either reduce their paid work or refrain from seeking it (*40*). An analysis of the General Household Survey in the United Kingdom found that informal care reduced the probability of working by 13% for men and 27% for women (*41*). In the United States members of families of children with developmental disabilities work fewer hours than members in other families, are more likely to have left their employment, have more severe financial problems, and are less likely to take on a new job (*42, 43*).
- **Excessive demands on children**. When adults acquire a disability, children are often asked to help (*44*). Male children may be expected to enter the workforce to compensate for a parent who is no longer working. Female children may be expected to contribute to domestic tasks or to help support the parent with a disability. These increased demands on children may impair their education, and their health (*45*). In Bosnia and Herzegovina children aged 11–15 years whose parents were experiencing health problems or a disability were 14% more likely than other children in that age group to drop out of school (*46*). There are many examples, mainly from Africa, of children having to drop out of school because of a parent developing AIDS. In Uganda, among children aged 15–19 years whose parents had died of AIDS, only 29% continued their schooling undisrupted, 25% lost school time, and 45% dropped out of school (*47*).
- **Greater difficulties as family members age**. As parents or other family members contributing to care grow older and become frail or die, it can be difficult for the remaining family to continue providing care. The increased life expectancy of children with intellectual disabilities, cerebral palsy, or multiple disabilities suggests that parents may eventually be unable to continue providing care for their disabled family member. This is often a hidden unmet need, as families may not have sought formal support when the disabled individual was younger, and may find it hard to seek help later in life. The needs of such families have not been adequately addressed in most countries (*48*), including such high-income countries as Australia (*49*) and the United States (*50*).

Policy responses to the support needs of informal caregivers can sometimes compete with the demands of people with disabilities for support for independent living and participation (*51*). The needs and rights of the informal caregiver should be separated from the needs and rights of the disabled person. A balance must be found, so that each person has independence, dignity, and quality of life. Caring, despite its demands, has many positive aspects that need to be brought out (*52*). People with disabilities who do not have families able to provide the necessary support and assistance should be a priority in formal support services.

Provision of assistance and support

Assistance and support are complex, because they are provided by different suppliers, funded in different ways, and delivered in different locations. In supply, the main divide is between informal care, provided by families and friends, and formal services, provided by government, non-profit organizations, and the for-profit sector. The cost of formal support can be met through state funding, raised through general taxation, through social insurance contributions by those covered by the scheme, through charitable or voluntary sector funding, through out-of-pocket payment to private service providers, or through a mixture of these methods. The services can be provided within a family setting or single occupancy, or congregate living in group homes or institutional settings.

While formal organized support services and programmes for people with disabilities are common in high-income countries, they are a fairly new concept in many low-income and middle-income countries. But even in countries with well-developed systems of support, informal care and support from families and friends predominates, being indispensable and cost-efficient. In all countries family support is essential (53). Across high-income countries families meet around 80% of the support needs of older people (52). In the United States more than 75% of people with disabilities receive assistance from unpaid informal caregivers (54). Among adults with developmental disabilities more than 75% live at home with family caregivers, and more than 25% of these caregivers are 60 years or older, with another 35% aged between 41 and 59 years. Fewer than 11% of people with developmental disabilities were living in supervised residential settings in 2006 (55).

Limited data are available on the economic value of informal care, overwhelmingly performed by women. In 2005–2006 the estimated value of all unpaid care in Australia was A$ 41.4 billion, the major part of all "welfare services resources", which amounted to around A$ 72.6 billion (56). A Canadian study found that private expenditure, largely related to time costs for provision of assistance, accounted for 85% of total home-care costs, which escalated as activity limitations increased (57).

Government-led service delivery was traditionally focused on institutional care. Governments have also provided day services such as home care and day centres for people living in the community. With the recent trend towards "contracting out" services, governments, particularly local ones, are shifting from being direct service providers to commissioning, retaining funding and regulatory functions such as assessment procedures, standard setting, contracting, monitoring, and evaluation.

Nongovernmental organizations – also known as private not-for-profit, voluntary, or civil society organizations – have often appeared where governments have failed to provide for specific needs. Their advantages can include their potential for innovation, specialization,

and responsiveness. NGOs often provide community-based and user-driven programmes to promote participation by people with disabilities in their communities (58, 59). For example, in South Africa the Disabled Children's Action Group was set up by parents of children with disabilities, predominantly from the black and coloured communities, in 1993. The aim of this low-cost, mutual support group is to promote inclusion and equal opportunities, particularly in education. It has 311 support centres, mostly in poorer areas, with 15 000 parent members and 10 000 children and young people actively involved. Its work has been supported by grants from international NGOs as well as national charities (60).

NGOs can partner with governments to deliver services for people with disabilities (61). They also frequently act as vehicles for testing new types of service provision and for evaluating the outcomes. But many are small, with limited reach, so their good practices cannot always be disseminated and replicated more widely. Disadvantages may arise because of their fragile financial base and because they may have different priorities to government.

Private for-profit suppliers of residential and community support services exist in most societies, and their services are either contracted by government, or paid directly by the client. They are often concentrated in particular areas of the care market, such as care for the elderly and home care. Where people with disabilities can afford to do so, they or their families may employ people to support them in activities of daily living.

In practice, people with disabilities receive a range of services from different providers. For example in Australia the Commonwealth–State/Territory Disability Agreement sets the national framework to fund, monitor, and support services for 200 000 people with a disability. Community access and respite services had a high proportion of people using nongovernment services. Employment services for people with disabilities were accessed almost exclusively through NGOs. Support services in the community were accessed mainly through government agencies (*56*).

Barriers to assistance and support

Lack of funding

Social safety net programmes in developing countries typically amount to between 1% and 2% of gross domestic product, and to about twice that in developed countries, although rates are variable (*62*). Upper middle-income and high-income countries often provide a combination of cash programmes and a variety of social welfare services. In contrast, in many developing countries, a significant share of safety net resources is often allocated to cash programmes targeted at the poor and vulnerable households, with only a fraction going to the provision of social welfare services to vulnerable groups, including individuals with disabilities or their families. In low-income settings, social welfare services are often the only safety net, but the spending is low and programmes are fragmented and of a very small scale, reaching only a fraction of the needy population.

The lack of effective financing for support – or its distribution within a country – is a major obstacle to sustainable services. For example, in India, in 2005–06, the spending on the welfare of people with disabilities – which focused on support to national disability institutions, non-government organizations providing services and spending on assistive devices – represented 0.05% of Ministry of Social Justice and Welfare allocations (*5*).

In countries that lack social protection schemes, funding assistance and support can be problematic. Even in high-income countries, funding long-term care for older people is proving difficult (*21*, *63*). An Australian study found that 61% of caregivers of people with profound or severe disabilities lacked any main source of assistance (*64*). In many middle-income and low-income countries governments cannot provide adequate services and commercial service providers are either not available or not affordable for most households (*65*).

Governments often do not support the voluntary sector to develop innovative services able to meet the needs of families and individuals with disabilities. In Beijing, China, in addition to existing government welfare institutions, a small number of nongovernmental housing support agencies have been set up for children and young people with a disability. A study of four of them showed that the main service was skills training (*6*). The government does not support these organizations financially, though the local government subsidizes the fee for a small number of the most disadvantaged children or orphans (*66*). Instead, the services rely on fees paid by families and donations, including international assistance. As a result, the services are likely to be less affordable to users and their quality and staffing arrangements will probably suffer (*67*). In India NGOs and independent living organizations are often successful in innovating and creating empowering services, but they can rarely scale them up to wider coverage (*5*).

Lack of adequate human resources

Personal support workers – also known as direct care workers or home aides – play a vital role in community-based service systems, but there is a shortage of such workers in many countries (*68–70*). As the proportion of older people in a country increases, the demand for personal support workers will grow. In the United States, for example, the demand for personal support workers far exceeds their availability. But their numbers are growing, and it has been estimated that the number of home health aides will increase by 56% between 2004 and 2014 and the number of personal and home care aides by 41% (*71*). A study in the United Kingdom estimated that 76 000 individuals were already working as personal assistants funded through direct payments schemes (*72*).

Many personal support workers are poorly paid and have inadequate training (*70, 73*). A United States study found that 80% of social care workers had no formal qualifications or training (*74*). Many workers may be working in social care temporarily, rather than as a career. A study in the United Kingdom found that only 42% of personal assistants had qualifications in social care (*72*). Combined with their high turnover, the result can be substandard care and a lack of a stable relationship with the service user.

Many support workers are economic migrants, lacking skills and a career ladder. They are vulnerable to exploitation, particularly given their precarious immigration status. The high demand for support workers in more affluent countries has led to an inflow of people, largely women, from neighbouring poorer countries – for instance, from the Plurinational State of Bolivia to Argentina or from the Philippines to Singapore. The knock-on effect of this migration – described as a "global care chain" (*75*) – is that in their home countries, other relatives have to step in to act as caregivers.

Inappropriate policies and institutional frameworks

From the 18th and 19th century onwards, the main framework for formal services was to provide support by placing persons with disabilities in institutions. Until the 1960s people with intellectual impairments, mental health conditions, and physical and sensory impairments usually lived in segregated residential institutions in developed countries (*76–78*). In developing countries institutions along similar lines were sometimes initiated by international NGOs, but the sector remained minimal compared with high-income countries (*79–81*).

Although it was once thought humane to meet the needs of people with disabilities in asylums, colonies, or residential institutions, these services have been widely criticized (*82, 83*). Lack of autonomy, segregation from the wider community, and even human rights abuses are widely reported (see Box 5.3).

People with disabilities worldwide have been demanding community-based services that offer greater freedom and participation. They have also promoted supportive relationships that allow them to exercise more control over their lives and to live in the community (*85*). The CRPD promotes policies and institutional frameworks that enable community living and social inclusion for people with disabilities.

Inadequate and unresponsive services

In some countries support services are available only to people living in sheltered housing projects or institutions and not to those living independently. Institution-based services have had limited success in promoting independence and social relationships (*86*). Where community services do exist, people with disabilities have lacked choice and control over when they receive support in their homes. Disabled people often see relationships with professionals, seldom disabled themselves, as unequal and patronizing (*87*). Such relationships have also led to an unwanted dependency (*88*).

Some recent reviews reveal that while community living shows significant improvements over institutional living, people with disabilities are still far from achieving a lifestyle comparable to that of people not disabled (*2*). For many people with intellectual impairments and mental health conditions, the main community service is attendance at a day centre, but a review of a range of studies failed to find good evidence of benefits (*89*). The community service often fails to provide an entry to employment, produce greater satisfaction (*85*), or deliver meaningful adult activities (*90*).

Poor service coordination

Where services are delivered by different suppliers – at local or national level, or from health, education, and housing, or from state, voluntary, and private suppliers – coordination has often been inadequate. Existing

145

Box 5.3. Mental health system reform and human rights in Paraguay

In 2003 Disability Rights International (DRI) documented life-threatening abuses against people detained in the state-run psychiatric hospital in Paraguay. These included the detention in tiny cells of two boys, aged 17 and 18 years, with diagnoses of autism. The boys had been held there, naked, for the previous four years, without access to toilets. The other 458 people in this institution also lived in atrocious conditions, which included:

- open sewage, rotting garbage, broken glass, and excrement and urine strewn around wards and common areas;
- inadequate staffing;
- a lack of proper medical attention and medical record-keeping;
- shortages of food and medicines;
- the detention of children with adults;
- a lack of adequate mental health services or rehabilitation.

DRI, along with the Center for Justice and International Law (CEJIL), filed a petition with the Inter-American Commission on Human Rights of the Organization of American States, requesting urgent intervention on behalf of those held in the institution. In response, the Commission called on the Paraguayan government to take all necessary steps to protect the lives, health, and safety of those detained in the psychiatric hospital.

Deinstitutionalization agreement

In 2005 DRI and CEJIL signed an historic agreement with the Paraguayan government to initiate mental health reform in the country. The agreement was the first in Latin America to guarantee the rights of people with mental health disabilities to live in the community and receive services and support there. Paraguay also took steps to address the unhygienic conditions and to separate children from adults. A home for eight long-term hospital residents was opened in the community. One of the boys who had been detained naked in his cell returned to live with his family. But the ethos of human rights abuses and the lack of proper treatment in the hospital remained largely unchanged.

In July 2008 the Commission found in favour of a new petition that made charges of a series of deaths, numerous cases of sexual abuse, and grievous injuries inside the institution, all in the preceding six months. It called on the government to take immediate action to protect those in the institution and to investigate the deaths and allegations of abuse.

Reforms in line with human rights

The result: for the first time, a Member State of the Pan American Health Organization (PAHO) formally committed itself to reform its public health system in accordance with regional human rights treaties and the recommendations of regional human rights bodies. The agreement stemmed in part from the technical collaboration of PAHO and WHO with the Paraguayan government on human rights and mental health.

Since the 2008 emergency measures, and following its ratification of the CRPD and the optional protocol, the Paraguayan government has taken positive steps towards mental health reform. The hospital's in-patient population has been reduced by almost half since 2003, and the government is expanding community-based services and support. Today 28 long-term hospital residents in group homes in the community, and a handful of "chronic patients" live independently, having joined the workforce. Another nine group homes are scheduled to open in the next two years.

Source (*84*).

services and support schemes may be operated, in any given place, by a range of public or private providers. In India different NGOs or agencies serve different impairment groups, but the lack of coordination between them undermines their effectiveness (*5*). Multiple assessments and different eligibility criteria make life more difficult for people with disabilities and their families, particularly in the transition between services for young people and those for adults (*91*). Lack of knowledge about a disability can be a barrier to referrals for effective support services and care coordination (*15*), as can a lack of communication between different health and social care agencies.

Awareness, attitudes, and abuse

People with disabilities and their families often lack information about the services available, are disempowered, or are unable or unwilling to express their needs. A Chinese study of caregivers of stroke survivors found a need for information about recovery and stroke prevention, and for training in moving and handling (*92*). A study of family care for children with intellectual disabilities in Pakistan revealed stigma in the community and lack of knowledge about effective interventions, causing distress for caregivers (*93*). A Belgian study of family caregivers of people with dementia found that lack of awareness of services was a major barrier to service use (*94*).

Empowerment through disability rights organizations, community-based rehabilitation organizations, self-advocacy groups, or other collective networks can enable individuals with disabilities to identify their needs and lobby for service improvement (*95*). Most countries that have developed support services have strong organizations of persons with disabilities and their families lobbying governments to reform policies on service delivery and to increase or at least maintain the resources allocated. In the United Kingdom support from a disabled people's organization is an important influence on people with disabilities signing up for direct payment schemes (*96*).

As explored in Chapter 1, negative attitudes are a cross-cutting issue in the lives of people with disabilities. Negative attitudes towards disability may have particular implications for the quality of assistance and support. Families hide or infantilize children with disabilities, and caregivers might abuse or disrespect the people they work with.

Negative attitudes and discrimination also undermine the possibility for people with disabilities to make friends, express their sexuality, and achieve the family life that non-disabled people take for granted (*97*).

People who need support services are usually more vulnerable than those who do not. People with mental health conditions and intellectual impairments are sometimes subject to arbitrary detention in long-stay institutions with no right of appeal, in contravention of the CRPD (*98, 99*). Vulnerability – both in institutions and in community settings – can range from the risk of isolation, boredom, and lack of stimulation, to the risk of physical and sexual abuse. Evidence suggests that people with disabilities are at higher risk of abuse, for various reasons, including dependence on a large number of caregivers and barriers to communication (*100*). Safeguards to protect people in both formal and informal support services are therefore particularly important (*101*).

Addressing the barriers to assistance and support

Achieving successful deinstitutionalization

A catalyst for the move from institutions to independent and community living was the adoption in 1993 of the United Nations *Standard Rules on the Equalization of Opportunities for Persons with Disabilities*, which promoted equal rights and opportunities for people with disabilities (*102*). Since these rules were issued, there has been a marked shift in many high-income countries and countries in transition, from large residential institutions and nursing homes to smaller settings within the community, along with the growth of the independent living movement (*103–105*). Countries such as Norway and Sweden have eliminated all institutional placements. Elsewhere – including Australia, Belgium, Germany, Greece, the Netherlands, and Spain – institutional care exists alongside alternative community living arrangements (*106*).

In a major transformation in eastern Europe, countries no longer rely predominantly on institutions (*107*). Alternative care services have been progressively developed – including day care, foster care, and home support for people with disabilities (*108*). Romania closed 70% of its institutions for children between 2001 and 2007, but for adults the process has been slower (*109*). Alongside deinstitutionalization, there has also been decentralization from central to local government and an expansion and diversification of social services and service providers.

Plans for closing an institution and moving residents to community settings should be started early. Adequate resources need to be available for the new support infrastructure before attempts are made to alter the balance of care (*110*). Deinstitutionalization takes time, especially if individuals are to prepare for their new lives in the community and be involved in decisions about their accommodation and support services. Some "double funding" of institutional and community systems will therefore be needed during the transition, which may take several years.

The lesson from deinstitutionalization in various countries is that it requires a range of institutional assistance and support services, including:

- health care
- crisis response systems
- housing assistance
- income support
- support for social networks of people living in the community.

Unless the agencies responsible for these services work together, there is a danger that individuals will not obtain adequate support at crucial times in their lives (*110*). People with mental health conditions may need support and service coordination to reduce vulnerability to homelessness (*111*). Some countries, including Denmark and Sweden, have excellent coordination between health care, social service providers, and the housing sector, allowing people with disabilities to find living arrangements that suit their needs.

Outcomes of deinstitutionalization

Improvements in the quality of life and personal functioning have been found in several studies of people who move out of institutions into community settings (*106, 112*). A study in the United Kingdom of people with intellectual impairments 12 years after leaving residential institutions showed that both quality of life and care were better in the community than in hospitals (*113*). Small-scale living arrangements offer people with intellectual impairments more friends, more access to mainstream facilities, and more chances to acquire skills – they also result in greater satisfaction (*85*). Evidence from a Chinese study shows that residents with intellectual impairments in small residential homes experienced better outcomes at lower cost than persons living in medium-size group homes or institutions (*114*).

In some countries, deinstitutionalization programmes have converted institutions into alternative facilities, such as:

- vocational training and resource centres;
- rehabilitation centres providing specialist secondary and tertiary services;
- smaller home units where people with complex impairments can live semi-independently with some support;
- respite facilities where people with disabilities can come for short breaks and training;
- clubs or similar centres for people with mental health issues to achieve peer support and respite;
- emergency sheltered accommodation, not only for people with disabilities but for all who may be vulnerable to abuse or exploitation.

Comparison of costs

The mix of evidence on the relative costs and effectiveness of institutional and community services shows that community services, if well planned and resourced, have better outcomes but may not be cheaper.

In the United States the cost of public institutions for people with intellectual disabilities is considerably higher than that of community-based services (*115*). However a review of evidence from 28 European countries found slightly higher costs for community-based services (*110*), but the study also found that the quality of life was generally better for people living outside institutions, particularly those who made the move from an institutional to a community setting. If well planned and adequately resourced, community-based services were much more cost-effective than institutional care. A personal assistance service evaluated by the Serbian Center for Independent Living found that the scheme was more cost-effective than institutional care (*116*).

The European review also revealed a link between cost and quality, with lower cost institutional systems tending to offer lower quality care. The conclusion: community systems of independent and supported living – when effectively set up and managed, and when well planned to prepare services and individuals for the major change in support arrangements – delivered better overall outcomes than institutions (*110*).

In the United Kingdom research which found that user-controlled personal assistance schemes were cheaper than government-provided home care contributed to the adoption of a system of direct payments. But recent evidence is more cautious (*117*). Further research is needed to know whether paid personal assistance, which may substitute for informal care, increases costs to governments more than alternative arrangements (*118–121*). User-controlled arrangements have the potential to promote individual independence and to improve quality of life, but they are unlikely to produce major savings.

Creating a framework for commissioning effective support services

Governments may decide to provide a range of support services for all those in need – or they may target people who cannot afford to pay out of their own resources. Mobilizing financial resources will in both cases involve some pooling of funds.

A "pooled" system of revenue generation to finance support systems can include various forms of prepayment, the most common being through national, regional or local taxation, social insurance (through employers), and private voluntary insurance. Each may require some financial contributions by people who use services or by their families ("user charges" or "co-payments"). Mechanisms where people pay for all services out of their own resources are the least equitable (*122*).

Many developed countries have support services covering all those who need them (*21*). In other countries access to public funding for support services depends on a means test, as in the United Kingdom, where about half of all spending on social support comes from private sources (*123*). Other strategies to contain government spending on support services in countries with developed care systems include:

- charges to users
- restrictions on eligibility
- case management to limit the use of services
- budget-limited programmes (*63*).

In countries in transition that have invested widely in residential care, reallocating resources can help build community support services. In low-income and middle-income countries, for example in Yemen, there have been good examples of social funds financing support services (*124*).

Funding services

There are many ways to pay providers, with the main government mechanisms including:

- retrospective fee-for-service payments;
- direct budgetary allocations to decentralized providers;
- performance-based contracting;
- consumer-directed services through devolution of budgets to people with disabilities or their families.

Each method has its incentives and limitations, and each therefore has the potential to influence how cost-effective and equitable the support system is. The success of a support system depends on the mix, volume, and deployment of staff and other resource inputs and the services they deliver. In turn, these depend on how funds are made available through the various commissioning arrangements. Devolved or direct payments to people with disabilities offer a relatively new commissioning option (125).

- In Sweden the Personal Assistance Reform Act of 1994 ensured that individuals with extensive disabilities would be entitled to cash payments from the national social insurance fund to pay for assistance. The weekly number of assistance hours is determined on the basis of need. About 70% of users buy services from local governments, and 15% have organized themselves into user cooperatives that provide services. The remainder purchase services from private companies or directly employ assistants (126). More than 15 000 individuals in Sweden use state aid to purchase services to meet their care needs (127).
- In the Netherlands the *Persoonsgebondenbudget* is a similar direct payment system. The most common service purchased is personal assistance – from an existing informal care provider or a nonprofessional private service provider. Introduced in 2003, when 50 000 people used the new style *Persoongebondenbudget*, 120 000 people were taking advantage of the scheme by 2010, when it was temporarily halted. The benefits include lower administrative costs and greater individualization of services. Evaluations have found high levels of satisfaction, better quality of life, and greater independence (128).
- In South Africa the Social Assistance Act of 2004 established a direct payment known as "grant in aid". Individuals who already receive old age, disability, or war veterans' benefits qualify for this additional money if they require full-time care. But the small monthly allowance is insufficient to pay for support. The scheme is currently being reviewed by the Department of Social Development (129).

Because support and assistance services have been provided almost entirely by families, formal support schemes could increase demand and substitute for informal care (121). Regulatory mechanisms, including eligibility criteria and sound and fair assessment procedures, are necessary to ensure the most equitable and cost-effective use of resources, and to allow delivery services to grow gradually.

Assessing individual needs

Assessment is vital to meet the needs of people with disabilities. In high-income countries assessment is a general process of deciding which categories of people can be granted entitlement, followed by evaluating individual need. It is generally carried out by formal systems for disability determination. In New Zealand, for instance, once eligibility for support services is established, access depends on (130):

- **A needs assessment.** This identifies and ranks the care and support needs of a person, without taking into account possible funding and services;
- **Service coordination or planning.** This identifies the most appropriate services and support options to meet the assessed needs, within the available funding;
- **Provision of services.** This is generally a support package of services for the person with disability, as well as for the family, where appropriate.

Assessment, historically, was based on eligibility according to medical criteria (124). The focus now is more on support needs to improve functioning, as reflected in the *International Classification of Functioning, Disability and Health* (ICF) (131). Colombia, Cuba, Mexico, and Nicaragua have recently introduced ICF-based disability assessment systems.

In many countries assessment has been separated from the delivery of services, to remove a conflict of interests. In the Netherlands, while independent assessment agencies feel that this makes the process more transparent and objective, care providers find it less accessible and efficient (*132*).

In the United Kingdom assessment has shifted from being service-led (fitting the individual to the available service) to needs-based (with services appropriate to meet the need), and then to a focus on outcome (with personalized social care through enhanced choice). Self-assessment is an important part of this process. It is not always easy for service users to articulate their needs, so supported decision making may be indicated (*47*).

Regulating providers

The state has an important role in regulating, setting standards, inspecting, monitoring, and evaluating.

In the United Kingdom the Comprehensive Area Assessment evaluates the success of local authorities in implementing government policy, managing public resources, and responding to the needs of their communities. Social care providers, whether public, private, or voluntary, must register with the Care Quality Commission and face regular assessment and inspections. Social care providers are judged by seven criteria:

- improving health and well-being.
- improving the quality of life
- making a positive contribution
- choice and control
- freedom from discrimination
- economic well-being
- personal dignity.

In countries where NGOs, assisted by foreign aid and local philanthropy, have been the main providers of support services, stable public regulatory frameworks and funding are needed to sustain and build on the services.

Regulatory frameworks should cover:
- quality standards
- contracting and funding procedures

- an assessment system
- allocation of resources (*108*).

In establishing regulatory frameworks, in whatever setting, people with disabilities and their families should be included, and service users should help in evaluating services (*133*). Service outcomes can improve when providers are accountable to consumers (*8*).

Supporting public-private-voluntary services

A variety of suppliers from different sectors (public, private, voluntary) provide support services.

In high-income countries, assistance and support services were set up mostly by charities and self-help groups, with later support from the state. This approach is still in use:

- In the past decade NGOs working on disability have been set up in the Balkan countries. Many are delivering services, often initially in pilots, with the support of state funding, such as the Serbian Social Innovation Fund (*134*). An example is the pilot project for interpreting in Novi Pazar, Serbia, run by the Association of Deaf and Hard of Hearing People.
- In India the National Trust Act – created as the result of a campaign for the rights of people with disabilities – has produced collaboration among a range of NGOs. The Act gives individuals with autism, cerebral palsy, intellectual impairment, or multiple impairments, as well as their families, access to government services to enable people with disabilities to live as independently as possible within their communities. It also encourages NGOs to collaborate, giving support to families who need it, and to facilitate the appointment of a legal guardian (*135*). Mechanisms under the Act offer training in personal assistance, to support people with a range of disabilities in the community.

Some countries have gone beyond simply supporting NGO services, by tendering services formerly provided by the state to the private not-for-profit sector. In Ireland, with funding from the government, NGOs provide nearly all services for people with intellectual disabilities (*136*). The main aims have been to provide access to specialist and complementary support services – and for the tendering to raise quality and drive down prices. This model, widely used in high-income countries, is being adopted in transition and middle-income countries. Governments retain the regulatory role of licensing suppliers and monitoring standards. But as countries shift to contracting, the processes for contracting and monitoring should be effective (*108*), to avoid neglect of clients or other abuses (*137*).

Where NGOs and disabled people's organizations develop a role as service providers in a mixed economy of care, this can lead to tensions with their client base if they have to cut costs to remain competitive, or if they become more responsive to their funders than those they work with, or if advocacy roles are neglected in favour of service provision (*138, 139*).

Many countries have seen an expansion of private provision in mental health, following a fall in public provision (*140*), but a systematic review in 2003 found that not-for-profit providers had better performances in access, quality, and cost-efficiency than for-profit mental health inpatient services (*141*).

Although systems for public-private partnership are well developed in high-income countries, the situation is quite different in low-income and middle-income countries. Support services are fairly recent, and there generally is little support from the state for NGOs and for-profit organizations.

Coordinating flexible service provision

People with disabilities have needs for assistance and support that are not neatly packaged into what a single provider can offer. Informal assistance and support are most effective when underpinned by a range of formal systems and services, whether public or private.

Formal assistance and support must be coordinated with health care, rehabilitation, and housing. For example, a range of residential support services – independent housing and congregate living in group homes and institutional settings – should be offered alongside other support services, with the type and level based on assessed need (*142*). Research shows that a comprehensive package of housing adaptations and assistive technology for older people would be cost-effective because of reductions in need for formal care (*143*).

Several high-income countries have moved from providing generic services to a more individualized and flexible system of service provision. This calls for a high level of interagency coordination to ensure effective and continual delivery of support.

In the United States the Illinois Home Based Support Services Program, a successful direct payment scheme, supports people with disabilities and their families to decide which services to buy, including respite care, personal assistance, home modifications, recreational and employment services, therapies, and transportation. Families that used this service were less likely to place family members in institutional care (*144*). Efficiencies resulted because families tended to not spend all the available funds, and home-based care costs were lower than those of institutionalization (*144*).

In a similar vein, several countries – including Australia, Canada, and several European countries – have started to look at individualized models of funding. In this approach, public funding from different sources is allocated according to an assessment of need. The combined personal budget is then placed under the control of the individual to buy services, often within certain constraints, ranging from assistive devices and therapy to personal assistance (*145–147*). Increasing the power of consumers, this can make services more accountable. In consumer-directed services the professionals are available when needed, but are not the dominant partner. Appropriate legal frameworks and infrastructure can help develop personal assistance schemes, not just for people with physical impairments but also people with intellectual impairments and mental health issues.

Consumer organizations also deliver community-based responses for mental health.

- In Zambia the Mental Health Users Network provides a forum for users of mental health services to support each other and exchange ideas and information (*148*).
- In the United States MindFreedom has "landing zones" for communities to provide support and housing to people so that they can avoid hospitalization or institutionalization (*99*).

Consumer-directed services are often less costly and just as safe as professional-directed services (*149–151*). Consumer-directed services probably substitute for informal care and can thus raise overall government costs (*118, 119*). The choice offered by such quasi-markets depends on supply, which may be lacking, especially in rural areas (*152*).

Consumer-directed models may not always improve efficiency and quality. Service users may find the choice and bureaucracy overwhelming. Full flexibility through direct payments and personal assistance involves responsibilities as an employer – with all the associated administrative duties, such as accounting and completing tax returns, that may be unwelcome to individuals. Some of these tasks can be undertaken by user cooperatives or agencies.

In practice, and depending on needs and preferences, people with disabilities may opt for varying levels of choice and control. In the United Kingdom, despite the growth of personal assistance schemes, the majority of people with disabilities still do not opt for direct payments (*153, 154*). So a range of models is needed, and further research should determine which models of personal assistance are most effective and efficient (*118–121*).

Support for informal caregivers

Informal care will continue to be important for people with disabilities (*155*). Apart from meeting assistance and support needs, it may well also be cost-effective to provide support to family members and others providing informal care, as suggested by the Illinois Home Based Support Services Program.

- **Respite services** – either in the home or outside the home – providing short-term breaks from caring (*156*). These have been developed in high-income countries and countries in transition, but unmet needs for respite are reported (*157, 158*).
- **Direct or indirect financial support**. Countries in transition, including the Republic of Moldova and Serbia, and parts of South America, where pensions have been provided for otherwise unpaid caregivers, and developing countries, such as South Africa, provide some cash benefit for caregivers in families with people with disabilities (*62, 159*).
- **Psychosocial support services** to improve family well-being.
- **Paid sick leave** and other support from employers to facilitate family caring.

Families can benefit from opportunities for autonomy and support services. Early family support programmes within the developmental disabilities system emerged in the 1960s in the Nordic countries and Australia (*160*) and in the late 1970s and early 1980s in the United States. Families in consumer-directed programmes are more satisfied with services, and have fewer unmet needs and fewer out-of-pocket expenses for disability services than those in other types of programme (*161, 162*).

Families may also need training in working with caregivers, roles, boundary setting, and empowering their relative with disability. They may also need information about available services. But a Japanese study found that providing information was not effective in reducing the burden on caregivers, whereas social communication did help (*163*).

User involvement

User involvement has become a criterion for judging the quality of service delivery. The

European Quality in Social Services initiative includes effective partnerships and participation among the principles governing its quality certification – a process complementary to national quality certification. Users can be involved in service delivery in different ways, including (*108, 138, 139*):

- in complaints procedures
- during evaluation and feedback
- as participants on management boards
- as members of advisory groups of people with disabilities
- in making decisions for themselves.

The concept of the "co-production" of support services has recently been promoted, bringing together the traditional organizations working on behalf of people with disabilities with organizations controlled by people with disabilities (*164*). It recognizes the contribution disabled people can make, based on their experiences, seeks to put disabled people in control of service developments and service delivery, and provides non-disabled people with the role of a supportive ally.

The advantages of co-produced service organizations are: the focus is on the needs of the users, and the combined resources improve the possibility of reducing disabling barriers and creating equality and interdependence (*165*). The principles of co-production and user involvement have been put into practice around the world by organizations of people with disability and by parents of children with disabilities, whether in formal service delivery or community-based rehabilitation (*166*).

Mechanisms for independent living

Randomized trials in high-income countries have compared personal assistance with usual care for children with intellectual impairments, adults with physical impairments, and older persons without dementia. Personal assistance was generally preferred over other services, had benefits for some recipients, and may benefit caregivers (*118–121*).

Personal assistance schemes are not limited to those with physical impairments. A range of approaches can benefit people with intellectual impairments or mental health conditions, including:

- **Advocates** – where the person is supported one-on-one by a trained and skilled individual to make and carry through a decision.
- **Circles of support** – networks of supporters and friends who know the person well and who can make decisions to which the person freely consents.
- **KeyRing** or living support networks – where people with intellectual impairments live in the community, but with a "community living worker" available to provide support and help make connections in the community.
- **User-controlled independent living trusts** – similar to circles of support, but with a legal structure that sets up the necessary framework of decision-making around the individual.
- **Service brokerage** – where a skilled supporter enables the person to choose services, helping with the assessment process and supporting implementation of assistance packages. An agency can act as the named employer of support on behalf of an individual, if required.

Despite evidence of the benefits of direct payments, mental health users are underrepresented in individualized funding arrangements in Australia, Canada, the United Kingdom, and the United States (*167*).

Because of the lack of funds, personal assistance is rarely publicly provided in low-income and middle-income settings. But some innovative programmes suggest that low-cost solutions can be effective and that independent living principles remain relevant (*3*).

- In 2003 in Brazil there were 21 centres for independent living, with the first in Rio de Janeiro, already been operating for 15 years

(166). As elsewhere, the independent living movement brings together people from different impairment groups, and offers services such as peer support, information, training and personal assistance, with staff who themselves have disabilities. However, unlike those in developed countries, centres for independent living do not tend to receive money from the state, but instead have to raise their own funds, such as through employment brokerage services.

- In the Philippines a national disabled peoples organization has developed a multisectoral programme in partnership with the Department of Education and the parents association. It supports the training of teachers and parents on providing appropriate personal assistance, so that children with severe impairments can attend local mainstream schools. It works with more than 13 000 children in rural areas, offering joint training workshops with preschool children, parents, and teachers *(168)*.

Building capacity of caregivers and service users

Training for support workers

Support workers, regardless of setting and service, need professional training (variously known as human services, social work, or social care) that takes into account the principles of the CRPD *(169)*. While many workers lack postschool education *(74)*, further and higher education programmes in social work and health and social care are increasingly available in high income countries. The United Kingdom offers a National Vocational Qualification in health and social care, achieved through demonstrating competency at work and possession of background knowledge. Often, people with disabilities can complement any formal training with on-the-job instruction.

How the training is conducted is as important as the content. In general, people with disabilities prefer the personal assistance model where they direct the tasks, rather than have the social care worker provide the services *(170)*. A new generation of support workers – including personal assistants, advocates, and those supporting people with intellectual difficulties – present a fresh approach to working with people with disabilities in the community and helping them attain their own goals and aspirations, based on respect for human rights rather than the traditional ethos of "care" *(171)*.

Support for users of assistance and support services

Funding arrangements for personal assistance schemes must take into account the additional tasks that users of the schemes may be called on to perform. People receiving direct payments, for instance, should be properly supported so that complexities in the system are not the cause of additional stress or isolation. People with disabilities who employ support workers need to know how to manage staff and fulfil their employer responsibilities. A study in the United Kingdom found that 27% of people with disabilities employing personal assistants found becoming an employer daunting, and 31% found it difficult to cope with the administration *(72)*.

Disabled peoples' organizations and caregivers' organizations help users benefit from consumer-directed services *(96)*. Individualized funding models are most effective when coupled with other support services *(117)*. Support is also needed to ensure that brokers and fund managers are not excessively directive and that the quality of care is good. Some disabled peoples' organizations – such as the Scottish Personal Assistant Employers' Network – have launched recruitment and training programmes aimed at personal support workers and their supervisors, as well as at their potential employers with disabilities and their families *(172)*. In low-income settings, community-based rehabilitation programmes may be able to provide training to people with disabilities and their families to manage their support needs and create links with self-help groups for information and advice.

Developing community-based rehabilitation and community home-based care

Community-based rehabilitation

In many low-income and middle-income countries, consumer-led, government-delivered, or NGO-delivered community-based rehabilitation (CBR) programmes are becoming a source of assistance and support for many people with disabilities and their families. Many focus on information provision, working closely with families, and facilitating disabled peoples' participation in the community (*173*). They can also counter tendencies towards overprotection by families. In all income settings, it may be useful for CBR workers, social workers, or community workers to bring together families who share similar experiences in supporting relatives with disabilities.

- In Lesotho the leaders of nine branches of the national association of parents of disabled children found that parents required support in how to teach, train and handle their child; information about the rights of people with disabilities and how to work with professionals; and information on how to create teaching aids and obtain equipment (*174*).
- RUCODE, an NGO in the state of Tamil Nadu, India, runs community-based day-care centres for children with intellectual disabilities and cerebral palsy, with the help of local government and parents. Each centre caters to around 10 children, with one teacher and one attendant at each centre and support from RUCODE staff. The community contributes the venue and provides lunch for the children.
- In Nepal CBR programmes are implemented in 35 districts by local NGOs, with the government providing funding, direction, advice, and monitoring at the national and district levels (*175*).

As the CBR model strengthens the quality of the relationship between people with disabilities and their families, it can bring significant support to people with disabilities and caregivers (*176*). Recently the principles of independent living have started to be introduced within community-based rehabilitation, which will help CBR services ensure greater self-determination for people with disabilities.

Community home-based care

Community home-based care is any support given, in their homes, to people who are ill and their families (*177*). The model, developed particularly to cope with HIV/AIDS, operates in many African and Asian countries, with care of orphans a special concern. A government community home-based care programme might provide food, transport, medication, respite care, cash allowances, and emotional and physical care.

Including assistance and support in disability policies and action plans

The inclusion of formal assistance and support services within a national disability policy and related action plan can improve community participation of persons with disabilities, for example:

- Australia's Disability Discrimination Act (1992) encourages organizations to create action plans to eliminate discrimination in provision of goods, services and facilities (*178*).
- New Zealand's Disability Strategy (2001) offers a framework for government to begin removing barriers to the participation of people with disabilities (*179*).
- Sweden's "From Patient to Citizen" national action plan (2000) has a vision of complete access and seeks to eliminate discrimination at all levels (*180*).

CBR programmes can also promote local action plans in low-income and middle-income countries (*181*).

Conclusion and recommendations

Many persons with disabilities need assistance and support to achieve a good quality of life and to participate in social and economic activities on an equal basis with others. Across the world most of the assistance and support services are provided informally by family members or social networks. While informal care is invaluable, it is sometimes unavailable, inadequate or insufficient. Formal provision of assistance and support services, by contrast, is insufficient, especially in low-income settings: state supply of services is generally underdeveloped, not-for-profit organizations have limited coverage, and private markets rarely offer enough support to meet the needs of people with disabilities. The result is significant unmet need for assistance and support services.

A multitude of stakeholders have roles in ensuring that adequate assistance and support services are accessible to persons with disabilities. Government's role is to ensure equal access to services including through making policies and implementing them; regulating service provision including setting standards and enforcing them; funding services for people with disabilities who cannot afford to purchase services; and if needed, organizing the provision of services. In planning and introducing formal assistance and support services, careful consideration should be given to avoiding disincentives for informal care. Service users and disabled peoples' organizations and other NGOs should increase awareness, lobby for the introduction of services, participate in policy development and monitor implementation of policies and service provision. Service providers should provide the highest quality of services. Through international cooperation, good and promising cost-effective practices should be shared and technical assistance provided to countries that are introducing assistance and support services.

This chapter has discussed some of the models of organizing, funding, and delivering formal assistance and support services. No single model of support services will work in all contexts and meet all needs. Person-centred services are preferable, so that individuals are involved in decisions about the support they receive and have maximum control over their lives. The following measures are recommended for countries introducing or developing assistance and support services.

Support people to live and participate in the community

Provide services in the community, not in residential institutions or segregated settings. For countries that have previously relied on institutional living:

- Plan adequately for the transition to a community-based service model, including human resources and sufficient funding for the transition phase.
- Progressively develop and reallocate resources to build community support services, including the possible transformation of institutions into alternative care services such as resource or day care centres.

Foster development of the support services infrastructure

- Include the introduction and development of formal assistance and support services – customized to different economic and social environments – in national disability action plans to improve participation of persons with disabilities.
- Support the development of a range of providers – state, not-for-profit providers, for-profit entities, and individuals – and models to meet, in a cost-effective manner, the diverse assistance and support needs of people with disabilities.
- Consider a variety of financing measures including: contracting out services to private providers, offering tax incentives, and devolving budgets to people with

disabilities and their families for direct purchases of services.

- In low-income and middle-income countries, support service provision through civil society organizations, which can expand the coverage and range of services. CBR programmes have been effective in delivering services to very poor and underserved areas.

Ensure maximum consumer choice and control

This is more likely to be achieved by formal services when:

- Services are individualized and flexible rather than "one size fits all" agency-based and controlled services.
- Consumers are involved in decisions on the type of support and direct the care tasks wherever possible rather than being a passive recipient of care.
- Providers are accountable to consumers and their relationship is regulated through a formal service arrangement.
- "Supported decision-making" is available for people who have difficulties making choices independently – for example, people with severe intellectual impairment or mental health conditions.

Support families as assistance and support providers

Separate the needs and rights of informal caregivers from the needs and rights of persons with disabilities. A balance must be found so that each person has independence, dignity, and quality of life.

Promote collaboration between families and family organizations, governmental and nongovernmental organizations, including disabled peoples' organizations, to provide support for families through a range of systems and services including by:

- Arranging for respite care, which can provide a short break from care and psychosocial counselling to improve family well-being.

- Providing direct or indirect financial support.
- Providing information about the services available for caregivers and people with disabilities.
- Organizing opportunities for families, who share similar experiences in supporting relatives with disabilities, to come together and offer mutual information and support.

Community-based rehabilitation workers, social workers, or community workers can provide these opportunities for families. Useful family-oriented approaches also include developing communities of care and social networks.

Step up training and capacity building

Effective assistance and support services require training of both care recipients and care providers, irrespective of whether the care is provided formally or informally.

- Formal support workers, regardless of setting and service, should be provided with relevant professional training, which takes into account the principles of the CRPD and preferably involves people with disabilities as trainers to sensitize and familiarize service providers with their future clients.
- Provide training to families on working with caregivers, defining roles, setting boundaries, and on how to empower their relative with disability.
- In low-income settings, community-based rehabilitation programmes can provide training to people with disabilities and their families to manage their support needs and create links with self-help groups for information and advice.
- Persons with disabilities directly employing support workers using allocated public funds may need training and assistance in recruitment, management and fulfilling their employer responsibilities.
- Training schemes for sign-language interpreters and advocacy workers will help improve supply of these vital personnel.

Improve the quality of services

To ensure that formal assistance and support services are of good quality, the following are recommended:

- Develop sound and fair disability assessment criteria and procedures, focusing on support needs to maintain and improve functioning. Use ICF as a guiding framework in developing disability assessment criteria.
- Develop clear eligibility criteria for assistance and support services and transparent decision-making processes. In resource-constrained environments, focus on people with disabilities most in need of support services – those without any informal caregiver and limited means.
- Set standards of services, enforce them, and monitor compliance.
- Monitor service provision.
- Keep updated records of users, providers, and services provided.
- Ensure coordination across different government agencies and service providers, possibly through introducing case management, referral systems, and electronic record-keeping.
- Establish complaints mechanisms.
- Introduce mechanisms to detect and prevent physical and sexual abuse in both residential and community settings.
- Ensure that support staff have appropriate training, proper levels of pay, status, and working conditions.
- Encourage the monitoring of service quality by disabled peoples' organizations and other NGOs.

References

1. *Convention on the Rights of Persons with Disabilities*. Geneva, United Nations, 2006 (http://www2.ohchr.org/english/law/disabilities-convention.htm, accessed 16 May 2009).
2. Verdonschot MM et al. Community participation of people with an intellectual disability: a review of empirical findings. *Journal of Intellectual Disability Research: JIDR*, 2009,53:303-318. doi:10.1111/j.1365-2788.2008.01144.x PMID:19087215
3. Takamine Y. The cultural perspectives of independent living and self-help movement of people with disabilities. *Asia Pacific Journal on Disability*, 1998, 1 (http://www.dinf.ne.jp/doc/english/asia/resource/z00ap/002/z00ap00208.html, accessed 15 July 2009).
4. Misra S, Orslene LE, Walls RT. Personal assistance services for workers with disabilities: views and experiences of employers. *Journal of Rehabilitation*, 2010,76:22-27.http://findarticles.com/p/articles/mi_m0825/is_1_76/ai_n50152435/accessed 5 April 2010.
5. *People with Disabilities in India: From Commitments to Outcomes*. Washington, World Bank, 2009 (http://imagebank.worldbank.org/servlet/WDSContentServer/IW3P/IB/2009/09/02/000334955_20090902041543/Rendered/PDF/502090WP0Peopl1Box0342042B01PUBLIC1.pdf, accessed 5 June 2010).
6. Fisher K, Jing L. Chinese disability independent living policy. *Disability & Society*, 2008,23:171-185. doi:10.1080/09687590701841216
7. Saetermoe C, Gómez J, Bámaca M, Gallardo C. A qualitative enquiry of caregivers of adolescents with severe disabilities in Guatemala City. *Disability and Rehabilitation*, 2004,26:1032-1047. doi:10.1080/09638280410001703512 PMID:15371040
8. *World Development Report: Making Services Work for Poor People*. Washington, World Bank, 2004.
9. *Principles for implementation of CRPD Article 12*. New York, International Disability Alliance, CRPD Forum, 2008 (http://www.internationaldisabilityalliance.org/representation/legal-capacity-working-group/, accessed 20 August 2009).
10. *From exclusion to equality: realizing the rights of persons with disabilities. Handbook for parliamentarians on the Convention on the Rights of Persons with Disabilities and its Optional Protocol*. Geneva, United Nations, 2007 (http://www.un.org/disabilities/default.asp?id=212, accessed 20 August 2009).
11. Jesperson M. Personal ombudsman in Skåne: a user-controlled service with personal agents. In: Stastny P, Lehmann P, eds. *Alternatives beyond psychiatry*. Shrewsbury, United Kingdom, Peter Lehmann Publishing, 2007:299–303.
12. Canadian Association for Community Living [web site]. (http://www.cacl.ca/, accessed 20 August 2009).
13. Nidus Personal Planning Resource Center and Registry [web site]. (http://www.rarc.ca/textual/home.htm, accessed 20 August 2009).
14. Personal Ombud programme in Skåne, Sweden [web site]. (http://www.po-skane.org/, accessed 20 August 2009).

15. Kroll T, Neri MT. Experiences with care co-ordination among people with cerebral palsy, multiple sclerosis, or spinal cord injury. *Disability and Rehabilitation*, 2003,25:1106-1114. doi:10.1080/0963828031000152002 PMID:12944150

16. *ICF Australian user guide*, version 1. Canberra, Australian Institute of Health and Welfare, 2003.

17. *Participation and activity limitation survey*. Ottawa, Statistics Canada, 2001.

18. *Household disability survey*. Wellington, Statistics New Zealand, 2001.

19. *Adult disability follow-back surveys*. Hyattsville, United States National Center for Health Statistics, 1998.

20. *Understanding the health-care needs and experiences of people with disabilities*. Menlo Park, Kaiser Family Foundation, 2003.

21. Brodsky J, Habib J, Hirschfeld M. *Key policy issues in long term care*. Geneva, World Health Organization, 2003.

22. Anonymous Disability advocate who speaks her mind. *China Development Brief*, 1 October, 2001 (http://www.chinadevelopmentbrief.com/node/182, accessed 28 November 2008).

23. Clark P, Macarthur J. Children with physical disability: gaps in service provision, problems joining in. *Journal of Paediatrics and Child Health*, 2008,44:455-458. doi:10.1111/j.1440-1754.2008.01327.x PMID:18557807

24. Napier J. Sign language interpreter training, testing, and accreditation: an international comparison. *American Annals of the Deaf*, 2004,149:350-359. doi:10.1353/aad.2005.0007 PMID:15646939

25. Yarger CC. Educational interpreting: understanding the rural experience. *American Annals of the Deaf*, 2001,146:16-30. PMID:11355073

26. Nkwangu R. Sign language and community based rehabilitation (CBR). In: Hartley S, Okune J, eds. *CBR: inclusive policy development and implementation*. Norwich, University of East Anglia, 2008:214–231.

27. Haualand H, Allen C. *Deaf people and human rights*. Helsinki, World Federation of the Deaf and Swedish National Association of the Deaf, 2009.

28. McConkey R. Fair shares? Supporting families caring for adult persons with intellectual disabilities. *Journal of Intellectual Disability Research*, 2005,49:600-612. doi:10.1111/j.1365-2788.2005.00697.x PMID:16011553

29. Nageswaran S. Respite care for children with special health care needs. *Archives of Pediatrics & Adolescent Medicine*, 2009,163:49-54. doi:10.1001/archpediatrics.2008.504 PMID:19124703

30. *World population ageing, 1950–2050*. New York, United Nations Department of Economic and Social Affairs, 2002 (http://www.un.org/esa/population/publications/worldageing19502050/index.htm, accessed 20 November 2008).

31. *Kenya at a glance*. New York, United Nations Children's Fund, 2008 (http://www.unicef.org/kenya/overview_4616.html, accessed 1 April 2010).

32. Ahmad OB, Lopez AD, Inoue M. The decline in child mortality: a reappraisal. *Bulletin of the World Health Organization*, 2000,78:1175-1191. PMID:11100613

33. Knodel J, Chayovan N. Intergenerational relationships and family care and support for Thai elderly. *Ageing International*, 2009,33:15-27. doi:10.1007/s12126-009-9026-7

34. Malhotra R, Kabeer N. *Demographic transition, inter-generational contracts and old age security: an emerging challenge for social policy in developing countries*. Brighton, University of Sussex, Institute of Development Studies, 2002 (IDS Working Paper No. 157).

35. Jenkins A et al. *The future supply of informal care 2003 to 2013: Alternative scenarios*. Canberra, Australian Institute for Health and Welfare, 2003.

36. Budlender D. *The statistical evidence on care and non-care work across six countries*. Geneva, United Nations Research Institute for Social Development, 2008.

37. Dahlberg L, Demack S, Bambra C. Age and gender of informal carers: a population-based study in the UK. *Health & Social Care in the Community*, 2007,15:439-445. doi:10.1111/j.1365-2524.2007.00702.x PMID:17685989

38. Rogers M, Hogan D. Family life with children with disabilities: the key role of rehabilitation. *Journal of Marriage and the Family*, 2003,65:818-833. doi:10.1111/j.1741-3737.2003.00818.x

39. Hartley S et al. How do carers of disabled children cope? The Ugandan perspective. *Child: Care, Health and Development*, 2005,31:167-180. doi:10.1111/j.1365-2214.2004.00464.x PMID:15715696

40. Esplen E. *Gender and care overview report*. Brighton, BRIDGE, Institute of Development Studies, University of Sussex, 2009 (http://www.bridge.ids.ac.uk/reports_gend_CEP.html#Care, accessed 16 June 2009).

41. Carmichael F, Charles S. The opportunity costs of informal care: does gender matter? *Journal of Health Economics*, 2003,22:781-803. doi:10.1016/S0167-6296(03)00044-4 PMID:12946459

42. Anderson L et al. Children with disabilities: social roles and family impacts in the NHIS-D. *DD Data Brief*, 2002, 4(1) (http://rtc.umn.edu/docs/dddb4-1.pdf, accessed 28 July 2009).

43. Parish SL et al. Economic implications of caregiving at midlife: comparing parents with and without children who have developmental disabilities. *Mental Retardation*, 2004,42:413-426. doi:10.1352/0047-6765(2004)42<413:EIOCAM>2.0.CO;2 PMID:15516174

44. Aldridge J, Sharpe D. *Pictures of young caring*. Loughborough, University of Loughborough, 2007.

45. Becker S, Becker F. *Service needs and delivery following the onset of caring amongst children and young adults: evidence-based review*. Nottingham, Young Caregivers International Research and Evaluation, Commission for Rural Communities, 2008 (http://www.ruralcommunities.gov.uk/files/CRC%20web36%20YCIRE.pdf, accessed 17 July 2009).

46. Mete C, ed. *Economic implications of chronic illness and disability in Eastern Europe and the Former Soviet Union*. Washington, World Bank, 2008.

47. Foster M et al. Personalised social care for adults with disabilities: a problematic concept for frontline practice. *Health & Social Care in the Community*, 2006,14:125-135. doi:10.1111/j.1365-2524.2006.00602.x PMID:16460362

48. Menon DK, Peshawaria R, Ganguli R. Public policy issues in disability rehabilitation in developing countries of South-East Asia. In: Thomas M, Thomas MJ, eds. *Selected readings in community based rehabilitation: disability and rehabilitation issues in South Asia*. Bangalore, APDRJ Group Publication, 2002.

49. Bigby C, Ozanne E, Gordon M. Facilitating transition: elements of successful case management practice for older parents of adults with intellectual disability. *Journal of Gerontological Social Work*, 2002,37:25-43. doi:10.1300/J083v37n03_04

50. Heller T, Caldwell J, Factor A. Aging family caregivers: policies and practices. *Mental Retardation and Developmental Disabilities Research Reviews*, 2007,13:136-142. doi:10.1002/mrdd.20138 PMID:17563896

51. Morris J. *Pride against prejudice*. London, Women's Press, 1991.

52. McKee KJ et al. COPE PartnershipThe COPE index–a first stage assessment of negative impact, positive value and quality of support of caregiving in informal carers of older people. *Aging & Mental Health*, 2003,7:39-52. doi:10.1080/1360786021000006956 PMID:12554314

53. Askheim O. Personal assistance: direct payments or alternative public service? Does it matter for the promotion of user control? *Disability & Society*, 2005,20:247-260. doi:10.1080/09687590500060562

54. Thompson L. *Long-term care: support for family caregivers*. Washington, Georgetown University, 2004.

55. Braddock D, Hemp R, Rizzolo M. *The state of the states in developmental disabilities*, 7th ed. Washington, American Association on Intellectual and Developmental Disabilities, 2008.

56. *Australia's welfare 2007*. Canberra, Australian Institute of Health and Welfare, 2007 (Cat. No. 93).

57. Guerriere DN et al. Costs and determinants of privately financed home-based health care in Ontario, Canada. *Health & Social Care in the Community*, 2008,16:126-136. doi:10.1111/j.1365-2524.2007.00732.x PMID:18290978

58. Holland D. Grass roots promotion of community health and human rights for people with disabilities in post-communist Central Europe: a profile of the Slovak Republic. *Disability & Society*, 2003,18:133-143. doi:10.1080/0968759032000052798

59. Kandyomunda B et al. The role of local NGOs in promoting participation in CBR. In: Hartley S, ed. *Community-based rehabilitation (CBR) as a participatory strategy in Africa*. Cornell University ILR School, New York, 2002.

60. *Disabled children's action group (DICAG) South Africa*. Manchester, United Kingdom, Enabling Education Network, 2001 (http://www.eenet.org.uk/key_issues/parents/stories/dicag.shtml, accessed 25 February 2008).

61. Fisher WF. Doing good? The politics and antipolitics of NGO practice. *Annual Review of Anthropology*, 1997,26:439-464. doi:10.1146/annurev.anthro.26.1.439

62. Weigand C, Grosh M. *Levels and patterns of safety net spending in developing and transition countries*. Washington, World Bank, 2008 (SP Discussion Paper No. 0817).

63. *Home-based long-term care: report of a WHO study group*. Geneva, World Health Organization, 2000.

64. Vecchio N. The use of support systems by informal caregivers: an Australian experience. *Australian Journal of Primary Health*, 2008,14:27-34.

65. Razavi S. *The political and social economy of care in a development context: contextual issues, research questions and policy options*. Geneva, United Nations Research Institute for Social Development, 2007.

66. Lu Y. *The limitations of NGOs: a preliminary study of non-governmental social welfare organisations in China*. London, Center for Civil Society, London School of Economics and Political Science, 2003 (CCS International Working Paper No. 13) (http://www.lse.ac.uk/collections/CCS/pdf/IWP/IWP13LuYiyi.pdf, accessed 25 November 2008).

67. Fu T. Good will is not enough. *China Development Brief*, 2002 (http://www.chinadevelopmentbrief.com/node/161, accessed 26 July 2006).

68. The Future Supply of Long-Term Care Workers in relation to The Aging Baby Boom Generation – Report to United States Congress. Washington, United States Department of Health and Human Services, 2003 (http://aspe.hhs.gov/daltcp/reports/ltcwork.pdf, accessed 27 May 2010).

69. Blok W. Social Work in Poland: a helping profession in need. *Social Work and Society Online News Magazine*, 2007 (http://www.socmag.net/?p=97, accessed 27 May, 2010).

70. Chu LW, Chi I. Nursing homes in China. *Journal of the American Medical Directors Association*, 2008,9:237-243. doi:10.1016/j.jamda.2008.01.008 PMID:18457798

71. *Occupational employment and wages, May 2005*. Washington, United States Bureau of Labor Statistics, 2006.

72. *Employment aspects and workforce implications of direct payments*. Leeds, United Kingdom, Skills for Care, 2008 (http://www.skillsforcare.org.uk, accessed 24 March 2010).

73. Jorgensen D et al. The providers' profile of the disability support workforce in New Zealand. *Health & Social Care in the Community*, 2009,17:396-405. doi:10.1111/j.1365-2524.2008.00839.x PMID:19220491

74. Mcfarlane L, Mclean J. Education and training for direct care workers. *Social Work Education*, 2003,22:385-399. doi:10.1080/02615470309140

75. Ehrenreich B, Hochschild A, eds. *Global women: nannies, maids and sex workers in the new economy*. London, Granta, 2003.

76. Scull A. *Museum of Madness: The Social Organization of Insanity in Nineteenth Century England*. New York, St. Martin's Press, 1979.

77. Wright D, Digby A, eds. *From Idiocy to Mental Deficiency: historical perspectives on people with learning disabilities*. London, Routledge, 1996.

78. Miller EJ, Gwynne GV. *A life apart: a pilot study for residential institutions for the physically handicapped and the young chronic sick*. London, Tavistock, 1972.

79. Zinkin P, McConachie H, eds. *Disabled children and developing countries*. London, Mac Keith Press, 1995.

80. Ingstad B, Whyte SR, eds. *Disability and culture*. Berkeley, University of California Press, 1995.

81. Turmusani M. *Disabled people and economic needs in the developing world: a political perspective from Jordan*. Aldershot, United Kingdom, Ashgate Publishing, 2003.

82. Parmenter TR. The present, past and future of the study of intellectual disability: challenges in developing countries. *Salud Pública de México*, 2008,50:Suppl 2s124-s131. PMID:18470339

83. Borbasi S et al. 'No going back' to institutional care for people with severe disability: reflections on practice through an interpretive study. *Disability and Rehabilitation*, 2008,30:837-847. doi:10.1080/09638280701419359 PMID:17852275

84. Disability Rights International [website]. (http://www.disabilityrightsintl.org/, accessed 8 March 2011).

85. Kozma A, Mansell J, Beadle-Brown J. Outcomes in different residential settings for people with intellectual disability: a systematic review. *American Journal on Intellectual and Developmental Disabilities*, 2009,114:193-222. doi:10.1352/1944-7558-114.3.193 PMID:19374466

86. Dobrzyńska E, Rymaszewska J, Kiejna A. [Needs of persons with mental disorders–definitions and literature review] *Psychiatria Polska*, 2008,42:515-524. PMID:19189596

87. Freidson E. *Profession of Medicine: a study of the sociology of applied knowledge*. Chicago, University of Chicago Press. 1988

88. Barnes C, Mercer G. *Independent Futures: creating user-led disability services in a disabling society*. Bristol, Policy Press, 2006.

89. Catty JS et al. Day centers for severe mental illness. *Cochrane database of systematic reviews (Online)*, 2007,1CD001710- PMID:17253463

90. Perrins K, Tarr J. The quality of day care provision to encourage the transition to adulthood for young women with learning difficulties. *Research in Post-Compulsory Education*, 1998,3:93-109. doi:10.1080/13596749800200027

91. Stewart S. The use of standardized and non-standardized assessments in a social services setting: implications for practice. *British Journal of Occupational Therapy*, 1999,62:417-423.

92. Mak AKM, Mackenzie A, Lui MHL. Changing needs of Chinese family caregivers of stroke survivors. *Journal of Clinical Nursing*, 2007,16:971-979. doi:10.1111/j.1365-2702.2006.01754.x PMID:17462048

93. Mirza I, Tareen A, Davidson LL, Rahman A. Community management of intellectual disabilities in Pakistan: a mixed methods study. *Journal of Intellectual Disability Research: JIDR*, 2009,53:559-570. doi:10.1111/j.1365-2788.2009.01176.x PMID:19504727

94. Roelands M, Van Oost P, Depoorter AM. Service use in family caregivers of persons with dementia in Belgium: psychological and social factors. *Health & Social Care in the Community*, 2008,16:42-53. doi:10.1111/j.1365-2524.2007.00730.x PMID:18181814

95. Charlton J. *Nothing about us without us: disability oppression and empowerment*. Berkeley and Los Angeles, University of California Press, 2000.

96. Riddell S et al. The development of direct payments: implications for social justice. *Social Policy and Society*, 2005,4:75-85. doi:10.1017/S1474746404002209

97. Shakespeare T, Gillespie-Sells K, Davies D. *The sexual politics of disability: untold desires*. London, Cassell, 1996.

98. Adams L. *The right to live in the community: making it happen for people with intellectual disabilities in Bosnia and Herzegovina, Montenegro, Serbia and Kosovo*. Sarajevo, Disability Monitor Initiative for South East Europe, Handicap International Regional Office for South East Europe, 2008.

99. Agnetti G. The consumer movement and compulsory treatment: a professional outlook. *International Journal of Mental Health*, 2008,37:33-45. doi:10.2753/IMH0020-7411370403

100. Sobsey D. *Violence and abuse in the lives of people with disabilities: the end of silent acceptance?* Baltimore, Brookes Publishing, 1994.

101. Brown H. *Safeguarding adults and children with disabilities against abuse*. Strasbourg, Council of Europe, 2002.

102. *The Standard Rules on the Equalization of Opportunities for Persons with Disabilities*. Adopted by the United Nations General Assembly, forty-eighth session, resolution 48/96, annex, of 20 December 1993. New York, United Nations, 1993 (http://www.un.org/esa/socdev/enable/dissre00.htm, accessed 27 July 2009).

103. Mansell J, Ericsson K, eds. *Deinstitutionalisation and community living: intellectual disability services in Britain, Scandinavia and the USA*. London, Chapman and Hall, 1996.

104. Braddock D, Emerson E, Felce D, Stancliffe RJ. Living circumstances of children and adults with mental retardation or developmental disabilities in the United States, Canada, England and Wales, and Australia. *Mental Retardation and Developmental Disabilities Research Reviews*, 2001,7:115-121. doi:10.1002/mrdd.1016 PMID:11389566

105. Laragy C. Individualised funding in disability services. In: Eardley T, Bradbury B, eds. *Competing visions: refereed proceedings of the National Social Policy Conference 2001*. Sydney, Social Policy Research Center, University of New South Wales, 2002:263–278.

106. Mansell J. Deinstitutionalisation and community living: progress, problems and priorities. *Journal of Intellectual & Developmental Disability*, 2006,31:65-76. doi:10.1080/13668250600686726 PMID:16782591

107. Better health, better lives: children and young people with intellectual disabilities and their families. Bucharest, World Health Organization Europe, 2010 (Background paper for the conference, 26–27 November) (http://www.euro.who.int/__data/assets/pdf_file/0003/126408/e94421.pdf, accessed 6 January 2011).

108. Chiriacescu D. *Shifting the paradigm in social service provision: making quality services accessible for people with disabilities in South East Europe*. Sarajevo, Disability Monitor Initiative for South East Europe, Handicap International Regional Office for South East Europe, 2008.

109. *Protection of disabled persons*. Bucharest, Romania Ministry of Labour, 2009 (http://www.mmuncii.ro/pub/imagemanager/images/file/Statistica/Buletin%20statistic/2009/handicap4_68.pdf, accessed 5 April 2010).

110. Mansell J et al. *Deinstitutionalisation and community living—outcomes and costs: report of a European study* [Volume 2: Main report]. Canterbury, Tizard Center, University of Kent, 2007.

111. Battams S, Baum F. What policies and policy processes are needed to ensure that people with psychiatric disabilities have access to appropriate housing? *Social Science & Medicine (1982)*, 2010,70:1026-1034. doi:10.1016/j.socscimed.2009.12.007 PMID:20116916

112. Davis D, Fox-Grage W, Gehshan S. *Deinstitutionalization of persons with developmental disabilities: a technical assistance report for legislators*. Denver, National Conference of State Legislatures, 2000 (http://www.mnddc.org/parallels2/pdf/00-DPD-NCS.pdf, accessed 28 July 2009).

113. Hallam A et al. Service use and costs of support 12 years after leaving hospital. *Journal of Applied Research in Intellectual Disabilities*, 2006,19:296-308. doi:10.1111/j.1468-3148.2006.00278.x

114. Chou YC et al. Outcomes and costs of residential services for adults with intellectual disabilities in Taiwan: A comparative evaluation. *Journal of Applied Research in Intellectual Disabilities*, 2008,21:114-125. doi:10.1111/j.1468-3148.2007.00373.x

115. Stancliffe R, Lakin C. *Costs and outcomes of community services for people with intellectual disabilities*. Baltimore, Brookes Publishing, 2004.

116. Dinkinć M, Momčilović J. *Cost of independence: cost-benefit analysis of investing in the organization of personal assistant service for persons with disabilities in Serbia*. Belgrade, Institute G17 Plus and Center for Independent Living, 2007.

117. Glendinning C et al. *Evaluation of the individual budgets pilot program*. York, University of York, 2008.

118. Mayo-Wilson E, Montgomery P, Dennis JA. Personal assistance for children and adolescents (0–18) with intellectual impairments. *Cochrane database of systematic reviews (Online)*, 2008,3CD006858- PMID:18646172

119. Montgomery P, Mayo-Wilson E, Dennis JA. Personal assistance for older adults (65+) without dementia. *Cochrane database of systematic reviews (Online)*, 2008,1CD006855- PMID:18254118

120. Mayo-Wilson E, Montgomery P, Dennis JA. Personal assistance for adults (19–64) with both physical and intellectual impairments. *Cochrane database of systematic reviews (Online)*, 2008,2CD006860- PMID:18425973

121. Mayo-Wilson E, Montgomery P, Dennis JA. Personal assistance for adults (19–64) with physical impairments. *Cochrane database of systematic reviews (Online)*, 2008,3CD006856- PMID:18646171

122. Carrin G, Mathauer I, Xu K, Evans DB. Universal coverage of health services: tailoring its implementation. *Bulletin of the World Health Organization*, 2008,86:857-863. doi:10.2471/BLT.07.049387 PMID:19030691

123. *Cutting the cake fairly: CSCI review of eligibility criteria for social care*. London, Commission for Social Care Inspection, 2008.

124. Cote A. Gate keeping: urgent need for reform to ensure fair and effective access to social protection entitlements. *Disability Monitor Initiative–Middle East Journal*, 2009,1:18-20.

125. Chisholm D, Knapp M. Funding of mental health services. In: Thornicroft G, ed. *Oxford textbook of community mental health*. Oxford, Oxford University Press, 2010.

126. Ratzka AD. *Independent living and attendant care in Sweden: a consumer perspective*. New York, World Rehabilitation Fund, 1986 (Monograph No. 34) (http://www.independentliving.org/docs1/ar1986spr.pdf, accessed 27 December 2007).

127. Lilja M, Mansson I, Jahlenius L, Sacco-Peterson M. Disability policy in Sweden. *Journal of Disability Policy Studies*, 2003,14:130-135. doi:10.1177/10442073030140030101

128. de Klerk M, Schellingerhout R. *Ondersteuning gewenst, Mensen met lichamelijke beperkingen en hun voorzieningen op het terrein van wonen, zorg, vervoer en welzijn (Support is Desired, people with physical disabilities and their support in the domains of living, care, transportation and well-being).* Den Haag, SCP, May 2006, (http://www.scp.nl/publicaties/boeken/9037702600/Ondersteuning_gewenst.pdf.

129. *You and your grants 2009/10.* Pretoria, South African Social Security Agency, 2009 (http://www.sassa.gov.za/applications/cms/documents/file_build.asp?id=100000081, accessed 26 July 2009).

130. *Disability support services: increasing participation and independence.* Wellington, Ministry of Health, 2002.

131. *International Classification of Functioning, Disability and Health.* Geneva, World Health Organization, 2001.

132. Algera M, Francke AL, Kerkstra A, van der Zee J. An evaluation of the new home-care needs assessment policy in the Netherlands. *Health & Social Care in the Community*, 2003,11:232-241. doi:10.1046/j.1365-2524.2003.00424.x PMID:12823428

133. Jones K, Netten A, Francis J, Bebbington A. Using older home care user experiences in performance monitoring. *Health & Social Care in the Community*, 2007,15:322-332. doi:10.1111/j.1365-2524.2006.00687.x PMID:17578393

134. Axelsson C, Granier P, Adams L. *Beyond de-institutionalization: the unsteady transition towards an enabling system in South East Europe.* Sarajevo, Disability Monitor Initiative for South East Europe, 2004.

135. Puri M. *Assisted decision making: does the National Trust Act deliver?* Disability India Network, n.d. (http://www.disabilityindia.org/natTrust.cfm, accessed 10 October 2008).

136. Mulvany F, Barron S, McConkey R. Residential provision for adult persons with intellectual disabilities in Ireland. *Journal of Applied Research in Intellectual Disabilities*, 2007,20:70-76. doi:10.1111/j.1468-3148.2006.00306.x

137. Mandelstam M. *Safeguarding vulnerable adults and the law.* London, Jessica Kingsley Publishers, 2009.

138. Acheson N. Service delivery and civic engagement: disability organisations in Northern Ireland *Voluntas*, 2001,12:279-293. doi:10.1023/A:1012395402144

139. Priestley M. *Disability Politics and Community Care.* London, Jessica Kingsley, 1998.

140. Hatfield B, Ryan T, Simpson V, Sharma I. Independent sector mental health care: a 1-day census of private and voluntary sector placements in seven Strategic Health Authority areas in England. *Health & Social Care in the Community*, 2007,15:407-416. doi:10.1111/j.1365-2524.2007.00698.x PMID:17685986

141. Rosenau PV, Linder SH. A comparison of the performance of for-profit and nonprofit U.S. psychiatric inpatient care providers since 1980. *Psychiatric Services (Washington, D.C.)*, 2003,54:183-187. PMID:12556598

142. McConkey R et al. Variations in the social inclusion of people with intellectual disabilities in supported living schemes and residential settings. *Journal of Intellectual Disability Research: JIDR*, 2007,51:207-217. doi:10.1111/j.1365-2788.2006.00858.x PMID:17300416

143. Lansley P et al. Adapting the homes of older people: a case study of costs and savings. *Building Research and Information*, 2004,32:468-483. doi:10.1080/0961321042000269429

144. Heller T, Caldwell J. Impact of a consumer-directed family support program on reduced out-of-home institutional placement. *Journal of Policy and Practice in Intellectual Disabilities*, 2005,2:63-65. doi:10.1111/j.1741-1130.2005.00010.x

145. Pijl M. Home care allowances: good for many but not for all. *Practice: Social Work in Action*, 2000,12:55-65.

146. Rabiee P, Moran N, Glendinning C. Individual budgets: lessons from early users' experiences, 2009. *British Journal of Social Work*, 2009,39:918-935. doi:10.1093/bjsw/bcm152

147. Carr S, Robins D. *The implementation of individual budget schemes in adult social care.* London, Social Care Institute for Excellence, 2009 (SCIE Research Briefing 20).

148. *Vulnerable groups in development: the case for targeting mental health conditions.* Geneva, World Health Organization, 2010.

149. Benjamin AE, Matthias R, Franke TM. Comparing consumer-directed and agency models for providing supportive services at home. *Health Services Research*, 2000,35:351-366. PMID:10778820

150. Kim WM, White GW, Fox MH. Comparing outcomes of persons choosing consumer-directed or agency-directed personal assistance services. *Journal of Rehabilitation*, 2006,72:32-43.

151. Clark MJ, Hagglund KJ, Sherman AK. A longitudinal comparison of consumer-directed and agency-directed personal assistance service programmes among persons with physical disabilities. *Disability and Rehabilitation*, 2008,30:689-695. doi:10.1080/09638280701463878 PMID:17852213

152. Spall P, McDonald C, Zetlin D. Fixing the system? The experience of service users of the quasi-market in disability services in Australia. *Health & Social Care in the Community*, 2005,13:56-63. doi:10.1111/j.1365-2524.2005.00529.x PMID:15717907

153. Priestley M et al. Direct payments and disabled people in the UK: supply, demand and devolution. *British Journal of Social Work*, 2007,37:1189-1204. doi:10.1093/bjsw/bcl063

154. Stevens M et al. Choosing services or lifestyles: assessing the role of increasing choice in UK social care services. *Journal of Social Policy*, forthcoming

155. Grassman EJ, Whitaker A, Larsson AT. Family as failure? The role of informal help-givers to disabled people in Sweden. *Scandinavian Journal of Disability Research*, 2009,11:35-49. doi:10.1080/15017410802253518

156. Dougherty S et al. *Planned and crisis respite for families with children: results of a collaborative study.* Arlington, Child Welfare League of America, ARCH National Respite Network and Resource Center, 2002 (http://www.archrespite.org/Collaborative%20Respite%20Report%20.pdf, accessed 15 April 2010).

157. Mansell I, Wilson C. Current perceptions of respite care: experiences of family and informal carers of people with a learning disability. *Journal of Intellectual Disabilities: JOID*, 2009,13:255-267. doi:10.1177/1744629509356725 PMID:20048347

158. *Breaking point: families still need a break.* London, Mencap, 2006 (http://www.mencap.org.uk/document.asp?id=297, accessed 15 April 2010).

159. Giménez DM. *Género, previsión y ciudadanía social en América Latina (Gender, pensions and social citizenship in Latin America).* Santiago, Economic Commission for Latin America and the Caribbean, 2005 (Serie Mujer y Desarrollo No. 46).

160. *Australia's welfare 1993: services and assistance.* Canberra, Australian Institute of Health and Welfare, 1993.

161. Caldwell J. Consumer-directed supports: economic, health, and social outcomes for families. *Mental Retardation*, 2006,44:405-417. doi:10.1352/0047-6765(2006)44[405:CSEHAS]2.0.CO;2 PMID:17132035

162. Glendinning C et al. *Individual budgets pilot program: impact and outcomes for caregivers.* York, University of York, 2009.

163. Yamada M, Hagihara A, Nobutomo K. Coping strategies, care manager support and mental health outcome among Japanese family caregivers. *Health & Social Care in the Community*, 2008,16:400-409. doi:10.1111/j.1365-2524.2007.00752.x PMID:18221487

164. Gillinson S, Green H, Miller P. *Independent living: the right to be equal citizens.* London, Demos, 2005.

165. Meyer J. A non-institutional society for people with developmental disability in Norway. *Journal of Intellectual & Developmental Disability*, 2003,28:305-308.

166. Bieler RB. Independent living in Latin America: progress in adapting a "First World" philosophy to the realities of the "Third World". In: Garcia Alonso JV, ed. *El movimiento de vida independiente: experiencias internacionales.* Madrid, Spain, Fundación Luis Vives, 2003:218–242 (http://www.disabilityworld.org/11-12_03/il/latinamerica.shtml, accessed 31 March 2010).

167. Spandler H, Vick N. Opportunities for independent living using direct payments in mental health. *Health & Social Care in the Community*, 2006,14:107-115. doi:10.1111/j.1365-2524.2006.00598.x PMID:16460360

168. Ilagan V. Breaking the barriers: enabling children with disabilities in the Philippines. *Development Outreach*, 2005 July (http://devoutreach.com/july05/SpecialReportBreakingtheBarriers/tabid/908/Default.aspx, accessed 6 April 2010).

169. Windley D, Chapman M. Support workers within learning/intellectual disability services perception of their role, training and support needs. *British Journal of Learning Disabilities*, 2010,38:310-318. doi:10.1111/j.1468-3156.2010.00610.x

170. *Determining the training needs of personal assistants working directly with personal assistance users.* London, Independent Living Alternatives, 2008 (http://www.ilanet.co.uk/id15.html, accessed 5 April 2010).

171. Finkelstein V. *Rethinking care in a society providing equal opportunities for all.* Geneva, World Health Organization, 2001.

172. Larson S, Hewitt A. *Staff recruitment, retention, training strategies for community human services organizations.* Baltimore, Brookes Publishing, 2005.

173. Kishorekumar BD. *Community based rehabilitation: an approach to empower the disabled.* Hyderabad, ICFAI Books, 2009.

174. McConkey R, Alant E. Promoting leadership and advocacy. In: Alant E, Lloyd LL, eds. *Augmentative and alternative communication and severe disabilities: beyond poverty.* London, Whurr Publishers, 2005:323–344.

175. Upadhyaya GP. *Policy, programs and activities to protect and promote the rights and dignity of persons with disabilities in Nepal.* Bangkok, Expert Group Meeting and Seminar on an International Convention to Protect and Promote the Rights and Dignity of Persons with Disabilities, 2003 (http://www.worldenable.net/bangkok2003/papernepal2.htm, accessed 25 November 2008).

176. Lysack C, Kaufert J. Comparing the origins and ideologies of the independent living movement and community based rehabilitation. *International Journal of Rehabilitation Research. Internationale Zeitschrift fur Rehabilitationsforschung. Revue Internationale de Recherches de Réadaptation*, 1994,17:231-240. PMID:8002130

177. *Community home-based care in resource limited settings: a framework for action.* Geneva, World Health Organization, 2002.

178. Australian Human Rights Commission [web site]. (www.hreoc.gov.au/disability_rights/, accessed 6 April 2010).

179. *New Zealand disability strategy.* Wellington, Ministry of Health, 2001 (www.odi.govt.nz/nzds, accessed 25 November 2008).

180. Handisam [website]. (http://www.handisam.se/Tpl/NormalPage____297.aspx, accessed 6 April 2010).

181. *CBR guidelines.* Geneva, World Health Organization, 2010.

Chapter 6

Enabling environments

"I have been forced to come up with practical solutions to face head-on with confidence an ill-equipped environment to live an active life with Muscular Dystrophy while, in parallel, campaigning for a more inclusive society. Among these private efforts, I have had to hire a driver/assistant who provides me with the support needed for transportation purposes. It is not an uncommon sight in Port-au-Prince to witness my assistant carrying me as we climb several flights of stairs, even at the tax office to pay my dues!"

Gerald

"After injury I felt that my social life has been affected so much, due to the difficulty of transportation and environment challenges, it is difficult to do the daily activities (visiting friends, going out…etc), as well as go to hospital appointments and rehabilitation. Before the injury I was an active member in the society, I had many friends and used to go out with them to do some activities and sports. But after the injury, it was difficult for me to go out with them, because the environment is not adapted for wheelchair users, either the streets, transportation, shops, restaurants, or other facilities."

Fadi

"I am joining a first gathering of a group that discusses professional topics in psychology. The meeting was very stressful and frustrating for me, since I was not able to follow the group discussion. After the session was over, I called the instructor, told her about my hearing problem, and asked her permission to pass a special microphone between the speakers, a microphone that transmits their voices straight to my hearing-aids. To my surprise the instructor refused my request and said that it was not good for the group because it would ruin the atmosphere of spontaneity."

Adva

"The hardest obstacle for my independence has been the attitude of the people. They think that we can't do many things. Also, the steps and architectural barriers. I had an experience in the Casa de la Cultura with the director. There were many steps and I couldn't enter so I sent someone to call for help and when the director came, surprised, he said 'what's happened, what's happened, why are you like this'. He thought that I was there to beg for money, and had not thought that I was working."

Feliza

"Until I was 19 years old, I had no opportunities to learn sign language, nor had Deaf friends. After I entered a university, I learned sign language(s) and played an active role as a board member of Deaf clubs. Since I completed graduate school, I worked as a bio-scientist in a national institute. I mainly communicate with my colleagues by hand-writing, while I use public sign language-interpreting service for some lectures and meetings. My Deaf partner and I have two Deaf children…my personal history gives me the distinct opinion that the sign language and Deaf culture are absolutely imperative for Deaf children to rise to the challenge."

Akio

6

Enabling environments

Environments – physical, social, and attitudinal – can either disable people with impairments or foster their participation and inclusion. The United Nations *Convention on the Rights of Persons with Disabilities* (CRPD) stipulates the importance of interventions to improve access to different domains of the environment including buildings and roads, transportation, information, and communication. These domains are interconnected – people with disabilities will not be able to benefit fully from improvements in one domain if the others remain inaccessible.

An accessible environment, while particularly relevant for people with disabilities, has benefits for a broader range of people. For example, curb cuts (ramps) assist parents pushing baby strollers. Information in plain language helps those with less education or speakers of a second language. Announcements of each stop on public transit may aid travellers unfamiliar with the route as well as those with visual impairments. Moreover, the benefits for many people can help generate widespread support for making changes.

To succeed, accessibility initiatives need to take into account external constraints including affordability, competing priorities, availability of technology and knowledge, and cultural differences. They should also be based on sound scientific evidence. Often, accessibility is more easily achievable incrementally – for example, by improving the features of buildings in stages. Initial efforts should aim to build a "culture of accessibility" and focus on removing basic environmental barriers. Once the concept of accessibility has become ingrained and as more resources become available, it becomes easier to raise standards and attain a higher level of universal design.

Even after physical barriers have been removed, negative attitudes can produce barriers in all domains. To overcome the ignorance and prejudice surrounding disability, education and awareness-raising is required. Such education should be a regular component of professional training in architecture, construction, design, informatics, and marketing. Policy-makers and those working on behalf of people with disabilities need to be educated about the importance of accessibility.

The information and communication environment is usually constructed by corporate bodies with significant resources, a global reach and – sometimes – experience with issues of accessibility. As a result new technologies with universal designs are usually adopted more quickly in the virtual rather than in the built environment. But even with the rapid

---

Box 6.1. Definitions and concepts

Accessibility – in common language, the ability to reach, understand, or approach something or someone. In laws and standards on accessibility, it refers to what the law requires for compliance.

Universal design – a process that increases usability, safety, health, and social participation, through design and operation of environments, products, and systems in response to the diversity of people and abilities (1).

Usability, though, is not the only goal of universal design, and "adaption and specialized design" are a part of providing customization and choice, which may be essential for addressing diversity. Other overlapping terms for the same general concept are "design for all" and "inclusive design".

Standard – a level of quality accepted as a norm. Sometimes standards are codified in documents such as "guidelines" or "regulations", both with specific definitions, with different legal implications in different legal systems. An example is Part M of the Building Regulations in the United Kingdom of Great Britain and Northern Ireland. Standards can be voluntary or compulsory.

Public accommodations – buildings open to and provided for the public, whether publicly owned (such as courts, hospitals, and schools) or privately owned (such as shops, restaurants, and sports stadia) as well as public roads.

Transportation – vehicles, stations, public transportation systems, infrastructure, and pedestrian environments.

Communication – "includes languages, text displays, Braille, tactile communication, large print, and accessible multimedia as well as written, audio, plain-language, human-reader and augmentative and alternative modes, means, and formats of communication, including accessible information and communication technology" (2). These formats, modes, and means of communication may be physical, but are increasingly electronic.

---

development of information and communication technology (ICT), accessibility can be limited by unaffordability and unavailability. As new technologies are created in rapid succession, there is a danger that access for people with disabilities will be overlooked and that expensive assistive technologies will be opted for, rather than universal design.

This chapter focuses on the environmental barriers to gaining access to buildings, roads, transport and information and communication and the measures needed to improve access (see Box 6.1).

Understanding access to physical and information environments

Access to public accommodations – **buildings and roads** – is beneficial for participation in civic life and essential for education, health care, and labour market participation (see

Box 6.2). Lack of access can exclude people with disabilities, or make them dependent on others (6). As an example, if public toilets are inaccessible, people with disabilities will find it difficult to participate in everyday life.

Transportation provides independent access to employment, education, and health care facilities, and to social and recreational activities. Without accessible transportation, people with disabilities are more likely to be excluded from services and social contact (7, 8). In a study in Europe, transport was a frequently cited obstacle to the participation of people with disabilities (9). In a survey in the United States of America lack of transportation was the second most frequent reason for a person with disability being discouraged from seeking work (10). The lack of public transportation is itself a major barrier to access, even in some highly developed countries (11).

A lack of accessible **communication and information** affects the life of many disabled people (12–14). Individuals with communication difficulties, such as hearing impairment or

Box 6.2. Political participation

Article 29 of the United Nations *Convention on the Rights of Persons with Disabilities* (CRPD) guarantees political rights to people with disabilities, first by highlighting the importance of accessible voting processes, electoral information and the right of people with disabilities to stand for election, and second, by advocating for people with disabilities to form and join their own organizations and participate in political life at every level.

Enabling environments are critical to promoting political participation. Physical accessibility of public meetings, voting booths and machines, and other processes is necessary if people with disabilities are to participate. Accessibility of information – leaflets, broadcasts, web sites – is vital if people are to debate issues and exercise informed choice. For example, sign language and closed captioning on party political broadcasts would remove barriers to deaf people and those with hearing loss. People who are confined to their home or live in institutions may need postal voting or proxy voting to exercise their franchise. The wider question of attitudes is also relevant to whether people with disabilities are respected as part of the democratic process – as voters, election observers, commentators or indeed elected representatives – or identify with mainstream society (*3*). In particular, people with intellectual impairments and mental health conditions often face discriminatory exclusion from the voting process (*4*).

The International Foundation for Electoral Systems has worked in different countries to promote voter registration and remove barriers to participation by people with disabilities as voters and as candidates, for example, a voter education programme in Iraq, registration and voting support in Kosovo (in association with OSCE) and initiatives in Armenia, Bangladesh, and other countries. In the United Kingdom the voluntary organization United Response has campaigned and developed resources to promote electoral participation of people with intellectual impairments (*5*).

In India, while the 1995 Disability Act guaranteed equal opportunities to disabled people, this had no impact on subsequent electoral processes. The disability movement in India campaigned vigorously for access to the political system, particularly in the run-up to the 2004 elections. The Supreme Court passed an interim order for state governments to provide ramps in all polling booths for the second round of voting in 2004, with Braille information to be available in future elections. In 2007 the Supreme Court passed an order by which the Election Commission was directed to instruct all the State Governments and Union Territories to make the following provisions for the 2009 General Elections:

- Ramps in all polling stations.
- Braille numbers by ballot buttons on Electronic Voting Machines.
- Separate queues for disabled people at polling stations.
- Electoral staff trained to understand and respect the needs of people with disabilities.

As a result of the campaigning and awareness-raising, the leading parties explicitly mentioned disability issues in their 2009 manifestos.

Increased political participation of people with disabilities may result in progress towards more disability-inclusive public policy. While progress has been achieved in making elections accessible, it is rare for people with disabilities to be elected to public positions. However, in countries including the United States, the United Kingdom, Germany, Ecuador, and Peru, persons with disabilities have held the highest office. In Uganda Section 59 of the Constitution of 1995 states that "Parliament shall make laws to provide for the facilitation of citizens with disabilities to register and vote," while Section 78 provides for representation of people with disabilities in Parliament. People with disabilities are elected through an electoral college system at all levels from village up to Parliament, giving influence which has resulted in disability-friendly legislation. Uganda has among the highest numbers of elected representatives with disabilities in the world.

Further information: http://www.electionaccess.org; http://www.ifes.org/disabilities.html; http://www.every-votecounts.org.uk.

speech impairment, are at a significant social disadvantage, in both developing and developed countries (15). This disadvantage is particularly experienced in sectors where effective communication is critical – such as those of health care, education, local government, and justice.

- People who are hard of hearing may need speech-reading, assistive listening devices, and good environmental acoustics in indoor settings (16). Deaf and deafblind people use sign languages. They need bilingual education in sign language and the national language, as well as sign language interpreters, including tactile or hands-on interpreters (17, 18). According to World Health Organization (WHO) estimates, in 2005, around 278 million people worldwide have moderate to profound hearing loss in both ears (19).
- People who are blind or have low vision require instruction in Braille, equipment to produce Braille materials, and access to library services that provide Braille, audio and large-print materials, screen readers, and magnification equipment (20, 21). About 314 million people around the world have impaired vision, due either to eye diseases or uncorrected refractive errors. Of this number, 45 million people are blind (22, 23).
- People with intellectual impairments need information presented in clear and simple language (24). People who have severe mental health conditions need to encounter healthworkers who have the communication skills and confidence to communicate effectively with them (25).
- Non-speaking individuals need access to "augmentative and alternative communication" systems and acceptance of these forms of communication where they live, go to school and work. These include communication displays, sign language and speech-generating devices.

Available empirical evidence suggests that people with disabilities have significantly lower rates of ICT use than non-disabled people (26–29). In some cases they may be unable to access even basic products and services such as telephones, television and the Internet.

Surveys on access to and the use of digital media in developed countries have found that disabled people are half as likely as non-disabled people to have a computer at home, and even less likely to have Internet access at home (30, 31). The concept of the digital divide refers not only to physical access to computers, connectivity, and infrastructure but also to the geographical, economic, cultural and social factors – such as illiteracy – that create barriers to social inclusion (31–36).

Addressing the barriers in buildings and roads

Prior to the CRPD the main instrument addressing the need for improved access was the United Nations *Standard Rules on Equalization of Opportunities for Persons with Disabilities*, which lacked enforcement mechanisms. A United Nations survey in 2005 of 114 countries found that many had policies on accessibility, but they had not made much progress (37). Of those countries, 54% reported no accessibility standards for outdoor environments and streets, 43% had none for public buildings, and 44% had none for schools, health facilities, and other public service buildings. Moreover, 65% had not started any educational programmes, and 58% had not allocated any financial resources to accessibility. Although 44% of the countries had a government body responsible for monitoring accessibility for people with disabilities, the number of countries with ombudsmen, arbitration councils, or committees of independent experts was very low.

The gap between creating an institutional and policy framework and enforcing it has been ascribed to various factors, including:
- lack of financial resources;
- a lack of planning and design capacity;

- limited research and information;
- a lack of cooperation between institutions;
- a lack of enforcement mechanisms;
- a lack of user participation;
- geographic and climatic constraints;
- a lack of a disability-awareness component in the training curricula of planners, architects and construction engineers.

Reports from countries with laws on accessibility, even those dating from 20 to 40 years ago, confirm a low level of compliance (38–41). A technical survey of 265 public buildings in 71 cities in Spain found that not a single building surveyed was 100% compliant (40), and another in Serbia found compliance rates ranging between 40% and 60% (40). There are reports from countries as diverse as Australia, Brazil, Denmark, India, and the United States of similar examples of non-compliance (39, 40, 42, 43). There is an urgent need to identify the most effective ways of enforcing laws and regulations on accessibility – and to disseminate this information globally.

Developing effective policies

Experience shows that voluntary efforts on accessibility are not sufficient to remove barriers. Instead, mandatory minimum standards are necessary. In the United States, for example, the first voluntary accessibility standard was introduced in 1961. When it became clear that the standard was not being used, the first law on accessibility, covering all federal buildings, was passed in 1968, after which standards were generally adhered to (44). In most countries that took measures early on, accessibility standards have evolved over time, especially in the domain of public accommodations. Recently some countries, such as Brazil, have extended their laws to private businesses that serve the public.

In new construction, full compliance with all the requirements of accessibility standards is generally feasible at 1% of the total cost (45–47). Making older buildings accessible requires

flexibility, because of technical constraints, issues of historic preservation and variability in the resources of the owners. Laws, such as the 1990 Americans with Disabilities Act in the United States and the Disability Discrimination Act of 1995 in the United Kingdom, introduced legal terms such as "reasonable accommodations", "without undue hardship", and "technically infeasible". These terms provided legally acceptable ways in which to accommodate the constraints in existing structures. The concept of "undue hardship", for example, allows more leeway to small businesses than to large corporations in making renovations that are costly because of the nature of existing structures.

Expanding the scope of buildings covered by laws and standards after introducing a first stage of accessibility may be a better approach than trying to make everything fully accessible. For developing countries, a strategic plan with priorities and a series of increasing goals can make the most of limited resources. Policy and standards might, in the first instance, treat traditional construction in low-income rural areas differently from other types of construction – focusing, perhaps, on ground-floor access and access to public toilets. After experimenting with different approaches for a limited period, more extensive standards might be introduced, based on knowledge of what works. The CRPD refers to this strategy as "progressive realization".

Improving standards

Standards for accessibility can create an enabling environment (38–40). Evaluations of existing standards have found generally low awareness about the existence of standards. For those aware of the standards, concerns were raised about their appropriateness, especially for resource-poor settings, including rural areas with traditional forms of construction and informal settlements. Relief workers, for instance, have reported accessibility standards to be inappropriate for the problems in refugee camps and reconstruction projects following natural disasters (48).

Contemporary standards have been developed through a largely consensual process. The participation of people with disabilities in developing standards is important for providing insight about the needs of users. But a systematic, evidence-based approach to standards is also needed. Evaluations of the technical accessibility provisions in high-income settings have found that wheelchair clearance and space requirements are often too low (49, 50). These shortcomings stem from the changing characteristics of assistive technology such as bigger wheelchairs, from the advances in knowledge about how to facilitate access, and from the time lag for incorporating new knowledge into standards.

The basic features of access in new construction should include:

- provision of curb cuts (ramps)
- safe crossings across the street
- accessible entries
- an accessible path of travel to all spaces
- access to public amenities, such as toilets.

A compilation of data on 36 countries and areas in Asia and the Pacific showed that 72% have accessibility standards for either the built environment or public transport or both. An assessment of the content of standards and coverage is required to understand the scope and application of these norms (51). Most accessibility standards concentrate on the needs of people with mobility impairments. The relevant standards, for instance, contain many criteria to ensure enough space and manoeuvring clearances for wheelchair and walking-aid users. It is also important to meet the needs of people with sensory impairments, primarily avoiding hazards and finding the right way. To this end, communication methods have been devised – including visual alarms and better contrasts on signs, Braille signage, tactile paving, and dual modes on interactive devices, such as automated teller machines in banks and ticket machines.

Accessibility standards rarely explicitly address the needs of people with cognitive impairments or mental health conditions.

Universal design guidelines do deal with matters such as better support for finding the way and for reducing stress which can be considered in accessibility standards (52).

Appropriate standards are needed for rural construction in developing countries. A study on accessibility in rural villages in Gujarat, India, found that current practices in affluent urban areas in India were not appropriate in these villages (53). Other studies on accessibility for persons with disability in developing countries have focused on hygiene and the use of water (54, 55) and proposed simple, low-cost solutions to make toilet facilities, water-carrying devices, water stands, and other facilities accessible.

Standards on accessibility are also needed in refugee camps and in informal settlements and reconstruction projects after a disaster. Studies of informal settlements in India and South Africa have found that the conditions there, as in poor rural areas, require different approaches to accessibility than urban areas – providing access to squat toilets and overcoming open drains, which create obstacles for wheelchair and pedestrian use. The serious security and privacy barriers in these communities are as important as independence in carrying out daily tasks (56). The Sphere Handbook, developed by more than 400 organizations around the world, sets out the minimum standards in a disaster response and includes approaches for meeting the needs of people with disabilities. In its 2010 update disability is addressed as an issue cutting across all the main sectors, including water supply, sanitation, nutrition, food aid, shelter, and health services (57).

Standards in industrialized countries have driven a "global convergence" in accessibility standards (8) rather than standards in developing countries reflecting cultural or economic conditions (58). Whether this accounts for the lack of implementation of accessibility laws and standards in many countries requires further research.

The International Organization for Standardization developed an international accessibility standard using a consensual approach, though not all regions of the world are represented on the committee (*59*). International and regional organizations can help improve standards by providing recommendations for member countries. The European Concept for Accessibility Network has taken this approach by publishing a technical manual to help organizations develop standards and regulations incorporating universal design (*60*).

An international effort is needed to develop standards appropriate for different stages of policy evolution, different levels of resources, and cultural differences in construction.

Enforcing laws and regulations

The reporting guidelines for the CRPD obliges States Parties to report on progress in achieving Article 9 (Accessibility). Systematic comparison is difficult, but several practices can lead to better enforcement:

- **Laws with mandatory access standards** are the most effective way to achieve accessibility. The first accessibility standard in the world – a voluntary one in the Unites States – demonstrated a very low level of adoption (*44*). Similar results are reported in other countries (*39–41, 61*). Standards and compliance should be regulated and mandated by law.
- **Good design reviews and inspections** ensure that accessibility will be provided from the day a building is completed. Accessibility standards thus need to be part of building regulations. The delays caused by the denial of permits for construction or occupancy should provide an incentive for builders and developers to meet the rules. If there are no design reviews or inspections, the law can require effective penalties for non-compliance, as well as a mechanism for identifying non-compliance and correcting the offence. Government funding agencies – including those that fund health care facilities, transportation, and schools – can also review plans as part of their approval process, using consistent standards.
- **Accessibility audits** can also be conducted by disability organizations – or even by individual citizens. Such audits can encourage compliance. In Malaysia, for example, groups working on behalf of disabled people are completing audits of major hotels (see Box 6.3).

The lead agency

A lead government agency can be designated to take responsibility for coordinating the activities of other bodies involved with accessibility, particularly those that fund the construction of public buildings and monitoring the implementation of laws, regulations, and standards. Furthermore, it could oversee the licensing of design professionals, businesses, and services to ensure that accessibility is part of professional training curricula.

Implementing accessibility programmes requires adequate funding for the lead agency and other responsible agencies. Appropriate financing mechanisms need to be developed at various budget levels to ensure efficient flow of funding. There may often be penalties for non-compliance in access legislation, but the law may not be enforced, because of a lack of resources (*38*).

Monitoring

Monitoring and evaluation of the implementation of accessibility laws and standards will provide information to make continual improvements in accessibility for people with disabilities. An impartial monitoring body, preferably outside government, could be designated and funded to provide periodic independent evaluations of progress on accessibility laws and standards and to recommend improvements, as with the United States National Council on Disability (*62, 63*). This body should have a significant membership of people with disabilities. Without such monitoring, there will be no pressure on governments to move towards full accessibility.

In addition to an official monitoring body, a network of local action organizations

---

Box 6.3. Buildings without barriers in Malaysia

In recent years Malaysian law has been changed to ensure that people with disabilities have the same rights and opportunities as others. Between 1990 and 2003 Malaysia introduced and revised the standard codes of practice on accessibility and mobility for people with disabilities. In 2008 the People with Disabilities Act was introduced. This legislation, harmonizing with the CRPD, promotes rights of access for persons with disabilities to public facilities, housing, transport, and ICT, as well as to education and employment, cultural life and sport.

The government priorities are to increase public awareness of the needs of disabled people and to encourage young designers to create more innovative and inclusive designs. Local authorities in the country require architects and builders to adhere to the Malaysian Standard Codes of Practice for building plans to be approved. After a building is constructed, an "access audit" examines its usability by disabled people. The purpose of this audit is:

- to increase awareness among planners and architects about barrier-free environments for people with disabilities;
- to ensure, in both new buildings and retrofitting, the use of universal design concepts and adherence to the standard codes relating to people with disabilities;
- to evaluate the degree of access to existing public buildings and recommend improvements.

University schools of architecture can be a focus of education and research efforts for both students and practicing professionals. The International Islamic University in Malaysia recently introduced "barrier-free architecture" as an elective subject in its Bachelor of Architecture programme. In addition, the new Kaed Universal Design Unit at the university's Kulliyyah School of Architecture and Urban Design seeks to:

- create awareness of design issues for children, disabled people and older people;
- conduct research and develop new technologies;
- disseminate information;
- educate the design profession and the public on design regulations.

---

is essential for supporting the process. Such a network can also share information and help local building officials to review building plans, ensuring that a lack of knowledge among officials and designers does not undermine the goals of the law.

- In Norway, after a monitoring exercise found that few local communities had carried out any accessibility planning, the government set up pilot projects around the country, to make local communities better able to provide accessibility for people with disabilities (*64*).
- In Winnipeg, Canada, a local action group worked with the municipal administration in an assessment of barriers, with recommendations for their removal (*65*).
- In Kampala, Uganda, following the development of accessibility standards in association with the government, a National Accessibility Audit Team was created by Uganda National Association on Physical Disability (*66*).

There is an important role for people with disabilities and other members of the general public to be vigilant and seek redress, through legal and administrative actions, when building owners do not fulfil their obligations under the law. A combination of regulation, persuasion, and powerful interest groups can be most effective (see **Box 6.3**) (*67*).

Education and campaigning

Education, along with technical assistance on enforcement procedures, is essential to improve awareness of the need for accessibility and understanding of universal design. Educational programmes should be targeted to all those involved in enforcing accessibility laws and standards – including people with disabilities, design educators and professionals (*68*), government regulators, business owners and managers, and building developers and contractors (see **Box 6.4**).

Box 6.4. Creating an environment for all in India

India had outlined provisions for accessibility in the Persons with Disabilities Act, 1995 and building by-laws on accessibility. Research in four districts of Gujarat, India – by a local development organization, UNNATI Organisation for Development Education – identified accessibility to physical spaces as a key area for mainstreaming the rights of people with disabilities. A project was launched to build awareness in the region on accessibility, increase the capacity for local action, and build strategic alliances for advocacy by:

- setting up an informal "access resource group", bringing together architects, builders, designers, engineers, people with disabilities, and development and rehabilitation professionals;
- staging public events highlighting what can be done to improve access; greater stress was placed on the message that "access benefits all". Campaigns had the greatest impact when user groups acted collectively for their rights;
- conducting media training;
- holding workshops on accessibility, including national policies on disability and access;
- producing educational materials.

Initially, the access group contacted public and private institutions to raise awareness on the need for better accessibility. Within two years, they were receiving requests for audits. In these audits, members of the access group worked with people with disabilities to formulate technical recommendations.

Between 2003 and 2008, 36 audits were conducted of parks, government offices, academic institutions, banks, transport services, development organizations, and public events. Modifications were made in about half the venues, including:

- providing accessible parking spaces, ramps, and lifts
- installing accessible toilets
- adjusting counter heights
- providing tactile maps and improving signage.

For example, with government support, the State Administrative Training Institute for government officials in Ahmedabad, the state capital, has become a model of accessible building. Programmes of modifications required regular follow-up to support the implementation of recommendations for standard specifications. The maintenance of access features was best achieved when both users and managers of a space were aware of the importance of these features.

The project has shown architects and builders how to comply with the access provisions in the Persons with Disabilities Act 1995 and local access by-laws. A design institute in Ahmedabad now offers an elective course on universal design. People with disabilities have seen benefits in greater dignity, comfort, safety, and independence. All the same, non-compliance has resulted in new barriers. Accessibility for people with visual impairments remains a problem, with signage standards not commonly followed due to limited information in accessible user-friendly formats.

Source (69).

Adopting universal design

Universal design is practical and affordable, even in developing countries (53, 54). Simple examples in lower income settings include:

- a seating platform next to a communal hand pump to provide an opportunity for rest and enable small children to reach the pump (54);
- ramped access and a concrete apron at the pump post to help wheelchair users, making it possible to bring large, wheeled water containers to the village pump and reduce the number of trips (53);
- a bench fitted over a pit latrine, making latrine use easier (54).

An important application for universal design is to provide for emergency evacuations from buildings. Experience from major disasters has shown that people with disabilities and older people are often left behind (*70*). Other problems can also arise, such as when people dependent on ventilators are moved by unprepared first responders (*71*). In many places, work is being done on finding better management approaches for emergencies by improving building design, providing training, and running preparedness exercises (*72, 73*). Universal design can also help in enabling communications and assistance during evacuations, with new technologies ensuring that people with sensory and cognitive impairments are kept informed about the emergency and not left behind.

Addressing the barriers in public transportation

Worldwide, initiatives to develop accessible public transportation systems focus primarily on:

- improving accessibility to public transportation infrastructure and services;
- setting up "special transport services" for people with disabilities;
- developing campaigns and education programmes to improve policies, practices, and the use of services.

Specific obstacles are related to each of these goals.

Lack of effective programmes. Even where laws on accessible transportation exist, there is limited degree of compliance with the laws, especially in developing countries (*7, 74*). The benefits of universal design features are often not well understood. For this reason, many policy initiatives are not incorporated – such as using raised boarding platforms at the entrance to buses to reduce the boarding times for all passengers, as well as increasing accessibility (*7*).

Obstacles to special transport services and accessible taxis. Special transport services (STS) are designed specifically for people with disabilities or for other groups of passengers unable to access public or private transportation independently. STSs and taxis are forms of "demand-responsive transport" providing service only when requested by the customer. But accessible vehicles are expensive to purchase, and the cost to the provider of operating the service is high. And if demand increases, for example due to population ageing, the economic burden of STS, if provided by a public agency, can become unsustainable (*75, 76*).

For the service user, availability is often limited because of eligibility requirements and travel restrictions. While taxis are potentially a very good way to supplement accessible public transit, most taxi services do not provide accessible vehicles. In addition, there have been many instances of discrimination by taxi operators against people with disabilities (*77, 78*).

Physical and information barriers. Typical barriers in transportation include inaccessible timetable information, a lack of ramps for vehicles, large gaps between platforms and vehicles, a lack of wheelchair anchoring in buses, and inaccessible stations and stops (*7, 79*).

Existing commuter rail systems and ferries are particularly difficult to make accessible because of variations in platform heights, platform gaps, and vehicle designs (*80*). Improved visual environments are needed to accommodate people with visual impairments and elderly people – for example, with colour-contrasting railings and better lighting (*8*).

Lack of continuity in the travel chain. The "travel chain" refers to all elements that make up a journey, from starting point to destination – including the pedestrian access, the vehicles, and the transfer points. If any link is inaccessible, the entire trip becomes difficult (*81*). Many mass transit providers, particularly in developing countries, have implemented accessibility only partially, for example by providing a limited number of accessible vehicles on each route, making improvements only to the main stations, and providing access only on new lines.

Without accessibility throughout the travel chain, the job is incomplete. Inaccessible links require taking an indirect route, creating the barrier of longer travel times. The goal must be for people to have access to all vehicles and the full service area, as well as the pedestrian environment (82). But progressive realization may be the most practical short-term response.

Lack of pedestrian access. A major obstacle to maintaining continuity of accessibility in the travel chain is an inaccessible pedestrian environment, particularly in the immediate surroundings of stations. Common problems here include:

- nonexistent or poorly maintained pavements;
- inaccessible overpasses or underpasses;
- crowded pavements in the vicinity of stations and stops;
- hazards for people with visual impairments and deafblind people;
- lack of traffic controls;
- lack of aids at street crossings for people with visual impairments;
- dangerous local traffic behaviours.

These can be a particular problem in low-income urban environments.

Lack of staff awareness and other barriers. Operators of transport often do not know how to use the accessibility features that are available or how to treat all passengers safely and courteously. Outright discrimination by operators, such as not stopping at a bus stop, is not uncommon. Operating rules may conflict with the need to assist people with disabilities. In many places there are no fixed procedures for identifying and resolving problems with the service. Overcrowding, a major problem, particularly in developing countries, contributes to disrespectful behaviour towards passengers with disabilities.

Improving policies

Including access to transportation as part of the overall legislation on disability rights is a step towards improving access. Standards for accessibility in developed countries, however, are not always affordable or appropriate in low-income and middle-income countries (7). Solutions should be found to meet challenges specific to developing country contexts. Where aid programmes provide significant funding to build new mass transit systems, access requirements can be included.

Coordinated political action, both national and local, is needed to pass laws and ensure that laws are enforced. Local action is particularly important, not only when new systems are planned, but also to keep a running check on operations. National organizations in many countries have expertise in accessible transportation. Because of their special knowledge, they often receive government funding to document and disseminate best practices and offer training programmes to transport providers and to local groups working on behalf of disabled people.

National laws and rules on funding can oblige local transit authorities to have advisory bodies consisting of people with disabilities.

Fare structures are a critical element of local transit policies: reduced or free fares for people with disabilities, funded by local or national government, are a feature of most accessible public transportation initiatives, as in the Russian Federation.

Providing special transport services and accessible taxis

Transportation agencies can be required by law to provide STS as part of their service. In such a case this may be an incentive for agencies to increase accessibility in the overall system due to the eventual high cost of providing STS. While STS initially appears less costly and easier to implement than removing barriers to mass transportation, relying on that alone for accessible transport leads to segregation. And in the longer term it may result in high and possibly unsustainable costs as the proportion of older people in the population increases.

Shared vans. Shared vans equipped with lifts, individually owned and operated by

179

licensed providers, can be a viable way to start an STS programme for fairly small initial public investment. In India a team of designers found inexpensive ways of making small vans accessible for people with disabilities, with costs as low as US$ 224 (*83*). Having a wider passenger base can help make shared van services more sustainable in the longer term. In Curitiba, Brazil, owner-operated vans with lifts pick up passengers for a flat-rate fare.

Accessible taxis. Accessible taxis are an important part of an integrated accessible transportation system because they are highly demand-responsive (*77, 84*). Taxis and STSs are now being combined in many places. Sweden relies extensively on taxis for its STS, as do other countries (*77, 85*). In developing countries, accessible taxis are slower to come on line. Licensing regulations can require taxi fleets not to discriminate against people with disabilities. They can also require some or all vehicles to be accessible. In the United Kingdom a special initiative to make taxis accessible has resulted in a fleet that is 52% accessible (*86*).

Flexible transport systems. Innovative universal design solutions could increase availability and affordability. Information technology is making it possible to optimize routes and assign passengers to specific vehicles in real-time while vehicles are on the road. Originally developed in Sweden using a fleet of shared ride vans and since introduced in some other European countries, these "flexible transport systems" (FTSs) provide services on demand, at about half the cost of a taxi and with greater flexibility in reservation times, availability, and routes (*85*). The cost of accessible taxis, though, and the infrastructure for an FTS, may be prohibitive for some developing countries (but note the examples of affordable van solutions from India and Brazil). As these innovations are adopted more widely, there should be attempts to make them cheaper and bring them to low-income and middle-income countries.

Universal design and removing physical barriers

Making every vehicle entrance-accessible in existing systems may require purchasing new vehicles and, in some cases, renovating stops and stations. In Helsinki, Finland, the existing tram system was made accessible by using both these methods. The stops in the middle of the road are on safety islands equipped with short ramps at each end, accessed from the middle of marked pedestrian crossings. The islands are at the same level as the low floors of the new vehicles. Passengers can now wait in a safer environment, and there is no need to mount steps to enter the vehicle.

Portable lifts or manual folding ramps can create access to existing vehicles. But such solutions should be viewed as temporary, because they require properly trained attendants available for every vehicle arrival or departure. Nor are elevated small platforms served by lifts or ramps the most effective solutions because of the difficulty of stopping a train or bus in exactly the right position.

Rail systems. Bus and tram systems can potentially be renovated at relatively low cost over time as new vehicles go into service. But renovating existing rail systems presents various technical difficulties, including (*80*):

- dealing with the size of the gaps between vehicle floors and the platforms, which may be different at every station (*87*);
- increasing space in vehicles for wheelchair access;
- providing access to tracks at different levels within stations.

Technologies for automated lifts, bridgeplates, and ramps overcome the problems with platforms. Some new accessible cars can be provided on each train, and their number can be increased over time. Old single-level cars can be renovated to provide space by removing existing seats or replacing them with folding seats. Elevators or inclined lifts to reach upper or lower platforms can also be installed. A useful starting initiative is to make the main stations fully accessible, along with accessible bus transportation from the accessible stations to the locations served by the inaccessible stations.

In time more stations can be made accessible. Following the Transportation Accessibility Improvement Law (2000), the Tokyo subway system has become significantly more accessible: in 2002, 124 of the 230 stations in the Tokyo area had lifts; by 2008, 188 had lifts. A web site offers information on accessible routes.

Bus rapid transit systems. Large cities – including Beijing (China) and New Delhi (India) – have embarked on major programmes to upgrade their public transport, often using rail (*88*). There is a global trend towards "bus rapid transit" which is particularly pronounced in developing countries of Central and South America and of Asia. Low-floor buses are often used to provide access. Accessible bus rapid transit systems have been constructed in Curitiba (Brazil), Bogotá (Colombia), Quito (Ecuador) and more recently Ahmedabad (India) and Dar es Salaam (United Republic of Tanzania) (*88*). When cities host important international events new transit lines are often added to accommodate the expected large numbers of people attending (*80*). Although there can be resistance to new services from existing taxi operators and local residents (*89*), these projects offer the opportunity to create a good model that can subsequently be applied more widely in the country.

Alternative forms of transport. Rickshaw and pedicab services, common in many Asian cities, are gaining in popularity on other continents. An Indian design team has developed a type of pedicab that is easier for people with disabilities to get in and out of, improving access for all users and providing more comfort for the driver (*83*). Installing separate lanes and paths for bicycles, tricycles, and scooters can improve safety and accommodate the larger tricycle-style wheelchairs often used in Asia.

Universal design. Universal design is increasingly being adopted in bus and rail

transit operations in high-income countries, as in Copenhagen's underground rail system (*76, 90, 91*). The most important universal design innovation is the low-floor transit vehicle, adopted for heavy rail, light rail, trams, and buses, providing almost level access from curbs and short-ramp access from street levels.

Other examples of universal design include:

- lifts or ramps on all transit vehicles – not only on a limited number;
- a raised pad at a bus stop with ramp access, making it easier for someone with mobility impairment to enter a bus, helping visually impaired and cognitively impaired individuals find the stop, and improving the safety of all those waiting for a bus (*79*);
- real-time information on waiting times;
- smart cards for fare collection, gates, and ticketing;
- visual and tactile warning systems at the edge of platforms – or full safety barriers along the entire platform;
- railings and posts painted in bright contrasting colours;
- audible signs to help people with visual impairments find gates and identify buses.
- web access to real-time information about accessible routes and temporary obstacles, such as a lift out of order (*80*).

Many of the universal design innovations mentioned above are generally too expensive for developing economies. Affordable universal design concepts are needed for low-income and middle-income countries. More research is needed to develop and test for effectiveness solutions that are inexpensive and appropriate for such countries. Some simple low-cost examples of universal design include:

- lower first steps;
- better interior and exterior handrails at entrances to buses;
- priority seating;
- improved lighting;
- raised paved loading pads where there are no pavements;
- the removal of turnstiles.

Box 6.5. Integrated public transport in Brazil

In 1970 the city of Curitiba, Brazil, introduced a modern transportation system designed from the start to replace a system of many poorly coordinated private bus lines. The aim was to provide public transport that would be so effective that people would find little need for private transport. The system was to provide full accessibility for people with disabilities, as well as benefits for the general population from the adoption of universal design. The new system includes:

- express bus lines with dedicated right-of-way routes into the city centre;
- conventional local bus routes connecting at major terminals;
- interline "connector" buses travelling around the perimeter of the city;
- "Parataxi" vans for door-to-terminal service for those requiring them.

All terminals, stops, and vehicles are designed to be accessible. At terminals used by different types of transport, local buses deliver passengers to the stops on the express bus system. The vehicles are large "bus-trains" – two-unit or three-unit articulated buses, each carrying 250–350 people. These bus-trains load and unload directly onto raised platforms with the help of mechanized bridge plates that span the platform gap. All express bus terminals have ramps or lifts.

Private individuals operate the "parataxi" vans. Originally, these were designed specifically for people with disabilities, as a means of getting from their homes to a station. There was not enough demand, though, to make the vans economically viable on this basis, and they are now available for all passengers.

The Curitiba system is a good example of universal design. It gives a high level of access, and the integrated system of local routes, interline routes, and express routes provides a convenient and seamless means of travelling. The vehicles for each type of line are colour-coded, making them easy to distinguish for those who do not read. Although there are newer rapid-transit systems in existence, lessons can be learned from Curitiba.

- Even in developing countries accessibility can be provided relatively easily throughout a transportation system if it is an integral part of the overall plan from the start.
- Platform boarding allows for the convenient and rapid movement of passengers and provides full accessibility.
- The construction of "tube" stations requires the express buses to stop at a distance from the edge of the platform, to avoid hitting the curved station walls. In Curitiba, the emphasis was on improving the boarding and alighting from vehicles for people with mobility impairments. While certain features help other people with disabilities to find their way around the system, more attention needs to be paid to people with sensory and cognitive impairments.

Curitiba's integrated system is a good model of a less expensive universal design approach (see Box 6.5). Delhi Metro also incorporated universal design features in the design phase at little extra cost (*43*).

Assuring continuity in the travel chain

Establishing continuity of accessibility throughout the travel chain is a long-term goal. Creating steady improvements over a longer period requires campaigning, intelligent policy-making with appropriate resource allocation, and effective monitoring. Methods for achieving the goal include (*8, 92*):

- determining the initial priorities, through consultations with people with disabilities and service providers;
- introducing accessibility features into regular maintenance and improvement projects;
- developing low-cost universal design improvements that result in demonstrable benefits to a wide range of passengers, thus gaining public support for the changes.

Improving the quality of pavements and roads, installing ramps (curb cuts), and ensuring access to transport facilities is a key aspect of the travel chain and indispensable for people with disabilities. Planning pedestrian access to stations involves a range of agencies – including highway departments, local business groups, parking authorities, and public safety departments – and would benefit from involvement by people with disabilities. Neighbourhood participation will contribute local knowledge – such as the location for pedestrian crossings on dangerous streets. Independent organizations with special expertise in pedestrian planning and design can help with local surveys and plans.

Improving education and training

Continual education of all those involved in transportation can make sure that an accessible system is developed and maintained (*92*). Education should start with training for managers, so that they understand their legal obligations. Front-line staff need training about the range of disabilities, discriminatory practices, how to communicate with people with sensory impairments, and the difficulties people with disabilities face when using transport (*93*). People with disabilities can usefully be involved in such training programmes and through the programmes establish valuable communications links with transport staff. Disabled people's groups also can collaborate with transport managers to set up "secret rider" programmes, in which people with various disabilities travel on transport as passengers to uncover discriminatory practices. Public awareness campaigns are a part of the educational process: posters, for instance, can teach passengers about priority seating.

Barriers to information and communication

Accessible information and communication technology covers the design and supply of information and communication technology products (such as computers and telephones) and services (telephony and television)

including web-based and phone-based services (*94–98*). It relates to the **technology** – for example, control and navigation, through twisting a knob or clicking a mouse, and to the **content** – the sounds, images, and language produced and delivered by the technology.

ICT is a complex and fast-growing industry, worth some US$ 3.5 trillion worldwide (*99*). An increasing number of basic functions of society are organized with and delivered by ICT (*100, 101*). Computer interfaces are used in many areas of public life – from banking machines to ticket dispensers (*102*). Automation is often promoted as a cost-saving measure by dispensing with human interfaces, yet this can disadvantage those persons with disabilities – and others – who will always need personal assistance with some tasks (*103*).

In particular, the Internet is increasingly a channel for conveying information about health, transport, education and many government services. Major employers rely on online application systems for recruitment. Accessing general information online enables people with disabilities to overcome any potential physical, communication and transport barriers in accessing other sources of information. ICT accessibility is therefore needed for people to participate fully in society.

People with disabilities, once they are able to access the web, value the health information and other services provided on it (*31*). For example, one survey of Internet users with mental health conditions found that 95% used the Internet for diagnostic-specific information, as opposed to 21% of the general population (*104*). Online communities can be particularly empowering for those with hearing or visual impairments or autistic spectrum conditions (*105*) because they overcome barriers experienced in face-to-face contact. People with disabilities who are isolated value the Internet in enabling them to interact with others and potentially to conceal their difference (*104, 106*). For example, in the United Kingdom the state broadcasting company has set up a web site called "Ouch!" for people with disabilities (*107*) and created special web materials for people with intellectual impairments.

Future innovations in ICT could benefit people with disabilities and older persons by helping them overcome barriers of mobility, communication, and so on (*108*). When designing and distributing ICT equipment and services, developers should ensure that people with disabilities gain the same benefits as the wider population and that accessibility is taken into account from the outset.

Inaccessibility

Mainstream ICT devices and systems, such as telephones, television, and the Internet, are often incompatible with assistive devices and assistive technology, such as hearing aids or screen readers. Overcoming this requires:

- designing the mainstream features for the widest possible range of user capabilities;
- ensuring the device is adaptable for an even wider range of capabilities;
- ensuring the device can connect with a wide range of user interface devices (*109*).

People with disabilities should have the same choice in everyday telecommunications as other people – in access, quality, and price (*28*).

- People with hearing and speech impairments, including the deafblind, need public or personal telephones with audio outputs adjustable in volume and quality, and equipment compatible with hearing aids (*28, 110*).
- Many people need text telephones or videophones with visual displays of text, or sign language in real-time telephone communications (*111*). A relay service with an operator is also required, so that users of text telephones and videophones can communicate with users of ordinary voice telephones.
- People who are blind or deafblind and cannot access visual displays at all require other options such as speech and audio and Braille (*112*). Those with low vision need visual presentations to be adjusted for font type and size, contrast, and use of colours.

- People with dexterity impairments and upper extremity amputees may experience difficulties with devices requiring fine manipulation, such as small keyboards (*113*). Switch interfaces, alternative keyboards or use of head and eye movement can be possible solutions to access computers.
- To use computers and access the web, some people with disabilities need screen readers, captioning services, and web page design features such as consistent navigation mechanisms (*114–116*).
- People with cognitive impairments, including age-related changes in memory, and older adults may find the various devices and online services difficult to understand (*117–120*). Plain language and simple operating instructions are important.

The lack of captioning, audio description and sign language interpretation limit information access for people who are deaf and hearing impaired. In a survey conducted by the World Federation of the Deaf, only 21 of 93 countries were found to provide captioning of current affairs programmes and the proportion of programmes with sign language was very low. In Europe only one tenth of national-language broadcasts of commercial broadcasters were provided with subtitles, only five countries provided programmes with audio description, and only one country had a commercial broadcaster that provided audio description (*28*). A report on the situation in Asia has found that closed captioning or sign-language interpretation of television news broadcasts is limited (*39*). Where it is available, it is usually confined to large cities.

Furthermore, television programmes distributed over the Internet are not required to have closed captioning or video description – even if they originally contained captions or description when they were shown on television. As the dissemination of television programmes expands, moving from broadcast to cable and Internet and from analogue to digital, there is greater uncertainty over regulatory frameworks and whether the same rights to have material subtitled still pertain.

Few public and even fewer commercial web sites are accessible (*28, 116, 121*). A United Nations "global audit" examined 100 home pages on the web drawn from five sectors in 20 countries. Of these, only three achieved "single-A" status, the most basic level of accessibility (*2*). A study in 2008 found that five of the most popular social networking sites were not accessible to people with visual impairment (*122*). Surveys showing that disabled people have a much lower rate of web use than non-disabled people indicate that the barriers are associated with having a visual or dexterity impairment (*31*). Those who are deaf or have difficulties with mobility do not experience the same barriers, if socioeconomic status is controlled for.

Lack of regulation

While many countries have laws covering ICT, the extent to which these cover accessible ICT is not well documented (*51, 123*). In developed countries, many ICT sectors are not covered by existing legislation. Some important gaps include business web sites, mobile telephony, telecommunications equipment, TV equipment, and self-service terminals (*124*). Rapid development in ICT often leaves existing regulation outdated – for example, mobile phones often are not covered under legislation on telephony. Furthermore, technological developments and convergence across sectors blurs what were previously clear cut distinctions – for example, telephony over the Internet often falls outside the scope of legislation regarding landlines.

Standards for the development of ICT are lagging behind the development of accessibility standards for public accommodations and public transport. A compilation of data on 36 countries and areas in Asia and the Pacific showed that only 8 governments reported that they had accessibility standards or guidelines for ICT while 26 reported to have accessibility standards for either the built environment or public transport or both (*51*).

From a legislative and policy perspective, sectoral approaches to ICT provide challenges. It may be impractical and inefficient to consider a wide range of sectoral legislation to be developed to address the full spectrum of ICT and their applications. Consistency of standards for the same product or for services across sectors would be more difficult to achieve with this type of vertical approach. Regulating services separately from equipment has also been found unhelpful in ensuring access to all supply chain components – content production, content transmission, and content rendering through end-user equipment (*124*). A key challenge is influencing decisions in the development of products and services far enough back in the supply chain to guarantee access.

Regulation of television and video does not always keep pace with technology and service developments. For example, video carried on computers and hand-held devices is not always accessible. The United States Telecommunications Act of 1996 regulated "basic" services, such as telephony. But it did not regulate "enhanced" services, such as the Internet. This allowed the Internet to flourish without regulation, neglecting access requirements. With services converging and the distinction between basic and enhanced services steadily eroding, this has left major gaps in regulation (*125*). One study of United States web designers found that they would make web sites accessible only if the government required them to (*126*). Deregulation and self-regulation potentially undermine the scope for government action to mandate disabled access (*127*).

Cost

The high cost of many technologies limits access for people with disabilities, particularly in low-income and middle-income countries. In particular, intermediate and assistive technology are often unaffordable or unavailable. For example, a United Kingdom study found that the most common reason for people with disabilities not using the Internet was cost – of the computer, of online access, and of assistive devices (*128*). A screen reader such as JAWS can cost US$ 1000 (*102*), though there are some open source versions, such as the Linux Screen Reader. Internet-based high-speed broadband technology has only made the differences more apparent. While this technology can deliver services that people with disabilities need, such as sign-language videophone, it is often not available, and when available, its cost makes it unaffordable for many (*129*).

Pace of technological change

Assistive technology for accessing ICT quickly becomes obsolete as new technology develops at an increasing rate (*130–132*). Almost every time new technology is introduced, people with disabilities do not obtain the full benefit (*125*).

Few ICTs are designed to be inherently accessible. Ways of resolving problems of access in one generation of computer hardware or software do not always carry over to the next generation. Mainstream software upgrades, for instance, make software from the previous generation obsolete – including peripherals, such as the screen readers used by disabled people.

Addressing the barriers to information and technology

Given the wide spectrum of ICT products, services, and sectors (commerce, health, education, and so on) a multisectoral and multi-stakeholder approach is required to ensure accessible ICT. Governments, industry and end-users all have a role in increasing accessibility (*28, 97, 109, 110, 127, 133, 134*). That includes raising awareness of need, adopting legislation and regulations, developing standards and offering training.

An example of a partnership working towards these aims is G3ict, which is a public-private partnership, part of the United Nations Global Alliance for ICT and Development.

Among other activities, G3ict is assisting policy-makers around the world to implement the ICT accessibility dimension of the CRPD, with the help of a special "e-accessibility toolkit". In collaboration with the International Telecommunications Union (ITU), G3ict is also developing the first digital accessibility and inclusion index for people with disabilities. This is a monitoring tool surveying countries that have ratified the CRPD to measure how far they have implemented the digital accessibility provisions defined in it, scoring on 57 data points (*135*).

Improved ICT accessibility can be achieved by bringing together market regulation and antidiscrimination approaches along with relevant perspectives on consumer protection and public procurement (*124*). In Australia a complaint from a deaf customer led to a change in the mainstream telecommunications legislation to include a duty on operators to provide necessary equipment under equivalent conditions. Competition, rather than regulation, can also drive improvements. In Japan a civil service magazine runs an "e-city" competition, and different municipalities strive to excel in information and communication categories that include criteria for accessibility (*136*).

Those producing and providing ICT-based products and services and those deploying ICT products and services have complementary roles in providing accessible ICT (*124*). Producers and providers can incorporate accessibility features in the products and services they design and sell, and governments, banks, educational institutes, employers, travel agents, and the like can ensure that the products that they procure and use do not present access barriers to employees or customers with disabilities.

Legislation and legal action

States that currently address ICT accessibility do so through both bottom-up and top-down legislative approaches as well as non-legislative mechanisms. Top-down approaches impose direct obligations on those producing ICT products and services, such as close captioning on TVs and relay features to enable people with hearing impairments to use the telephone system. Bottom-up approaches include consumer protection and non-discrimination legislation that explicitly cover the accessibility of ICTs and protect the rights of users and consumers. For example, the Republic of Korea combines both approaches with the 2007 Korea Disability Discrimination Act and the 2009 National Informatization Act, which together provide information access rights and reasonable accommodation.

Evidence from a benchmarking study in Europe showed that countries with strong legislation and follow-up mechanisms tend to achieve higher levels of ICT access (*137*).

Legislation, such as the United States Television Circuitry Decoder Act, can be a way of ensuring that television manufacturers are required to include technology supporting closed captioning in addition to obliging cable providers to guarantee interoperability between the captioning services and receiver equipment (*126*). Legislation can also ensure subtitling of programmes. For example, the Danish Act on Radio and Television Broadcasting (2000) creates an obligation for public service television channels to promote access for disabled people, by subtitling (*138*).

Accessibility to public web sites can be addressed through a broad range of legislation directed towards the equality of persons with disabilities or as part of wider legislation on eGovernment or ICT. Vague antidiscrimination legislation, the main legislative approach for business web sites, is unlikely to be effective. Where legislation exists, regulatory gaps can be addressed through revisions such the United States 21ˢᵗ Century Communications and Video Accessibility Act and the Federal Communications Commission ruling that Voice Over Internet Protocol (the delivery of voice communications over the Internet which can improve access for visually impaired users) falls under Section 255 of the 1996 Telecommunications Act. The legislative approach can be supported by a range of support measures – awareness-raising, training, monitoring, reporting, providing technical guidelines and standards, and labelling – for providers of public web sites, as in some European countries (*124*).

Legal challenges under disability discrimination laws have led to improvements in telecommunications service in several countries. In Australia, for instance, the decision in 1995 in *Scott and DPI v. Telstra* defined telecommunications access as a human right (*100*). Title IV of the Americans with Disabilities Act directed providers of telephone services to provide relay systems for customers with hearing or speech impairments at no additional cost, and compliance has been very high (*126*).

Legal action can ensure compliance. In Australia, a landmark legal case involved a man who sued the Organizing Committee of the 2000 Olympic Games in Sydney on the grounds that its web site was not accessible. In response, the Organizing Committee claimed it would be excessively costly to make the required improvements. Even so, the Organizing Committee was found culpable by the Human Rights Equal Opportunities Commission and was fined. In Canada a complaint was filed against Air Canada because of its inaccessible ticketing kiosk. Although this was acknowledged to be a barrier, the Canadian Transport Agency rejected the complaint, because, while it doesn't comply with universal design principles, a check-in clerk could also issue boarding passes (*102*).

Where enforcement mechanisms rely on people with disabilities taking legal action, this can be expensive and time-consuming and require considerable knowledge and confidence on the part of plaintiffs. Research is not available to show how many cases are brought, how many succeed, and how the process can be improved (*126*).

Box 6.6. Laws on accessible technology

Access to information and communication needs to be addressed in a wide range of laws to ensure full access for persons with disabilities, as in the United States.

Procurement. Section 508 of the Rehabilitation Act requires electronic and information technology – such as federal web sites, telecommunications, software, and information kiosks – to be usable by people with disabilities. Federal agencies may not purchase, maintain, or use electronic and information technology that is not accessible to people with disabilities, unless creating accessibility poses an undue burden (*139*). Other jurisdictions, including states and municipalities, as well as some institutions such as colleges and universities, have adopted all or parts of Section 508.

Closed captioning. Section 713 of the Communications Act (1996) obliges distributors of video programming to provide closed captioning on 100% of new, non-exempt English-language video programmes.

Emergency services. Title II of the Americans with Disabilities Act (1990) requires direct teletypewriter access to public safety answering points. Section 255 of the Communications Act (1996) requires common carriers to provide emergency access to public safety answering points.

Hearing-aid compatible telephones. Section 710 of the Communications Act (1996) requires all essential telephones and all telephones manufactured in or imported into the United States to be hearing-aid compatible. The obligation applies to all wireline and cordless telephones and to certain wireless digital telephones. Hearing-aid compatible telephones provide inductive and acoustic connections, allowing individuals with hearing aids and cochlear implants to communicate by telephone.

Telecommunications equipment and services. Section 255 of the Communications Act (1996) requires telecommunication service providers and manufacturers to make their services and equipment accessible to and usable by people with disabilities, if these things can be readily achievable.

Telecommunications relay services. Section 225 of the Communications Act (1996) establishes a nationwide system of telecommunications relay services. The law requires that common carriers make annual contributions based on their revenues to a federally administered fund supporting the provision of these services. Telecommunication relay service providers must connect relay calls initiated by users dialling 7-1-1. This requirement simplifies access to telecommunications relay services. The user does not have to remember the toll-free number for every state, but simply dials 7-1-1 and is automatically connected to the default provider in that state (*140*).

Television decoders. The Television Decoder Circuitry Act (1990) requires television receivers with picture screens 13 inches (330 mm) or greater to contain built-in decoder circuitry to display closed captions. The Federal Communications Commission also applies this requirement to computers equipped with television circuitry sold with monitors with viewable pictures of at least 13 inches. The requirement of built-in decoder circuitry applies to digital television sets with a screen measuring 7.8 inches (198 mm) in height and to stand-alone digital television tuners and digital set-top boxes. The Act also requires closed-captioning services to be available as new video technology is developed.

Source (*140*).

Progress in achieving accessible ICT has been slow despite legislation (see Box 6.6) (*103*). As previously discussed, both top-down and bottom-up legislation is required. Other approaches, such as financial incentives for the development of accessible technologies and services, might also be fruitful. Further research and information is needed on the types of legislation and other measures that would be most appropriate to reach the various sectors and dimensions of information and communication access across different contexts is needed.

Standards

Article 9 of the CRPD calls for the development of universal design and technical standards. Guidelines and standards have generally related to product safety, though ease of use has become more important. Standards

Box 6.7. DAISY (Digital Accessible Information SYstem)

The DAISY consortium of talking-book libraries is part of the global transition from analogue to digital talking books. The aim of the consortium, launched in 1996, is to make all published information available – in an accessible, feature-rich, and navigable format – to people with print-reading disabilities. This should be done at the same time as, and at no greater cost than, for people who are not disabled. In 2005, for example, *Harry Potter and the Half-Blood Prince* was made available in DAISY format to visually impaired children on the day the story was originally published.

The consortium also works in developing countries on building and improving libraries, training staff, producing software and content in local languages, and creating networks of organizations (*141*). It also seeks to influence international copyright laws and best practices to further the sharing of materials.

DAISY collaborates with international standards organizations on standards that have the widest adoption around the world and that are open and non-proprietary. It develops tools that can produce usable content, and has intelligent reading systems. DAISY DTBOOK-XML, for instance, is a single-source document for the distribution of several formats such as hard-copy print book, EPUB e-text book, Braille book, talking book, and large-print book.

AMIS (Adaptable Multimedia Information System), available in Afrikaans, Chinese, English, French, Icelandic, Norwegian, and Tamil, is a free, open-source, self-voicing system that can be downloaded from the DAISY site.

In Sri Lanka the Daisy Lanka Foundation is creating 200 local-language and 500 English-language digital talking books, including school curriculum textbooks and university materials. The books, produced by sighted and blind students working in pairs, will be disseminated through schools for the blind and a postal library. This will allow access to a wider range of materials for the blind than currently available in Braille. Local-language talking books will also help those who are illiterate or have low vision.

organizations now take greater account of usability factors and stakeholder involvement in developing standards for ICT (*127*). Designers and manufacturers argue for voluntary standards, claiming that mandatory guidelines could restrict innovation and competition. However, unless enshrined in legislation, there may be limited compliance with standards.

Certification for accessible ICT and labelling are possible supports to improving access. The United States Rehabilitation Act Amendments of 1998 require the Access Board to publish standards for information and communication technology, including technical and functional performance criteria. Because of the size of the American market, effective regulation in the United States can drive accessibility improvements in technologies, which are then reproduced worldwide (see Box 6.6).

Different countries have achieved different levels of access, and not all technologies in developing countries have reached the access available elsewhere (*97, 109, 110, 130, 132, 141, 142*). Web Content Accessibility Guidelines

(WCAG) 1.0 remains the standard in most countries, although there is a shift towards WCAG 2.0. Efforts are under way to harmonise standards – for example, between the United States Section 508 and WCAG 2.0 accessibility requirements (*143*).

Two important developers of technical standards for accessible ICT products and services are the W3C Web Accessibility Initiative (*144, 145*) and the DAISY Consortium (*146*) (see Box 6.7).

Policy and programmes

Government telecommunications policies in several countries have improved in recent years, especially for landline phones. Where sectoral policies exist cross-cutting coordination may be indicated (*124*). Horizontal approaches may be able to address the barriers inherent in a sectoral approach. Policies on ICT accessibility in Australia, Canada, and the United States have set standards for other countries (*28, 147*). Sweden uses universal service obligations to ensure that telecommunications operators provide special services for people with disabilities. The Swedish National Post and Telecom Agency also offers speech support for people with speech and language difficulties and discussion groups for deaf-blind people (*148*).

While access to television is a fundamental problem for people who are deaf or blind, features to enable access exist (*110*). Some of these features require technological improvements to equipment – for example enabling closed captioning. Other features require policy decisions by broadcasters – for example, providing sign language interpretation for news programmes or other broadcasts (*17, 138*). Video services with audio descriptions can make the visual images of media available to those who are blind or who have low vision. Emergency alerts can be communicated by sound and caption. Radio programming is particularly helpful for people who are visually impaired.

Public sector channels are often more easily regulated or persuaded to offer accessible broadcasts (*149*). In Europe news programmes with sign language interpretation are provided in countries including Ireland, Italy, Finland, and Portugal (*138*). In Thailand and Viet Nam daily news programmes are broadcast with sign language interpretation or closed captioning. In India a weekly news programme broadcasts in sign language. China, Japan, and the Philippines encourage broadcasters to provide such programming (*39*). Elsewhere:

- In Colombia public service television is obliged to include closed captioning, subtitles, or sign language.
- In Mexico there exists a requirement for captioning.
- In Australia, where there are captioning requirements for both analogue and digital television, the target for captioning on prime time television is 70% of all programmes broadcast between 18:00 and midnight.

Further progress is possible as illustrated by Japan (Ministry of Internal Affairs and Communications) having set a target of captioning 100% of programmes where captioning is technically possible, for both live and pre-produced programmes, by 2017.

Several countries have initiatives to improve ICT accessibility such as:

- Sri Lanka has several ICT accessibility projects, including improving payphone access for people with disabilities (*110*).
- In Japan the Ministry of Internal Affairs and Communications (known until 2004 as the Ministry of Public Management, Home Affairs, Posts and Telecommunications) has set up a system to evaluate and correct access problems on web sites. The ministry also helps other government organizations make web sites more accessible for people with disabilities including older persons.
- South Africa has a National Accessibility Portal that can handle many languages. The portal is accessed by computers in service centres with accessible equipment and through a telephone interface (*142, 150*). The portal serves as a one-stop shop for information, services and communications for people with disabilities, caregivers, the medical profession, and others providing services in the field of disability.

Procurement

Procurement policies in the public sector can also promote ICT accessibility (*109, 142*). Some governments have comprehensive legislation on ICT accessibility, including procurement policies requiring accessible equipment, such as Section 508 of the United States Rehabilitation Act (*140, 147, 151*). Government procurement policies can create incentives for the industry to adopt technical standards for universally designed technology (*35, 97, 132, 134, 152, 153*). The European Parliament and other bodies within the European Union have passed resolutions on web accessibility and are harmonizing public procurement policies (*124*). The European Union included ICT accessibility in its European Action Plan, which also covered investment in the research and development of accessible ICT and suggested strengthening the provisions on accessibility (*151*). Tools are available for promoting accessible procurement, for example the Canadian Accessible Procurement Toolkit (*154*) and the United States Buy Accessible Wizard (*155*).

Universal design

Different people with disabilities prefer different solutions to access barriers, and choice is a key principle in developing accessibility (*102*).

Accessible telephone handsets for landline phones are increasingly available. In developed countries telecommunications suppliers offer telephone equipment with features including: volume control, a voice-aid facility, large buttons, and visual signal alerts; a range of teletypewriters, including a Braille teletypewriter and one with a large visual display; and adaptors for cochlear implant users.

Access innovations in mobile telephony include:

- Hand-held devices, using mobile phones as platforms, can deliver a range of services, including (*156*):
  - aids for finding the way for blind people
  - route guidance for people with motor disabilities
  - video sign-language communication for deaf people
  - memory aids for older users and people with cognitive disabilities.
- The "VoiceOver", a screen reader that "speaks" whatever appears on the display of the "iPhone" mobile device, lets visually impaired users make calls, read e-mail, browse web pages, play music, and run applications (*157*).
- The cognitive accessibility of mobile phones can be increased for people with intellectual impairments (*158*). A special phone has been designed for those who find the ordinary mobile device too complicated, with a large back-lit keyboard and simple menus and access options (*159*).

- In Australia the mobile telephone industry has launched a global information service for reporting the accessibility features of mobile phones (*160*). Australia and the United States also require that accessible information be provided with telecom equipment.
- Deaf people often use SMS (texting on mobile telephones) for face-to-face as well as long distance communication (*161*).
- In Japan the Raku Raku phone has been universally designed, with a large screen, dedicated buttons, read aloud menus, voice input text messages, and an integrated DAISY player. More than 8 million have been sold, particularly for the ageing population, previously an untapped market for mobile phone manufacturers (*162*).

Disabled people's organizations have called for universal design in computers and the web – a proactive rather than reactive approach to accessible technology (*163*). For example, screen-reader users often do not like the offer of a "text only" version of web sites, because they are less commonly updated: it is preferable to make the graphic version accessible (*164*). Raising the Floor proposes a radical new approach: building alternative interface features and services directly into the Internet, so that any users who need accessibility features can invoke the exact features they need on any computer they encounter, anywhere, anytime (*165*). Accessibility features in such operating systems as Microsoft Windows and Mac OS X already offer basic screen reading facilities, but awareness of those features is sometimes low.

Guidelines for designers and operators of web sites on how to deliver accessible content to hand-held mobile devices are also being produced by W3C (*166*).

Action by industry

There is a strong business case for removing barriers and promoting usability (*167*). This requires focusing on "pull" factors, rather than the "push" factor of regulation, as well as challenging myths that accessibility is complex, uncool, expensive, and for the few (*168*). Accessibility can offer market benefits, particularly with an ageing population. Accessible web sites and services can be easier for all customers to use – hence, the term "electronic curb cuts" (*167*).

By the end of 2008 the number of mobile phone subscribers reached 4 billion (*169*). In Africa, for example, the number of mobile telephone users increased from 54 million to almost 350 million between 2003 and 2008 – far in excess of the number of landline users (*169*). One of the largest mobile providers in China is offering a special SIM card to users with disabilities. The discounted monthly fee of the service and the low charge for text messages makes it affordable for hard-of-hearing or deaf users. Card users can recharge their account by sending a text message. The company also has an audio version of its news service that allows people with visual impairment to listen to news reports (*170*).

A United Kingdom grocery supplier with an online service has produced an accessible site in close consultation with the Royal National Institute of Blind People and a panel of visually impaired shoppers (*171*). The site offers an alternative to the high-graphic content of the mainstream version of the site. Originally designed for visually-impaired users, the site attracts a much wider audience – with many fully sighted people finding the accessible site easier to use than other sites. Spending through the site is £13 million a year, almost 400 times the original cost of £35 000 to develop the accessible site. And as a result of the access improvements, the site, at no extra cost, will be easy to use with personal digital assistants, web TV, and pocket computers with low-speed connections and limited screen sizes.

Recent research on barriers to inclusive design in communications equipment, products, and services – and on ways to address these barriers – suggests areas for improvement (*172*):

- procurement processes that require tenderers to consider accessibility and usability;
- better communication with stakeholders;
- marketing of accessible products and services as an ethical choice;
- wider access to information and mechanisms for sharing knowledge about the needs of older and disabled people.

Removing operational barriers can also enable companies to benefit from the expertise of disabled workers. For example, major corporations have led the way in ensuring that employees can access assistive technologies and promote ICT accessibility. One company achieved a 40% reduction in bandwidth costs after introducing an accessible intranet solution. Getting disabled access right can enhance reputation, as well as potentially saving costs or improving sales (*143*).

Role of nongovernmental organizations

Disabled people's organizations have campaigned for better access to ICT, based on a rights-based approach (*102*). This has included advocating for more regulation, trying to influence manufacturers and service providers to ensure access, and resorting to legal challenges in cases of non-compliance (*127*). Active involvement in nongovernmental organizations in oversight and enforcement has been identified as helpful in improving access (*124*).

Whether through organizations or as individuals, people with disabilities should be involved in the design, development, and implementation of ICTs (*102*). These steps would reduce costs and widen markets by ensuring that more people can use ICTs from the start (*126*).

Nongovernmental organizations can also undertake programmes to help persons with disabilities access to ICT – including offering related training to ensure digital literacy and skills. For example, the New Delhi branch of the Indian National Association for the Blind established a computer training and technology centre with accessible and affordable ICT for blind people and has been running initial and update courses for free since 1993. Courseware was developed in Braille, audio, large-print, and electronic-text formats to cater to people with visual impairment. Projects included developing Braille transcription software, search engines, and text-to-speech software in Hindi. Visually impaired students became trainees at the computer company sponsoring the centre. This model of training is being used in other countries. In Ethiopia the Adaptive Technology Center for the Blind, with support from United Nations Educational, Scientific and Cultural Organization (UNESCO), created a computer training centre for people who are blind or visually impaired to gain skills in the use of ICT and improve their employment opportunities (*173*).

Conclusion and recommendations

Environments can either disable people with health problems or foster their participation and inclusion in social, economic, political, and cultural life. Improving access to buildings and roads, transportation, and information and communication can create an enabling environment which benefits not only disabled people but many other population groups as well. Negative attitudes are a key environmental factor which needs to be addressed across all domains.

This chapter argues that the prerequisites for progress in accessibility are: creation of a "culture of accessibility;" effective enforcement of laws and regulations; and better information on environments and their accessibility. To succeed, accessibility initiatives need to take into account affordability, availability of technology, knowledge, cultural differences, and the level of development. Solutions that work in technologically sophisticated environments may be ineffective in low-resource settings. The best strategy for achieving accessibility is usually incremental improvement. Initial efforts should focus on removing basic environmental barriers. Once the concept of accessibility has become ingrained, and as more resources become available, it becomes easier to raise standards and attain a higher level of universal design.

Making progress in accessibility requires engagement of international and national actors, including international organizations, national governments, technology and products designers and producers, and persons with disabilities and their organizations. The following recommendations highlight specific measures that can improve accessibility.

Across domains of the environment

- Accessibility policies and standards should meet the needs of all people with disabilities.
- Monitor and evaluate the implementation of accessibility laws and standards. An impartial monitoring body, preferably outside government, and with a significant membership of disabled people, could be designated and funded to track progress on accessibility and recommend improvements.
- Awareness-raising is needed to challenge ignorance and prejudice surrounding disability. Personnel working in public and private services should be trained to treat disabled customers and clients on an equal basis and with respect.
- Professional bodies and educational institutions can introduce accessibility as a component in training curricula in architecture, construction, design, informatics, marketing, and other relevant professionals. Policy-makers and those working on behalf of people with disabilities need to be educated about the importance and public benefits of accessibility.
- International organizations can play an important role by:
  - Developing and promoting global accessibility standards for each domain of the physical environment that are widely relevant, taking into account constraints such as cost, heritage, and cultural diversity.

193

- Funding development projects that comply with relevant accessibility standards and promote universal design.
- Supporting research to develop an evidence-based set of policies and good practices in accessibility and universal design, with particular emphasis on solutions appropriate in low-income settings.
- Developing indices on accessibility and reliable methods of data collection to measure progress in improving accessibility.

■ Industry can make important contributions by promoting accessibility and universal design in the early stages of the design and development of products, programmes, and services.

■ Persons with disabilities and their organizations should be involved in accessibility efforts – for example, in the design and development of policies, products and services to assess the need of users, but also for monitoring progress and responsiveness.

Public accommodations – building and roads

■ Adopt universal design as the conceptual approach for the design of buildings and roads that serve the public.

■ Develop and mandate minimum national standards. Full compliance should be required for new construction of building and roads that serve the public. This comprises features such as ramps (curb cuts) and accessible entries; safe crossings across the street; an accessible path of travel to all spaces and access to public amenities, such as toilets. Making older buildings accessible requires flexibility.

■ Enforce laws and regulations by using design reviews and inspections; participatory accessibility audits; and by designating a lead government agency responsible for implementing laws, regulations, and standards.

■ For developing countries a strategic plan with priorities and a series of increasing goals can make the most of limited resources. Policy and standards should be flexible to account for differences between rural and urban areas.

Transportation

■ Introduce accessible transportation as part of the overall legislation on disability rights.

■ Identify strategies to improve the accessibility of public transport, including:
  - Applying universal design principles in the design and operation of public transport, for example in the selection of new buses and trams or by removing physical barriers when renovating stops and stations.
  - Requiring transportation agencies, in the short-term, to provide STS such as shared vans or accessible taxis.
  - Making public transport systems more flexible for the user by optimizing the use of information technology.
  - Make provisions for alternative forms of transport such as tricycles, wheelchairs, bicycles, and scooters by providing separate lanes and paths.

■ Establish continuity of accessibility throughout the travel chain by improving the quality of pavements and roads, pedestrian access, installing ramps (curb cuts), and ensuring access to vehicles.

■ To improve affordability of transport, subsidize transport fares for people with disabilities who may not be able to afford them.

■ Educate and train all parties involved in transportation: managers need to understand their responsibilities and front-line staff need to ensure customer care. Public awareness campaigns can assist the educational process: posters, for example, can teach passengers about priority seating.

Access standards and universal design innovations implemented in developed countries are not always affordable or appropriate in low-income and middle-income countries.

Country-specific solutions can be found. Low-cost examples include: lower first steps, better interior, and exterior handrails at entrances to buses, priority seating, improved lighting, raised paved loading pads where there are no pavements, and the removal of turnstiles.

Accessible information and communication

- Consider a range of bottom-up and top-down legislative and policy mechanisms including: consumer protection, non-discrimination legislation covering information and communication technologies and direct obligations on those developing ICT systems, products, and services.

- In the public and private sector adopt policies on procurement which take into consideration accessibility criteria.
- Support the development of telephone relay, sign language, and Braille services.
- When designing and distributing ICT equipment and services, developers should ensure that people with disabilities gain the same benefits as the wider population.
- Producers and providers should incorporate accessibility features in the products and services they design and sell.
- Support the education and training of persons with disabilities to take advantage of ICT – including training to ensure digital literacy and skills.

References

1. *Universal design*. Syracuse, Global Universal Design Commission, 2009 (http://tinyurl.com/yedz8qu, accessed 18 January 2010).
2. *United Nations global audit of web accessibility*. New York, United Nations, 2006 (http://www.un.org/esa/socdev/enable/gawanomensa.htm, accessed 17 February 2010).
3. Schur L et al. Enabling democracy: disability and voter turnout. *Political Research Quarterly*, 2002,55:167-190.
4. Redley M. Citizens with learning disabilities and the right to vote. *Disability & Society*, 2008,23:375-384. doi:10.1080/09687590802038894
5. *Making democracy accessible*. London, United Response, 2011 (http://www.unitedresponse.org.uk/press/campaigns/mda/, accessed 17 March 2011).
6. Meyers AR et al. Barriers, facilitators, and access for wheelchair users: substantive and methodologic lessons from a pilot study of environmental effects. *Social Science & Medicine (1982)*, 2002,55:1435-1446. doi:10.1016/S0277-9536(01)00269-6 PMID:12231020
7. Roberts P, Babinard J. *Transport strategy to improve accessibility in developing countries*. Washington, World Bank, 2005.
8. Venter C et al. Towards the development of comprehensive guidelines for practitioners in developing countries. In: *Proceedings of the 10th International Conference on Mobility and Transport for Elderly and Disabled Persons (TRANSED 2004), Hamamatsu, 23–26 May 2004* (http://tinyurl.com/yb7lgpk, accessed 10 February 2010).
9. Leonardi M et al. *MHADIE background document on disability prevalence across different diseases and EU countries*. Milan, Measuring Health and Disability in Europe, 2009 (http://www.mhadie.it/publications.aspx, accessed 21 January 2010).
10. Loprest P, Maag E. *Barriers to and supports for work among adults with disabilities: results from the NHIS-D*. Washington, The Urban Institute, 2001.
11. Gonzales L et al. Accessible rural transportation: an evaluation of the Traveler's Cheque Voucher Program. *Community Development: Journal of the Community Development Society*, 2006,37:106-115. doi:10.1080/15575330.2006.10383112
12. *Country report: Bolivia*. La Paz, Confederación Boliviana de la Persona con Discapacidad, 2009 (http://www.yorku.ca/drpi/, accessed 25 August 2009).
13. *State of disabled people's rights in Kenya*. Nairobi, African Union of the Blind, 2007 (http://www.yorku.ca/drpi/, accessed 25 August 2009).
14. Swadhikaar Center for Disabilities Information, Research and Resource Development. *Monitoring the human rights of people with disabilities. Country report: Andhra Pradesh, India*. Toronto, Disability Rights Promotion International, 2009 (http://www.yorku.ca/drpi/India.html, accessed 10 February 2010).
15. Olusanya BO, Ruben RJ, Parving A. Reducing the burden of communication disorders in the developing world: an opportunity for the millennium development project. *JAMA: Journal of the American Medical Association*, 2006,296:441-444. doi:10.1001/jama.296.4.441 PMID:16868302

16. *Accessibility guidelines*. Stockholm, International Federation of Hard of Hearing, 2008 (http://www.ifhoh.org/pdf/accessibilityguidelines2009.pdf, accessed 30 August 2009).

17. *Deaf people and human rights*. Stockholm, World Federation of the Deaf, Swedish National Association of the Deaf, 2009.

18. *How do people who are deaf-blind communicate?* London, Royal National Institute of the Deaf, 2009 (http://tinyurl.com/ydkwvfl, accessed 30 August 2009).

19. *Deafness and hearing impairment: fact sheet N°300*. Geneva, World Health Organization, 2010 (http://www.who.int/mediacentre/factsheets/fs300/en/index.html, accessed 1 July 2010).

20. Rowland W. Library services for blind: an African perspective. *IFLA Journal*, 2008,34:84-89. doi:10.1177/0340035208088577

21. *Annual report 2008–2009*. New Delhi, All India Confederation of the Blind, 2009 (http://www.aicb.org.in/AnnualReport/AnualReport2009.pdf, accessed 30 August 2009).

22. Resnikoff S et al. Global data on visual impairment in the year 2002. *Bulletin of the World Health Organization*, 2004,82:844-851. PMID:15640920

23. Resnikoff S et al. Global magnitude of visual impairment caused by uncorrected refractive errors in 2004. *Bulletin of the World Health Organization*, 2008,86:63-70. doi:10.2471/BLT.07.041210 PMID:18235892

24. Renblad K. How do people with intellectual disabilities think about empowerment and information and communication technology (ICT)? *International Journal of Rehabilitation Research. Internationale Zeitschrift fur Rehabilitationsforschung. Revue Internationale de Recherches de Réadaptation*, 2003,26:175-182. PMID:14501568

25. Iezzoni LI, Ramanan RA, Lee S. Teaching medical students about communicating with patients with major mental illness. *Journal of General Internal Medicine*, 2006,21:1112-1115. doi:10.1111/j.1525-1497.2006.00521.x PMID:16970561

26. Kaye HS. *Computer and Internet use among people with disabilities*. Washington, United States Department of Education, National Institute on Disability and Rehabilitation Research, 2000a (Disability Statistics Report 13).

27. Waddell C. *Meeting information and communications technology access and service needs for persons with disabilities: major issues for development and implementation of successful policies and strategies*. Geneva, International Telecommunication Union, 2008 (http://www.itu.int/ITU-D/study_groups/SGP_2006-2010/events/2007/Workshops/documents/05-success-policies.pdf, accessed 25 August 2009).

28. *Measuring progress of eAccessibility in Europe*. Brussels, European Commission, 2007 (http://ec.europa.eu/information_society/newsroom/cf/itemdetail.cfm?item_id=4280, accessed 27 August 2009).

29. Steinmetz E. *Americans with disabilities: 2002*. Washington, United States Census Bureau, 2006 (Household Economic Studies, Current Population Reports P70–107) (http://www.census.gov/hhes/www/disability/sipp/disab02/awd02.html, accessed 10 February 2010).

30. Kaye HS. *Disability and the digital divide*. Washington, United States Department of Education, National Institute on Disability and Rehabilitation Research, 2000b.

31. Dobransky K, Hargittai E. The disability divide in Internet access and use. *Information Communication and Society*, 2006,9:313-334. doi:10.1080/13691180600751298

32. *Bridging the digital divide: issues and policies in OECD countries*. Paris, Organisation for Economic Co-operation and Development, 2001 (http://www.oecd.org/dataoecd/10/0/27128723.pdf, accessed 18 August 2009).

33. Wolff L, MacKinnon S. What is the digital divide? *TechKnowLogia*, 2002, 4(3):7–9 (http://info.worldbank.org/etools/docs/library/57449/digitaldivide.pdf, accessed 19 August 2009).

34. Korean Society for Rehabilitation. *Review paper: Korea*. Paper presented at a regional workshop on "Monitoring the implementation of the Biwako Millennium Framework for action towards an Inclusive, barrier-free and right-based society for persons with disabilities in Asia and the Pacific," Bangkok, 13–15 October 2004 (http://www.worldenable.net/bmf2004/paperkorea.htm, accessed 21 August 2009)

35. The accessibility imperative: implications of the Convention on the Rights of Persons with Disabilities for information and communication technologies. *Georgia, G3ict, 2007*.

36. World Summit on the Information Society. Geneva, 18–22 May 2009 [web site]. (http://www.itu.int/wsis/implementation/2009/forum/geneva/agenda_hl.html, accessed 3 August 2009).

37. South-North Centre for Dialogue and Development. *Global survey on government action on the implementation of the standard rules on the equalization of opportunities for persons with disabilities*. Amman, Office of the UN Special Rapporteur on Disabilities, 2006:141.

38. *Regional report of the Americas 2004*. Chicago, International Disability Rights Monitor, 2004 (http://www.idrmnet.org/content.cfm?id=5E5A75andm=3, accessed 9 February 2010).

39. *Regional report of Asia 2005*. Chicago, International Disability Rights Monitor, 2005 (http://www.idrmnet.org/content.cfm?id=5E5A75andm=3, accessed 9 February 2010).

40. *Regional report of Europe 2007*. Chicago, International Disability Rights Monitor, 2007 (http://www.idrmnet.org/content.cfm?id=5E5A75andm=3, accessed 9 February 2010).

41. Michailakis D. *Government action on disability policy: a global survey*. Stockholm, Institute on Independent Living, 1997 (http://www.independentliving.org/standardrules/UN_Answers/UN.pdf, accessed 10 February 2010).

42. Mazumdar S, Geis G. Architects, the law and accessibility: architects' approaches to the ADA in arenas. *Journal of Architectural and Planning Research*, 2003,20:199-220.

43. *People with disabilities in India: from commitments to outcomes*. Washington, World Bank. 2009.

44. *Design for all Americans*. Washington, National Commission on Architectural Barriers, United States Government Printing Office, 1968 (http://tinyurl.com/ye32n2o, accessed 10 February 2010).

45. Schroeder S, Steinfeld E. *The estimated cost of accessibility*. Washington, United States Department of Housing and Urban Development, 1979.

46. Ratzka A. *A brief survey of studies on costs and benefits of non-handicapping environments*. Stockholm, Independent Living Institute, 1994.

47. Steven Winter Associates. *Cost of accessible housing*. Washington, United States Department of Housing and Urban Development, 1993.

48. Whybrow S et al. Legislation, anthropometry, and education: the Southeast Asian experience. In: Maisel J, ed. *The state of the science in universal design: emerging research and development*. Dubai, Bentham Science Publishers, 2009.

49. Van der Voordt TJM. Space requirements for accessibility. In: Steinfeld E, Danford GS, eds. *Measuring enabling environments*. New York, Kluwer Academic Publishers, 1999:59–88.

50. Steinfeld E, Feathers D, Maisel J. *Space requirements for wheeled mobility*. Buffalo, IDEA Center, 2009.

51. *Disability at a glance 2009: a profile of 36 Countries and areas in Asia and the Pacific*. Bangkok, United Nations Economic and Social Commission for Asia and the Pacific, 2009.

52. Castell L. Building access for the intellectually disabled. *Facilities*, 2008,26:117-130. doi:10.1108/02632770810849463

53. Raheja G. *Enabling environments for the mobility impaired in the rural areas*. Roorkee, India, Department of Architecture and Planning, Indian Institute of Technology, 2008.

54. Jones H, Reed R. *Water and sanitation for disabled people and other vulnerable groups: designing services to improve accessibility*. Loughborough, Loughborough University, Water and Development Centre, 2005 (http://wedc.lboro.ac.uk/knowledge/details.php?book=978-1-84380-090-3, accessed 10 February 2010).

55. Jones H, Reed R. *Supply and sanitation access and use by physically disabled people: reports of fieldwork in Cambodia, Bangladesh, Uganda*. London, Department for International Development, 2003.

56. Tipple G et al. *Enabling environments: reducing barriers for low-income disabled people*. Newcastle, Global Urban Research Unit, Newcastle University, 2009 (http://www.ncl.ac.uk/guru/research/project/2965, accessed 10 February 2010).

57. *Humanitarian charter and minimum standards in disaster response*. Geneva, The Sphere Project, 2004 (http://www.sphere-project.org/handbook/pages/navbook.htm?param1=0, accessed 3 February 2010).

58. Rapoport A, Watson N. *Cultural variability in physical standards: people and buildings*. New York, Basic Books, 1972.

59. *Information technology: accessibility considerations for people with disabilities. Part 3: Guidance on user needs mapping.*, Geneva, International Organization for Standardization, 2008 (ISO/IEC DTR 29138-3). (http://www.jtc1access.org/documents/swga_341_DTR_29138_3_Guidance_on_User_Needs_Mapping.zip, accessed 3 September 2009).

60. Aragall F. *Technical assistance manual 2003*. Luxembourg, European Concept for Accessibility, 2003 (http://tinyurl.com/yez3bv3, accessed 22 November 2009).

61. *Report of the special rapporteur on disability of the Commission for Social Development, 44th Session*. New York, Economic and Social Council, Commission for Social Development, 2006 (E/CN.5/2006/4).

62. *Promises to keep: a decade of federal enforcement of the Americans with Disabilities Act*. Washington, National Council on Disability, 2000.

63. *Implementation of the Americans with Disabilities Act: challenges, best practices and opportunities for success*. Washington, National Council on Disability, 2007.

64. Bringa OR. Norway's planning approach to implement universal design. In: Preiser WFE, Ostroff E, eds. *Universal design handbook*. New York, McGraw Hill, 2001:29.1–29.12.

65. Ringaert L. User/expert involvement in universal design. In: Preiser WFE, Ostroff E, eds. *Universal design handbook*. New York, McGraw Hill, 2001:6.1–6.14.

66. *Accessibility standards launched*. Kampala, Uganda National Action on Physical Disability, 2010 (http://www.unapd.org/news.php?openid=16, accessed 1 July 2010).

67. Ayres I, Braithwaite J. *Responsive regulation: transcending the deregulation debate*. Chicago, University of Chicago Press, 1995.

68. Lewis JL. Student attitudes towards impairment and accessibility: an evaluation of awareness training for urban planning students. *Vocations and Learning*, 2009,2:109-125. doi:10.1007/s12186-009-9020-y

69. *Civil society engagement for mainstreaming disability in development process report of an action research project initiated in Gujarat with multi-stakeholder partnership*. Gujarat, UNNATI and Handicap International, 2008.

70. *World Disasters Report—focus on discrimination*. Geneva, International Federation of the Red Cross and Red Crescent Societies, 2007 (http://www.ifrc.org/Docs/pubs/disasters/wdr2007/WDR2007-English.pdf, accessed 3 July 2010).

71. Steinfeld E. Evacuation of people with disabilities. *Journal of Security Education*, 2006,1:107-118. doi:10.1300/J460v01n04_10

72. *Emergency management research and people with disabilities: a resource guide*. Washington, United States Department of Education, 2008 (http://www.ed.gov/rschstat/research/pubs/guide-emergency-management-pwd.pdf, accessed 22 November 2009).

73. *Resources in emergency evacuation and disaster preparedness*. Washington, United States Access Board, 2009 (http://www.access-board.gov/evac.htm, accessed 18 August 2009).

74. Kuneida M, Roberts P. *Inclusive access and mobility in developing countries*. Washington, World Bank, 2006 (http://siteresources.worldbank.org/INTTSR/Resources/07-0297.pdf, accessed 10 February 2010).

75. Stahl A. *The provision of transportation for the elderly and handicapped in Sweden*. Lund, Institutionen för Trafikteknik, Lunds Tekniska Högskola, 1995.

76. Wretstrand A, Danielson H, Wretstrand K. Integrated organization of public transportation: accessible systems for all passengers. In: *Proceedings of the 11th International Conference on Mobility and Transport for Elderly and Disabled Persons (TRANSED 2007), Montreal, 18–22 June 2007* (http://www.tc.gc.ca/policy/transed2007/pages/1286.htm, accessed 6 February 2008).

77. Oxley P. *Improving access to taxis*. Geneva, International Road Transport Union, 2007 (http://www.internationaltransport-forum.org/europe/ecmt/pubpdf/07TaxisE.pdf, accessed 10 February 2010).

78. *Accessible taxis*. Dublin, National Council for the Blind of Ireland, 2003 (http://www.ncbi.ie/information-for-architects-engineers/accessible-taxi-report, accessed 28 July 2009).

79. Rickert T. *Bus rapid transit accessibility guidelines*. Washington, World Bank, 2006 (http://siteresources.worldbank.org/DISABILITY/Resources/280658-1172672474385/BusRapidEngRickert.pdf, accessed 10 February 2010).

80. Steinfeld E. Universal design in mass transportation. In: Preiser WFE, Ostroff E, eds. *Universal design handbook*. New York, McGraw Hill, 2001:24.1–24.25.

81. Maynard A. Can measuring the benefits of accessible transport enable a seamless journey? *Journal of Transport and Land Use*, 2009,2:21-30.

82. Iwarsson S, Jensen G, Ståhl A. Travel chain enabler: development of a pilot instrument for assessment of urban public bus transport accessibility. *Technology and Disability*, 2000,12:3-12.

83. Singh M, Nagdavane N, Srivastva N. Public transportation for elderly and disabled. In: *Proceedings of the 11th International Conference on Mobility and Transport for Elderly and Disabled Persons (TRANSED 2007), Montreal, 18–22 June 2007* (http://www.tc.gc.ca/policy/transed2007/pages/1288.htm, accessed 6 February 2007).

84. Moakley T. Advocacy for accessible taxis in New York City. In: *Proceedings of the 11th International Conference on Mobility and Transport for Elderly and Disabled Persons (TRANSED 2007), Montreal, 18–22 June 2007* (http://www.tc.gc.ca/policy/transed2007/pages/1257.htm, accessed 10 February 2010).

85. Nelson J, Masson B. *Flexible friends*. Swanley, ITS International, 2009 (http://www.itsinternational.com, accessed 28 July 2009).

86. Frye A, Macdonald D. Technical challenges of accessible taxis. In: *Proceedings of the 11th International Conference on Mobility and Transport for Elderly and Disabled Persons (TRANSED 2007), Montreal, 18–22 June 2007* (http://www.tc.gc.ca/policy/transed2007/pages/1078.htm, accessed 20 July 2009).

87. Daamen W, De Boer E, De Kloe R. The gap between vehicle and platform as a barrier for the disabled. In: *Proceedings of the 11th International Conference on Mobility and Transport for Elderly and Disabled Persons (TRANSED 2007), Montreal, 18–22 June 2007* (http://www.tc.gc.ca/policy/transed2007/pages/1251.htm, accessed 10 February 2010).

88. Wright L. *Planning guide: bus rapid transit*. Eschborn, Deutsche Gesellschaft für Technische Zusammenarbeit, 2004.

89. Dugger C. A bus system reopens rifts in South Africa. *New York Times*, 21 February 2010 (http://www.nytimes.com/2010/02/22/world/africa/22bus.html, accessed 14 March 2010).

90. Burkhardt JE. High quality transportation services for seniors. In: *Proceedings of the 11th International Conference on Mobility and Transport for Elderly and Disabled Persons, Montréal, 18–22 June 2007* (http://www.tc.gc.ca/policy/transed2007/pages/1298.htm, accessed 2 February 2008).

91. Bendixen K. *Copenhagen Metro: design for all—a must that calls for visibility*. Dublin, EIDD, 2000 (http://tinyurl.com/yz838pz, accessed 30 January 2010).

92. Meriläinen A, Helaakoski R. *Transport, poverty and disability in developing countries*. Washington, World Bank, 2001.

93. Rickert T. *Transit Access training toolkit*. Washington, World Bank, 2009. (http://siteresources.worldbank.org/DISABILITY/Resources/280658-1239044853210/5995073-1239044977199/TOOLKIT.ENG.CD.pdf, accessed 1 February 2010).

94. Mueller J et al. Assessment of user needs in wireless technologies. *Assistive Technology: the official journal of RESNA*, 2005,17:57-71. doi:10.1080/10400435.2005.10132096 PMID:16121646

95. Gould M. Assessing the accessibility of ICT products. In: *The accessibility imperative*. New York, Global Initiative for Inclusive Information and Communication Technologies, 2007:41–48 (http://www.g3ict.com/resource_center/g3ict_book_-_the_accessibility_imperative, accessed 27 August 2009).

96. Cooper RA, Ohnabe H, Hobson DA. *An introduction to rehabilitation engineering*. New York, Taylor and Francis, 2007.

97. Conference ITU. *Geneva, 21 April 2008*. Geneva, International Telecommunication Union, 2008 (http://www.itu.int/dms_pub/itu-t/oth/06/12/T06120060010001PDFE.pdf, accessed 27 August 2009).

98. Ashok M, Jacko JA. Dimensions of user diversity. In: Stephanidis C, ed. *The universal access handbook*. London, Taylor and Francis, 2009.

99. *WITSA on the first day of WCIT 2008*. San Francisco, CA, All Business, 2008 (http://www.allbusiness.com/economy-economic-indicators/economic-conditions-growth/10540743-1.html, accessed 27 August 2009).

100. Goggin G, Newell C. *Digital disability: the social construction of disability in new media*. Lanham, Rowman and Littlefield, 2003.

101. Helal S, Mokhtari M, Abdulrazak B, eds. *The engineering handbook of smart technology for aging, disability and independence*. Hoboken, John Wiley and Sons, 2008.

102. D'Aubin A. Working for barrier removal in the ICT area: creating a more accessible and inclusive Canada. *The Information Society*, 2007,23:193-201. doi:10.1080/01972240701323622

103. Goggin G, Newell C. The business of digital disability. *The Information Society*, 2007,23:159-168. doi:10.1080/01972240701323572

104. Cook JA et al. Information technology attitudes and behaviors among individuals with psychiatric disabilities who use the Internet: results of a web-based survey. *Disability Studies Quarterly*, 2005,25:www.dsq-sds.org/article/view/549/726accessed 1 July 2010).

105. Jaeger PT, Xie B. Developing online community accessibility guidelines for persons with disabilities and older adults. *Journal of Disability Policy Studies*, 2009,20:55-63. doi:10.1177/1044207308325997

106. Löfgren-Mårtenson L. Love in cyberspace: Swedish young people with intellectual disabilities and the Internet. *Scandinavian Journal of Disability Research*, 2008,10:125-138. doi:10.1080/15017410701758005

107. *Ouch! It's a disability thing*. London, British Broadcasting Company, 2010 (http://www.bbc.co.uk/ouch/, accessed 21 January 2010).

108. Gill J, ed. *Making Life Easier: how new telecommunications services could benefit people with disabilities*. Cost 219ter, 2005 (http://www.tiresias.org/cost219ter/making_life_easier/index.htm, accessed 1 July 2010).

109. *Meeting information and communications technology access and service needs for persons with disabilities: major issues for development and implementation of successful policies and strategies*. Geneva, International Telecommunication Union, 2008.

110. *Report on ICT accessibility for persons with disabilities*. Geneva, Telecommunication Development Bureau, International Telecommunication Union, 2008 (Document RGQ20/1/011-E).

111. *Electronic and information technology accessibility standards (Section 508)*. Washington, United States Access Board, 2000 (http://www.access-board.gov/sec508/standards.htm#Subpart_a, accessed 3 February 2010).

112. Kinzel E, Jackoo JA. Sensory impairments. In: Stephanidis C, ed. *The universal access handbook*. London, Taylor and Francis, 2009.

113. Keates S. Motor impairments and universal access. In: Stephanidis C, ed. *The universal access handbook*. London, Taylor and Francis, 2009.

114. Seeman L. *Inclusion of cognitive disabilities in the web accessibility movement*. Presentation at the 11th International World Wide Web Conference, Honolulu, HI, 7–11 May 2002. (http://www2002.org/CDROM/alternate/689/, accessed 25 August 2009).

115. Job Accommodation Network [web site]. (http://www.jan.wvu.edu/, accessed 10 February 2010).

116. Hanson VL et al. Accessing the web. In: Stephanidis C, ed. *The universal access handbook*. London, Taylor and Francis, 2009.

117. Lewis C. Cognitive disabilities. In: Stephanidis C, ed. *The universal access handbook*. London, Taylor and Francis, 2009.

118. Kurniawan S. Age-related differences in the interface design process. In: Stephanidis C, ed. *The universal access handbook*. London, Taylor and Francis, 2009.

119. *Seniorwatch 2: assessment of the senior market for ICT*. Brussels, European Commission, 2008a.

120. *ICT and ageing: users, markets and technologies*. Brussels, European Commission, 2009.

121. *The web: access and inclusion for disabled people*. Manchester, Disability Rights Commission, 2004 (http://joeclark.org/dossiers/DRC-GB.html, accessed 25 August 2009).

122. *State of the eNation reports*. Reading, AbilityNet, 2008 (http://www.abilitynet.org.uk/enation, accessed 27 August 2009).

123. Global Initiative for Inclusive Information and Communication Technologies [web site]. (http://www.g3ict.com/about, accessed 25 August 2009).

124. Accessibility to ICT products and services by Disabled and elderly People: Towards a framework for further development of UE legislation or other coordination measures on eAccessibility. *European Commission, Bonn, 2008b.*

125. Kennard WE, Lyle EE. With freedom comes responsibility: ensuring that the next generation of technologies is accessible, usable and affordable. [The Journal of Communications Law and Policy]*CommLaw Conspectus*, 2001,10:5-22.

126. Jaeger PT. Telecommunications policy and individuals with disabilities: issues of accessibility and social inclusion in the policy and research agenda. *Telecommunications Policy*, 2006,30:112-124. doi:10.1016/j.telpol.2005.10.001

127. Stienstra D, Watzke J, Birch GE. A three-way dance: the global good and accessibility in information technologies. *The Information Society*, 2007,23:149-158. doi:10.1080/01972240701323564

128. Piling D, Barrett P, Floyd M. *Disabled people and the Internet: experiences, barriers and opportunities*. York, Joseph Rowntree Foundation, 2004.

129. Davidson CM, Santorelli MJ. *The Impact of Broadband on People with Disabilities*. Washington, United States Chamber of Commerce, 2009.

130. Stephanidis C. Universal access and design for all in the evolving information society. In: Stephanidis C, ed. *The universal access handbook*. London, Taylor and Francis, 2009:1–10.

131. Emiliani PL. Perspectives on accessibility: from assistive technologies to universal access and design for all. In: Stephanidis C, ed. *The universal access handbook*. London, Taylor and Francis, 2009:2–17.

132. Vanderheiden GC. Standards and guidelines. In: Stephanidis C, ed. *The universal access handbook*. London, Taylor and Francis, 2009.

133. Seelman KD. Technology for full citizenship: challenges for the research community. In: Winters J, Story MF, eds. *Medical instrumentation: accessibility and usability considerations*. New York, CRC Press, 2007.

134. Kemppainen E, Kemp JD, Yamada H. Policy and legislation as a framework of accessibility. In: Stephanidis C, ed. *The universal access handbook*. London, Taylor and Francis, 2009.

135. Leblois A. The digital accessibility and inclusion index. Paper prepared for the Office of the High Commissioner for Human Rights, 2008 (www2.ohchr.org/.../GlobalinitiativeforinclusiveICT150909.doc, accessed 1 July 2010).

136. Yamada H. ICT accessibility standardization and its use in policy measures. New York, Global Initiative for Inclusive Information and Communication Technologies, 2007 (http://g3ict.org/resource_center/publications_and_reports/p/productCategory_books/subCat_4/id_58, accessed 1 July 2010)

137. *MeAC – measuring progress of eAccessibility in Europe: assessment of the status of eAccessibility in Europe*. Bonn, European Commission, 2007.

138. Timmermans N. *The status of sign languages in Europe*, Strasbourg, Council of Europe Publishing, 2005.

139. Blanck P et al. *Disability civil rights law and policy*. St. Paul, Thomson/West, 2004.

140. Coalition of Organizations for Accessible Technology [web site]. (http://www.coataccess.org/node/2, accessed 30 August 2009).

141. Manocha D. Critical issues for developing countries in implementing the Convention on the Rights of Persons with Disabilities. In: *The accessibility imperative*. New York, Global Initiative for Inclusive Information and Communication Technologies, 2007:198–204 (http://www.g3ict.com/resource_center/g3ict_book_-_the_accessibility_imperative, accessed 27 August 2009).

142. ITU Regional Workshop on ICT Accessibility for Persons with Disabilities for Africa Region, Lusaka, 15–16 July, International Telecommunication Union, 2008 [web site]. (http://www.itu.int/ITU-D/sis/PwDs/Seminars/Zambia/index.html, accessed 12 February 2010).

143. Ashington N. *Accessible Information and Communication Technologies: benefits to business and society*. OneVoice for Accessible ICT, 2010 (www.onevoiceict.org, accessed 30 June 2010).

144. *Introduction to web accessibility*. World Wide Web Consortium, 2005 (http://www.w3.org/WAI/intro/accessibility.php, accessed 20 August 2009).

145. *Shared web experiences: barriers common to mobile device users and people with disabilities*. World Wide Web Consortium, 2005 (http://www.w3.org/WAI/mobile/experiences, accessed 20 August 2009).

146. DAISY Consortium [web site]. (http://www.daisy.org/about_us/, accessed 29 August 2009).

147. *Assistive technology links*. Ottawa, Industry Canada, 2009 (http://www.at-links.gc.ca/as, accessed 7 September 2009).

148. e-Accessibility policy toolkit for persons with disabilities: a joint ITU/G3ict toolkit for policy makers implementing the Convention on the Rights of Persons with Disabilities [website]. (http://www.e-accessibilitytoolkit.org/, accessed 20 January 2010).

149. Gregg JL. Policy-making in the public interest: a contextual analysis of the passage of closed-captioning policy. *Disability & Society*, 2006,21:537-550. doi:10.1080/09687590600786793

150. South African National Accessibility Portal [web site]. (http://portal.acm.org/citation.cfm?id=1456669, accessed 25 August 2009).

151. Situation of disabled people in the European Union: the European action plan 2008–2009. *Communication from the Commission to the Council, the European Parliament, the European Economic and Social Committee and the Committee of the Regions*. Brussels, Commission of the European Communities, 2007 (COM (2007) 738 final).

152. Seelman KD. Technology for individuals with disabilities: government and market policies. In: Helal S, Mokhtari M, Abdulrazak B, eds. *The engineering handbook of smart technology for aging, disability and independence*. Hoboken, John Wiley and Sons, 2008:61–80.

153. Engelen J. eAccessibility standardization. In: Stephanidis C, ed. *The universal access handbook*. London, Taylor and Francis, 2009.

154. *Accessible Procurement Toolkit*. Industry Canada, Ottawa, 2010 (http://www.apt.gc.ca/, accessed 17 March 2011)

155. GSA BuyAccessible.gov [web site]. (http://www.buyaccessible.gov/, accessed 17 March 2011)

156. Kaikkonen A, Kaasinen E, Ketola P. Handheld devices and mobile phones. In: Stephanidis C, ed. *The universal access handbook*. London, Taylor and Francis, 2009.

157. *An iPhone the Blind can get behind*. Brooklyn, Abledbody, 2009 (http://abledbody.com/profoundlyyours/2009/06/08/an-iphone-the-blind-can-get-behind/, accessed 29 August 2009).

158. Stock SE et al. Evaluation of cognitively accessible software to increase independent access to cellphone technology for people with intellectual disability. *Journal of Intellectual Disability Research: JIDR*, 2008,52:1155-1164. doi:10.1111/j.1365-2788.2008.01099.x PMID:18647214

159. Jitterbug [web site]. (http://www.jitterbug.com/Default.aspx, accessed 20 August 2009).

160. Mobile accessibility [web site]. Mobile Manufacturers Forum, 2009. (http://www.mobileaccessibility.info/, accessed 25 August 2009).

161. Power MR, Power D, Horstmanshof L. Deaf people communicating via SMS, TTY, relay service, fax, and computers in Australia. *Journal of Deaf Studies and Deaf Education*, 2007,12:80-92. doi:10.1093/deafed/enl016 PMID:16950864

162. Irie T, Matsunaga K, Nagano Y. Universal design activities for mobile phone: Raku Raku phone. *Fujitsu Science and Technology Journal*, 2005, 41(1):78–85 (http://www.fujitsu.com/downloads/MAG/vol41-1/paper11.pdf, accessed 1 July 2010).

163. Stephandis C, Emiliani PL. "Connecting" to the information society: a European perspective. *Technology and Disability*, 1999,10:21-44.

164. Theofanos MF, Redish J. Guidelines for accessible and usable web sites: observing users who work with screen readers. *Interaction*, 2003,X:38-51.http://www.redish.net/content/papers/interactions.htmlaccessed 1 July 2010.

165. Raising the Floor [web site]. (http://raisingthefloor.net/about, accessed 27 August 2009).

166. Rabin J. McCathieNevile C, eds. *Mobile web best practices 1.0: basic guidelines: W3C recommendation 29 July 2008*. World Wide Web Consortium, 2008 (http://www.w3.org/TR/mobile-bp/, accessed October 2008).

167. Tusler A. How to make technology work: a study of best practices in United States electronic and information technology companies. *Disability Studies Quarterly*, 2005,25:www.dsq-sds.org/article/view/551/728accessed 1 July 2010.

168. Maskery H. Crossing the digital divide—possibilities for influencing the private-sector business case. *The Information Society*, 2007,23:187-191. doi:10.1080/01972240701323614

169. *Information Economy Report 2009: trends and outlook in turbulent times*. Geneva, United Nations Conference on Trade and Development, 2009.

170. *China Mobile provides special services for the Beijing Paralympics*. Beijing, China Mobile, 2008 (http://www.chinamobile.com/en/mainland/media/press080910_01.html, accessed 30 January 2010).

171. Employers Forum on Disability. Realising Potential [web site]. (www.realising-potential.org/case-studies/industry/e-commerce.html, accessed 12 April 2011).

172. *Access and inclusion: digital communications for all*. London, Ofcom, 2009. (http://stakeholders.ofcom.org.uk/binaries/consultations/access/summary/access_inc.pdf, accessed 30 January 2010).

173. Adaptive Technology Center for the Blind [web site]. (www3.sympatico.ca/tamru/, accessed, accessed 30 January 2010).

Chapter 7

Education

"I joined a mainstream school near my house for easy access. Although I could go to school on my wheelchair and could go back home with ease if any need arose, there was not any type of accessibility within the school. There were stairs everywhere and no access to classes by any other means. The best thing that could be done was to place my classroom on first floor which meant that I had 15 steps to conquer to get into or out of my class. This was usually done by having two people carry me up and down everyday. To make things really worse there were no accessible toilets. This meant that I either had not to use the toilet the whole day or go back home and lose my classes for the day."

Heba

"I am 10 years old. I go to a regular school; I am in the 4th grade. We have a wonderful teacher, and she does everything to make me feel comfortable. I use a wheelchair to get around and have a special desk and a special wheelchair at school. When there was no elevator in the school, my mother helped me to go up the stairs. Now there is an elevator, and I can go up by myself and I like it a lot. We also have a teacher who uses a wheelchair, just like me."

Olga

"[Being in an inclusive school] makes us learn how we can help each other and also understand that education is for everybody. In my former school both pupils and teachers used to laugh at me when I failed to say something, since I couldn't pronounce words properly and they wouldn't let me talk. But in this school if students laugh at me, teachers stop them and they ask forgiveness."

Pauline

"I did not have formal education. There just wasn't facilities. It didn't make me feel good. But I can't do much about that now. I just stayed at home. I was more or les self taught. I can read and articulate myself quite well. But the opportunities I would have wanted never occurred, so I was only able to reach a certain level, I could not get any further. Ideally I would have gone to university, studied history."

James

"By the time I reached Standard 6, I'd lost almost all of my sight. My dad didn't want me to go to school once I was completely blind – I think he was afraid for me – but an NGO convinced him to let me continue. After I graduated primary school my father was happy for me to continue on to high school. The NGO provided the funding for my four years of high school and they helped me with my cane, a Brailler, books, computer… things like that…"

Richard

"I want to go to school because I want to learn, and I want to be educated, and I want to define my life, to be independent, to be strong, and also to live my life and be happy."

Mia

7

Education

Estimates for the number of children (0–14 years) living with disabilities range between 93 million (*1, 2*) and 150 million (*3*). Many children and adults with disabilities have historically been excluded from mainstream education opportunities. In most countries early efforts at providing education or training were generally through separate special schools, usually targeting specific impairments, such as schools for the blind. These institutions reached only a small proportion of those in need and were not cost-effective: usually in urban areas, they tended to isolate individuals from their families and communities (*4*). The situation began to change only when legislation started to require including children with disabilities in educational systems (*5*).

Ensuring that children with disabilities receive good quality education in an inclusive environment should be a priority of all countries. The United Nations *Convention on the Rights of Persons with Disabilities* (CRPD) recognizes the right of all children with disabilities both to be included in the general education systems and to receive the individual support they require (see Box 7.1). Systemic change to remove barriers and provide reasonable accommodation and support services is required to ensure that children with disabilities are not excluded from mainstream educational opportunities.

The inclusion of children and adults with disabilities in education is important for four main reasons.

- Education contributes to human capital formation and is thus a key determinant of personal well-being and welfare.
- Excluding children with disabilities from educational and employment opportunities has high social and economic costs. For example, adults with disabilities tend to be poorer than those without disabilities, but education weakens this association (*8*).
- Countries cannot achieve Education for All or the Millennium Development Goal of universal completion of primary education without ensuring access to education for children with disabilities (*9*).
- Countries that are signatories to the CRPD cannot fulfil their responsibilities under Article 24 (see Box 7.1).

For children with disabilities, as for all children, education is vital in itself but also instrumental for participating in employment and other areas of social activity. In some cultures, attending school is part of becoming a complete person. Social relations can change the status of people with

Box 7.1. The rights and frameworks

The human right of all people to education was first defined in the United Nations' Universal Declaration of Human Rights of 1948 and further elaborated in a range of international conventions, including the Convention on the Rights of the Child and more recently in the CRPD.

In 1994 the World Conference on Special Needs Education in Salamanca, Spain produced a statement and framework for action The Salamanca Declaration encouraged governments to design education systems that respond to diverse needs so that all students can have access to regular schools that accommodate them in child-centred pedagogy (5).

The Education for All Movement is a global movement to provide quality basic education for all children, youth and adults (6). Governments around the world have made a commitment to achieve, by 2015, the six EFA goals: expand early childhood care and education; provide free and compulsory education for all; promote learning and life skills for young people and adults; increase adult literacy by 50%; achieve gender parity by 2005, gender equality by 2015; and improve the quality of education (6).

In Article 24 the CRPD stresses the need for governments to ensure equal access to an "inclusive education system at all levels" and provide reasonable accommodation and individual support services to persons with disabilities to facilitate their education (7).

The Millennium Development Goal of universal primary completion stresses attracting children to school and ensuring their ability to thrive in a learning environment that allows every child to develop to the best of their abilities.

disabilities in society and affirm their rights (10). For children who are not disabled, contact with children with a disability in an inclusive setting can, over the longer term, increase familiarity and reduce prejudice. Inclusive education is thus central in promoting inclusive and equitable societies.

The focus of this chapter is on the inclusion of learners with disabilities in the context of quality Education for All – a global movement that aims to meet the learning needs of all children, youth, and adults by 2015 and on the systemic and institutional transformation needed to facilitate inclusive education.

Educational participation and children with disability

In general, children with disabilities are less likely to start school and have lower rates of staying and being promoted in school (8, 11). The correlations for both children and adults between low educational outcomes and having a disability is often stronger than the correlations between low educational outcome and

other characteristics – such as gender, rural residence, and low economic status (8).

Respondents with disability in the *World Health Survey* experience significantly lower rates of primary school completion and fewer mean years of education than respondents without disability (see Table 7.1). For all 51 countries in the analysis, 50.6% of males with disability have completed primary school, compared with 61.3% of males without disability. Females with disability report 41.7% primary school completion compared with 52.9% of females without disability. Mean years of education are similarly lower for persons with disability compared with persons without disability (males: 5.96 versus 7.03 years respectively; females: 4.98 versus 6.26 years respectively). In addition, education completion gaps are found across all age groups and are statistically significant for both sub-samples of low-income and high-income countries.

Turning to country-specific examples, evidence shows young people with disabilities are less likely to be in school than their peers without disabilities (8). This pattern is more pronounced in poorer countries (9). The gap in primary school attendance rates between disabled and non-disabled children ranges from

Table 7.1. Education outcomes for disabled and not disabled respondents

Individuals	Low-income countries		High-income countries		All countries	
	Not disabled	Disabled	Not disabled	Disabled	Not disabled	Disabled
Male						
Primary school completion	55.6%	45.6%*	72.3%	61.7%*	61.3%	50.6%*
Mean years of education	6.43	5.63*	8.04	6.60*	7.03	5.96*
Female						
Primary school completion	42.0%	32.9%*	72.0%	59.3%*	52.9%	41.7%*
Mean years of education	5.14	4.17*	7.82	6.39*	6.26	4.98*
18–49						
Primary school completion	60.3%	47.8%*	83.1%	69.0%*	67.4%	53.2%*
Mean years of education	7.05	5.67*	9.37	7.59*	7.86	6.23*
50–59						
Primary school completion	44.3%	30.8%*	68.1%	52.0%*	52.7%	37.6%*
Mean years of education	5.53	4.22*	7.79	5.96*	6.46	4.91*
60 and over						
Primary school completion	30.7%	21.2%*	53.6%	46.5%*	40.6%	32.3%*
Mean years of education	3.76	3.21	5.36	4.60*	4.58	3.89*

Note: Estimates are weighted using WHS post-stratified weights, when available (probability weights otherwise) and age-standardized.
* *t*-test suggests significant difference from "Not disabled" at 5%.
Source (*12*).

10% in India to 60% in Indonesia, and for secondary education, from 15% in Cambodia to 58% in Indonesia (see Fig. 7.1). Household data in Malawi, Namibia, Zambia, and Zimbabwe show that between 9% and 18% of children of age 5 years or older without a disability had never attended school, but between 24% and 39% of children with a disability had never attended (*13–16*).

Enrolment rates also differ according to impairment type, with children with physical impairment generally faring better than those with intellectual or sensory impairments. For example in Burkina Faso in 2006 only 10% of deaf 7- to 12-year olds were in school, whereas 40% of children with physical impairment attended, only slightly lower than the attendance rate of non-disabled children (*17*). In Rwanda only 300 of an estimated 10 000 deaf children in the country were enrolled in primary and secondary schools, with another 9 in a private secondary school (*18*).

In India a survey estimated the share of disabled children not enrolled in school at more than five times the national rate, even in the more prosperous states. In Karnataka, the best performing major state, almost one quarter of children with disabilities were out of school, and in poorer such states as Madhya Pradesh and Assam, more than half (*11*). While the best-performing districts in India had high enrolment rates for children without disabilities – close to or above 90%, school attendance rates of children with disabilities never exceeded 74% in urban areas or 66% in rural. Most special education facilities are in urban areas (*19*, *20*), so the participation of children with disabilities in rural areas could be much worse than the aggregated data imply (*19*, *21*).

Partly as a result of building rural schools and eliminating tuition fees, Ethiopia nearly

Fig. 7.1. Proportion of children aged 6–11 years and 12–17 years with and without a disability who are in school

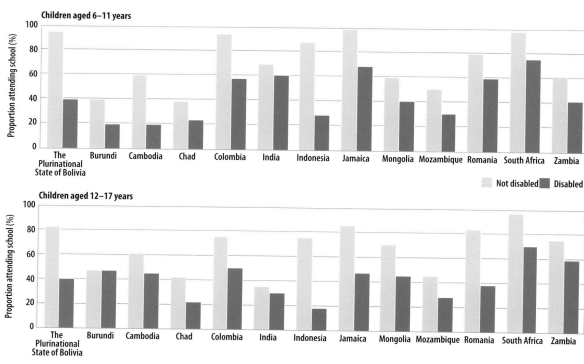

Source (8).

doubled its net enrolment ratio, from 34% in 1999 to 71% in 2007 (22). But there are no reliable data on the inclusion or exclusion of disadvantaged groups in education (23). A national baseline survey in 1995 estimated the number of children with disabilities of school age at around 690 000 (24). According to Ministry of Education data, there were 2276 children with disabilities in 1997 – or just 0.3% of the total – attending 7 special boarding schools, 8 special day schools and 42 special classes. Ten years later there were still only 15 special schools, but the number of special classes attached to regular government schools had increased to 285 (25).

Even in countries with high primary school enrolment rates, such as those in eastern Europe, many children with disabilities do not attend school. In 2002 the enrolment rates of disabled children between the ages of 7 and 15

years were 81% in Bulgaria, 58% in the Republic of Moldova, and 59% in Romania, while those of children not disabled were 96%, 97%, and 93%, respectively (26). Fig. 7.2 confirms the sizable enrolment gap for disabled young people between the ages of 16 and 18 years in selected countries of eastern Europe.

So, despite improvements in recent decades, children and youth with disabilities are less likely to start school or attend school than other children. They also have lower transition rates to higher levels of education. A lack of education at an early age has a significant impact on poverty in adulthood. In Bangladesh the cost of disability due to forgone income from a lack of schooling and employment, both of people with disabilities and their caregivers, is estimated at US$ 1.2 billion annually, or 1.7% of gross domestic product (27).

Understanding education and disability

What counts as disability or special educational need and how these relate to difficulties children experience in learning is a much debated topic for policy-makers, researchers, and the wider community (*28*).

Data on children with disabilities who have special education needs are hampered by differences in definitions, classifications, and categorizations (*29, 30*). Definitions and methods for measuring disability vary across countries based on assumptions about human difference and disability and the importance given to the different aspects of disability – impairments, activity limitations and participation restriction, related health condition, and environmental factors (see Chapter 2). The purpose and underlying intentions of classification systems and related categorization are multiple including: identification; determining eligibility; administrative; and guiding and monitoring interventions (*29, 30*). Many countries are moving away from medically-based models of identification of health condition and impairments, which located the difference in the individual, towards interactional approaches within education, which take into consideration the environment, consistent with the *International Classification of Functioning, Disability and Health* (ICF) (*28, 29*).

There are no universally agreed definitions for such concepts as **special needs education** and **inclusive education**, which hampers comparison of data.

The category covered by the terms special needs education, special educational needs, and special education is broader than education of children with disabilities, because it includes children with other needs – for example, through disadvantages resulting from gender, ethnicity, poverty, war trauma, or orphanhood (*8, 31, 32*). The Organization for Economic Co-operation and Development (OECD) estimates that between 15% and 20%

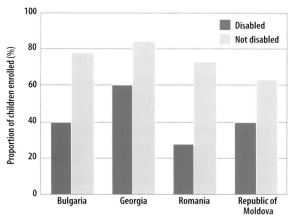

Fig. 7.2. School enrolment rates of children aged 16–18 years in selected European countries

Source (*26*).

of learners will have a special educational need at some point in their school career (*33*). This chapter focuses on the education of learners with disabilities, rather than on those covered in the broader definition of special needs. But not every person with a disability necessarily has a special educational need.

The broad sense of inclusion is that the education of all children, including those with disabilities, should be under the responsibility of the education ministries or their equivalent, with common rules and procedures. In this model education may take place in a range of settings – such as special schools and centres, special classes in integrated schools or regular classes in mainstream schools – following the principle of "the least restrictive environment". This interpretation assumes that all children can be educated and that regardless of the setting or adaptations required, all students should have access to a curriculum that is relevant and produces meaningful outcomes.

A stricter sense of inclusion is that all children with disabilities should be educated in regular classrooms with age-appropriate peers. This approach stresses the need for the whole school system to change. Inclusive education entails identifying and removing barriers and providing reasonable accommodation, enabling every learner to participate and achieve within mainstream settings.

Policy-makers need increasingly to demonstrate how policies and practice lead to greater inclusion of children with disability and improved educational outcomes. Current statistical data collected on the numbers of disabled pupils with special educational needs by setting provide some indications on the situation in countries and can be useful for monitoring trends in provision of inclusive education – if there is a clear understanding of which groups of pupils are included in data collection (28). Data and information useful in informing and shaping policy would focus more on the quality, suitability, or appropriateness of the education provided (28). Systematic collection of qualitative and quantitative data, which can be used longitudinally, is required for countries to map their progress and compare relative developments across countries (28).

Approaches to educating children with disabilities

There are different approaches around the world to providing education for people with disabilities. The models adopted include special schools and institutions, integrated schools, and inclusive schools.

Across European countries 2.3% of pupils within compulsory schooling are educated in a segregated setting – either a special school or a separate class in a mainstream school (see Fig. 7.3). Belgium and Germany rely heavily on special schools in which children with special needs are separated from their peers. Cyprus, Lithuania, Malta, Norway, and Portugal appear to include the majority of their students in regular classes with their same-age peers. A review of other OECD countries shows similar trends, with a general movement in developed countries towards inclusive education, though with some

exceptions (31). In developing countries the move towards inclusive schools is just starting.

The inclusion of children with disabilities in regular schools – inclusive schools – is widely regarded as desirable for equality and human rights. The United Nations Educational, Scientific and Cultural Organization (UNESCO) has put forward the following reasons for developing a more inclusive education system (35).

- **Educational**. The requirement for inclusive schools to educate all children together means that the schools have to develop ways of teaching that respond to individual differences, to the benefit of all children.
- **Social**. Inclusive schools can change attitudes towards those who are in some way "different" by educating all children together. This will help in creating a just society without discrimination.
- **Economic**. Establishing and maintaining schools that educate all children together is likely to be less costly than setting up a complex system of different types of schools specializing in different groups of children.

Inclusive education seeks to enable schools to serve all children in their communities (36). In practice, however, it is difficult to ensure the full inclusion of all children with disabilities, even though this is the ultimate goal. Countries vary widely in the numbers of children with disabilities who receive education in either mainstream or segregated settings, and no country has a fully inclusive system. A flexible approach to placement is important: in the United States of America, for example, the system aims to place children in the most integrated setting possible, while providing for more specialized placement where this is considered necessary (37). Educational needs must be assessed from the perspective of what is best for the individual (38) and the available financial and human resources within the country context. Some disability advocates have made the case that it should be a matter of individual

Fig. 7.3. Delivery of education by type of model for selected European countries

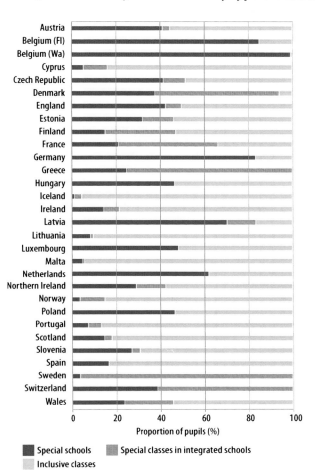

Special schools ■   Special classes in integrated schools ▩
Inclusive classes ▤

Note: The data refer to pupils who have been officially identified as having SEN. However, many more pupils may receive support for their special educational needs but they are not "counted". The only comparable data is the percentage of pupils who are educated in segregated settings. The European Agency for Development in Special Needs Education has an operational definition for segregation: "education where the pupil with special needs follows education in separate special classes or special schools for the largest part (80% or more) of the school day", which most countries agree upon and use in data collection.

Denmark: data only collected for pupils with extensive support needs who are generally educated in segregated settings; up to 23 500 receive support in the mainstream schools. Finland: data do not include 126 288 learners with minor learning difficulties (e.g. dyslexia) who receive part-time special needs education in the mainstream schools. Ireland: no data available for pupils with SEN in mainstream secondary schools. Germany and the Netherlands: no data available on numbers of pupils in special classes in mainstream schools. Hungary, Luxembourg and Spain: "special schools" includes special classes in mainstream schools. Poland: special classes in mainstream schools do not exist. Sweden, Switzerland: data indicate that pupils are educated in segregated settings, however data are not collected on those who receive support in inclusive settings.

Source (28, 34).

choice whether mainstream or segregated settings meet the needs of the child (39, 40).

Deaf students and those with intellectual impairments argue that mainstreaming is not always a positive experience (41, 42). Supporters of special schools – such as schools for the blind, deaf, or deafblind – particularly in low-income countries, often point to the fact that these institutions provide high-quality and specialized learning environments. The World Federation of the Deaf argues that often the best environment for academic and social development for a Deaf child is a school where both students and teachers use sign language for all communication. The thinking is that simple placement in a regular school, without

meaningful interaction with classmates and professionals, would exclude the Deaf learner from education and society.

Outcomes

The evidence on the impact of setting on education outcomes for persons with disabilities is not conclusive. A review of studies on inclusion published before 1995 concluded that the studies were diverse and not of uniformly good quality (43). While placement was not the critical factor in student outcomes, the review found:

▪ slightly better academic outcomes for students with learning disabilities placed in special education settings;

- higher dropout rates for students with emotional disturbances who were placed in general education;
- better social outcomes for students with severe intellectual impairments who were taught in general education classes.

While children with hearing impairments gained some academic advantage in mainstream education, their sense of self suffered. In general, students with mild intellectual impairments appeared to receive the most benefit from placement in supportive general education classes.

A review of research from the United States on special needs education concluded that the impact of the educational setting – whether special schools, special classes, or inclusive education – on educational outcomes could not be definitely established (44). It found that:

- most of the studies reviewed were not of good quality methodologically, and dependent measures varied widely across studies;
- the researchers often had difficulty separating educational settings from the types and intensity of services;
- the research was frequently conducted before critical policy changes took place;
- much of the research focused on how to implement inclusive practices, not on their effectiveness.

There are some indications that the acquisition of communication, social, and behavioural skills is superior in inclusive classes or schools. Several researchers have documented such positive outcomes (45–48). A meta-analysis of the impact of setting on learning found a "small-to-moderate beneficial effect of inclusive education on the academic and social outcomes of special needs students" (49). A small number of studies have confirmed the negative impact of placement in regular education where individualized supports are not provided (50, 51).

The inclusion of students with disabilities is generally not considered to have a negative impact on the educational performance of students without disabilities (52–54). Concerns

about the impact of inclusion of children with emotional and behavioural difficulties were more often expressed by teachers (53).

But where class sizes are large and inclusion is not well resourced, the outcomes can be difficult for all parties. There will be poor outcomes for children with disabilities in a general class if the classroom and teacher cannot provide the support necessary for their learning, development, and participation. Their education will tend to end when they finish primary school, as confirmed by the low rates of progression to higher levels of education (55). In Uganda, when universal primary education was first introduced, there was a large influx of previously excluded groups of children, including those with disabilities. With few additional resources schools were overwhelmed, reporting problems with discipline, performance, and drop-out rates among students (56).

A proper comparison of learning outcomes between special schools and the inclusion of children with disabilities in mainstream schools has not been widely carried out, beyond the few smaller studies already mentioned. In developing countries, almost no research comparing outcomes has been conducted. There is thus a need for better research and more evidence on social and academic outcomes. Box 7.2 presents data from a longitudinal study in the United States on the educational and employment outcomes of different groups of students with disabilities.

Barriers to education for children with disabilities

Many barriers may hinder children with disabilities from attending school (59–61). In this chapter they are categorized under systemic and school-based problems.

System-wide problems

Divided ministerial responsibility

In some countries education for some or all children with disabilities falls under separate

Box 7.2. Transition from school to work in the United States

All secondary education students with documented disabilities in the United States are protected by Section 504 of the Vocational Rehabilitation Act and the American Disabilities Act. A subgroup of students with disabilities also meets the eligibility requirements under Part B of the Individuals with Disabilities Education Act (IDEA). In the former category are students whose disability does not adversely affect their ability to learn, and who can progress through school with reasonable accommodations that enable them to have access to the same resources and learning as their peers. The students eligible under Part B of the IDEA are entitled to a "free and appropriate public education", which is defined through their individualized education plan. This case study refers to students with such a plan.

The National Longitudinal Transition Study 2 (NLTS2) provides data about students with disabilities covered by IDEA. The NLTS2 was launched after a nationally representative survey in 2000 of a sample of 11 272 students aged 13–16 years who were receiving special education. Of this sample of disabled students, 35% were living in disadvantaged households with annual incomes of US$ 25 000 or less. In addition, 25% were living in single-parent households. Of all sample students, 93.9% were attending regular secondary schools in 2000, 2.6% were attending special schools, and the remainder attending alternative, vocational, or other schools.

Graduation rates

The following figure shows the proportion of students aged 14–21 years who finished high school and the proportion who dropped out, over 10 years.

Proportion of exiting students with disabilities, aged 14–21 years, who graduated, received a certificate, or dropped out, 1996–2005

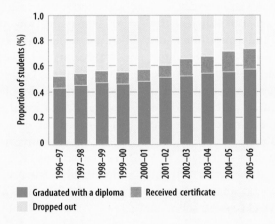

Source (57).

Post-school outcomes

According to NLTS2, 85% of young people with disabilities were engaged in employment, post-secondary education, or job training in the four years since leaving school. Of the sample students, 45% had enrolled in some type of post-secondary education, compared with 53% of students in the general population. Among those in post-secondary education, 6% had enrolled in business, vocational, or technical schools, 13% in a two-year college course, and 8% in a four-year college or university. Of young people within the same age ranges in the general population, 12% were enrolled in two-year colleges and 29% in four-year institutions (58).

About 57% of the young people with disabilities aged 17–21 years were employed at the time of the 2005 follow-up, compared with the 66% among the same age group in the general population. Young people with intellectual impairments or multiple impairments were the least likely to be engaged in school, work, or preparation for work.

continues ...

... continued

Young people with learning, cognitive, behavioural, or emotional impairments were 4–5 times more likely to have been involved with the criminal justice system than young people in the general population.

Young people with intellectual impairments were the least likely to have graduated with a diploma and had the lowest employment rates among all disability categories. Dropouts were far less likely to be engaged in post-school work or education and 10 times more likely than students with disabilities who finished high school to have been arrested.

Of the students with visual or hearing impairments, more than 90% received a regular diploma and were twice as likely as other students with a disability to have enrolled in some type of post-secondary school.

For some students, such as those with emotional disturbances, the educational outcomes are disturbingly low. Research is required to find forms of curricula, pedagogies, and assessment methods that take better account of students' diverse needs within education and in the transition to work.

ministries such as Health, Social Welfare, or Social Protection (El Salvador, Pakistan, Bangladesh) or distinct Ministries of Special Education. In other countries (Ethiopia and Rwanda) responsibilities for the education for disabled children are shared between ministries (*25*).

In India children with disabilities in special schools fall under the responsibility of the Ministry of Social Justice and Empowerment, while children in mainstream schools come under the Department of Education in the Ministry of Human Resource Development (*32*). This division reflects the cultural perception that children with disabilities are in need of welfare rather than equality of opportunity (*11*). This particular model tends to further segregate children with disabilities, and shifts the focus from education and achieving social and economic inclusion to treatment and social isolation.

Lack of legislation, policy, targets, and plans

While there are many examples of initiatives to include children with disabilities in education, a lack of legislation, policy, targets and plans tends to be a major obstacle in efforts to provide Education for All (*62*). The gaps in policy that are commonly encountered include a lack of financial and other targeted incentives for children with disabilities to attend school – and a lack of social protection and support

services for children with disabilities and their families (*63*).

A review of 28 countries participating in the Education for All Fast Track Initiative Partnership found that 10 had a policy commitment to include children with disabilities and also had some targets or plans on such issues as data collection, teacher training, access to school buildings, and the provision of additional learning materials and support (*64*). For example Ghana has enrolment targets, including one that all children with "nonsevere special educational needs" should be educated in mainstream schools by 2015. Djibouti and Mozambique mention targets for children in regular schools. Kenya is committed to increasing the gross enrolment rate of disabled children to 10% by 2010 and also has targets for training teachers and providing equipment. However, while a further 13 countries mentioned disabled children they provided little detail of their proposed strategies and five countries did not refer to disability or inclusion at all.

Inadequate resources

Limited or inappropriate resources are regarded as a significant barrier to ensuring inclusive education for children with disabilities (*65*). A study in the United States found that the average cost for educating a child with a disability was 1.9 times the cost for a child without a disability, with the multiplier ranging from 1.6 to 3.1 depending on the type and extent of the disability (*66*). In most developing countries it is difficult to reach all those in need even when educational systems are well planned and support inclusion.

National budgets for education are often limited and families are frequently unable to afford the costs of education (*9, 17, 67*). There are shortages of resources such as few schools, inadequate facilities, insufficient qualified teachers and a lack of learning materials (*6*). An assessment in 2006 on the status of El Salvador's capacity to create inclusive educational opportunities for students with disabilities found that there was limited funding to provide services to all students with disabilities (*68*).

The Dakar Framework for Action recognizes that achieving Education for All will require increased financial support by countries and increased development assistance from bilateral and multilateral donors (*67*). But this has not always been forthcoming, restricting progress (*17*).

School problems

Curriculum and pedagogy

Flexible approaches in education are needed to respond to the diverse abilities and needs of all learners (*69*). Where curricula and teaching methods are rigid and there is a lack of appropriate teaching materials – for example, where information is not delivered in the most appropriate mode such as sign language and teaching materials are not available in alternative formats such as Braille – children with disabilities are at increased risk of exclusion (*69*). Assessment and evaluation systems are often focused on academic performance rather than individual progress and therefore can also be restrictive for children with special education needs (*69*). Where parents have anxieties about the quality of mainstream schools, they are more likely to push for segregated solutions for their children with disabilities (*17*).

Inadequate training and support for teachers

Teachers may not have the time or resources to support disabled learners (*70*). In resource-poor settings classrooms are frequently overcrowded and there is a severe shortage of well trained teachers capable of routinely handling the individual needs of children with disabilities (*71, 72*). The majority of teachers lack sign-language skills creating barriers for Deaf pupils (*73*). Other supports such as classroom assistants are also lacking. Advances in teacher education have not necessarily kept pace with the policy changes that followed the Salamanca Declaration. For example, in India the pre-service training of regular teachers includes no familiarization with the education of children with special needs (*64*).

Physical barriers

Physical access to school buildings is an essential prerequisite for educating children with disabilities (*65*). Those with physical disabilities are likely to face difficulties in travelling to school if, for example, the roads and bridges are unsuitable for wheelchair use and the distances are too great (*17*). Even if it is possible to reach the school, there may be problems of stairs, narrow doorways, inappropriate seating, or inaccessible toilet facilities (*74*).

Labelling

Children with disabilities are often categorized according to their health condition to determine their eligibility for special education and other types of support services (*29*). For example, a diagnosis of dyslexia, blindness, or deafness can facilitate access to technological and communication support and specialized teaching (*75*). But assigning labels to children in education systems can have negative effects including stigmatization, peer rejection, lower self-esteem, lower expectations, and limited opportunities (*29*). Students may be reluctant about revealing their disability due to negative attitudes, thus missing out on needed support services (76). A study in two states of the United States examined the responses of 155 preschool teachers to the inclusion of children with disabilities (77). Two distinct versions of a questionnaire were created, including short sketches describing children with disabilities. One included a "labelling" version that used terms such as cerebral palsy. The other did not use labels, but simply described the children. The teachers who completed the non-labelling version were more positive about including disabled children than those who completed the labelling version. This suggested that a label can lead to more negative attitudes and that adults' attitudes were critical in developing policies on the education of children with disabilities.

Attitudinal barriers

Negative attitudes are a major obstacle to the education of disabled children (78, 79). In some cultures people with disabilities are seen as a form of divine punishment or as carriers of bad fortune (80, 81). As a result, children with disabilities who could be in school are sometimes not permitted to attend. A community-based study in Rwanda found that perceptions of impairments affected whether a child with a disability attended school. Negative community attitudes were also reflected in the language used to refer to people with disabilities (82, 83).

The attitudes of teachers, school administrators, other children, and even family members affect the inclusion of children with disabilities in mainstream schools (74, 84). Some school teachers, including head teachers, believe they are not obliged to teach children with disabilities (84). In South Africa it is thought that school attendance and completion are influenced by the belief of school administrators that disabled students do not have a future in higher education (85). A study comparing Haiti with the United States found that teachers in both countries generally favoured types of disabilities they perceived to be easier to work with in mainstream settings (36).

Even where people are supportive of students with disabilities, expectations might be low, with the result that little attention is paid to academic achievement. Teachers, parents, and other students may well be caring but at the same time not believe in the capacity of the children to learn (86, 87). Some families with disabled students may believe that special schools are the best places for their children's education (76).

Violence, bullying, and abuse

Violence against students with disabilities – by teachers, other staff, and fellow students – is common in educational settings (20). Students with disabilities often become the targets of violent acts including physical threats and abuse, verbal abuse, and social isolation. The fear of bullying can be as great an issue for children with disabilities as actual bullying (88). Children with disabilities may prefer to attend special schools, because of the fear of stigma or bullying in mainstream schools (88). Deaf children are particularly vulnerable to abuse because of their difficulties with spoken communication.

Addressing barriers to education

Ensuring the inclusion of children with disabilities in education requires both systemic and school level change (89). As with other complex change, it requires vision, skills, incentives, resources, and an action plan (90). One of the most important elements in an inclusive educational system is strong and continuous leadership at the national and school levels – something that is cost-neutral.

System-wide interventions

Legislation

The success of inclusive systems of education depends largely on a country's commitment to adopt appropriate legislation, develop policies and provide adequate funding for implementation. Since the mid-1970s Italy has had legislation in place to support inclusive education for all children with disabilities resulting in high inclusion rates and positive educational outcomes (*33, 91, 92*).

New Zealand shows how government ministries can promote an understanding of the right to education of disabled students by:

- publicizing support available for disabled children
- reminding school boards of their legal responsibilities
- reviewing information provided to parents
- reviewing complaints procedures (*93*).

A survey of low-income and middle-income countries found that if political will is lacking, legislation will have only a limited impact (*31*). Other factors leading to a low impact include insufficient funding for education, and a lack of experience in educating people with disabilities or special educational needs.

Policy

Clear national policies on the education of children with disabilities are essential for the development of more equitable education systems. UNESCO has produced guidelines to assist policy-makers and managers to create policies and practices supportive of inclusion (*94*). Clear policy direction at the national level has enabled a wide range of countries to undertake major educational reforms – including Italy, the Lao People's Democratic Republic, Lesotho, and Viet Nam (see Box 7.3).

In 1987 Lesotho started work on a series of policies on special education. By 1991 it had established a Special Education Unit and launched a national programme of inclusive education (*95*). A 1993 study carried out in a quarter of the country's primary schools, involving interviews with more than 2649 teachers, found that 17% of children in Lesotho had disabilities and special educational needs (*95*). The national programme for inclusive education was launched in 10 pilot schools, one in each district of the country. Training in inclusive teaching was developed for teachers in these schools, and for student teachers, with the help of specialists and people with disabilities themselves. A recent study on inclusive education in Lesotho found variability in the way that teachers addressed the needs of their children (*96*). There was a positive effect on the attitudes of teachers, and without a formal policy it is unlikely that improvements would have occurred.

National plans

Creating or amending a national plan of action and establishing infrastructure and capacity to implement the plan are key to including children with disabilities in education (*79*). The implications of Article 24 of the CRPD are that institutional responsibility for the education of children with disabilities should remain within the Ministry of Education (*97*), with coordination, as appropriate, with other relevant ministries. National plans for Education For All should:

- reflect international commitments to the right of disabled children to be educated;
- identify the number of disabled children and assess their needs;
- stress the importance of parental support and community involvement;
- plan for the main aspects of provision – such as making school buildings accessible, and developing the curriculum, teaching methods, and materials to meet a diversity of needs;
- increase capacity, through the expansion of provision and training programmes;
- make available sufficient funds;

Box 7.3. Inclusion is possible in Viet Nam – but more can be done

In the early 1990s Viet Nam launched a major programme of reform to improve the inclusion of students with disabilities in education. The Centre for Special Education worked with an international nongovernmental organization to set up two pilot projects, one rural and one urban. Local steering committees for each project were active in raising awareness in the community and conducting house-to-house searches for children who were missing from official school lists. The pilot projects identified 1078 children with a wide range of impairments who were excluded.

Training was provided to administrators, teachers, and parents on:

- the benefits of inclusive education
- special education services
- individualized educational programmes
- carrying out accommodation and environmental modifications
- assessment
- family services.

In addition, technical assistance was given in such areas as mobility training for blind students and training for parents on exercises to improve mobility for children with cerebral palsy.

Four years later, an evaluation found that 1000 of the 1078 children with disabilities had been successfully included in general education classes in local schools – an achievement welcomed by both teachers and parents. With international donor support a similar programme was conducted in three other provinces. Within three years attendance rates in regular classes of children with disabilities increased from 30% to 86%, and eventually 4000 new students were enrolled in neighbourhood schools.

Follow-up evaluations found that teachers were more open to including students with disabilities than previously – and were better equipped and more knowledgeable about inclusive practices. Teachers and parents had also raised their expectations of children with disabilities. More important, the children were better integrated into their communities. The average cost of the programme for a student with disabilities in the inclusive setting was US$ 58 per year, compared with US$ 20 for a student without disabilities and US$ 400 for education in segregated settings. This sum did not cover specialized equipment – such as hearing aids, wheelchairs, and Braille printers, which many students with disabilities required and whose cost was prohibitive for most families.

Despite the progress, only around 2% of preschool and primary schools in Viet Nam are inclusive, and 95% of children with disabilities still do not have access to school (*90*). But the success of the pilot projects has helped change attitudes and policies on disability and has led to greater efforts on inclusion. The Ministry of Education and Training has committed itself to increase the percentage of children with disabilities being educated in regular classes. New laws and policies that support inclusive education are being implemented.

- conduct monitoring and evaluation, and improve the qualitative and quantitative data on students (*64*).

Funding

There are basically three ways to finance special needs education, whether in specialized institutions or mainstream schools:

- through the national budget, such as setting up a Special National Fund (as in Brazil), financing a Special Education Network of Schools (as in Pakistan), or as a fixed proportion of the overall education budget (0.92% in Nicaragua and 2.3% in Panama);
- through financing the particular needs of institutions – for materials, teaching aids, training, and operational support (as in Chile and Mexico);
- through financing individuals to meet their needs (as in Denmark, Finland, Hungary, and New Zealand).

Other countries, including Switzerland and the United States, use a combination of funding methods that include national financing that can be used flexibly for special needs education at the local level. The criteria for eligibility of funding can be complex. Whichever funding model is used, it should:

- be easy to understand
- be flexible and predictable
- provide sufficient funds
- be cost-based and allow for cost control
- connect special education to general education
- be neutral in identification and placement (*98, 99*).

One system for comparing data on resources between countries categorizes students according to whether their needs arise from medical conditions, behavioural, or emotional conditions, or socioeconomic or cultural disadvantages (*31*). The resources dedicated to children with medical diagnoses remain the most constant across ages. Those allocated to children with socioeconomic or cultural disadvantages are more heavily concentrated among younger age groups, and drop off sharply by secondary school (*100*). The decline in resources for these categories may reflect higher drop-out rates for these groups, especially in the later stages of secondary school, implying that the system is not meeting their educational needs.

Table 7.2 summarizes the data for a range of Central and South American countries, making comparisons with similar data from New Brunswick province in Canada, the United States, and the median of the OECD countries. It is clear that the Central and South American countries are providing resources for students with disabilities in the pre-primary and primary years. But there is a rapid fall-off of provision in the early secondary school period and no provision at all in the later secondary period. This contrasts with the OECD countries, which provide education for students with disabilities across the full age range, even though the provision is reduced at older ages.

Table 7.2. Percentage of students with disabilities receiving educational resources by country and by level of education

Country	Compulsory education (%)	Pre-primary (%)	Primary (%)	Lower secondary (%)	Upper secondary (%)
Belize	0.95	–	0.96	–	–
Brazil	0.71	1.52	0.71	0.06	–
Chile	0.97	1.31	1.17	1.34	–
Colombia	0.73	0.86	0.84	0.52	N/A
Costa Rica	1.21	4.39	1.01	1.48	N/A
Guyana	0.15	N/A	0.22	N/A	N/A
Mexico	0.73	0.53	0.98	0.26	–
Nicaragua	0.40	0.64	0.40	–	–
Paraguay	0.45	N/A	0.45	N/A	N/A
Peru	0.20	0.94	0.30	0.02	N/A
Uruguay	1.98	–	1.98	–	–
United States of America	5.25	7.38	7.39	3.11	3.04
New Brunswick province, Canada	2.89	–	2.19	3.80	3.21
Median of OECD countries	2.63	0.98	2.43	3.11	1.37

Note: Mexico is an OECD country. Only partial data are available for countries listed in *italics*.
N/A not applicable.
– not available/never collected.
Source (*31, 101*).

Ensuring children with disabilities are able to access the same standard of education as their peers often requires increased financing (*17*). Low-income countries will require long-term predictable financing to achieve this. In the Lao People's Democratic Republic, Save the Children and the Swedish International Development Cooperation Agency provided long-term funding and technical support for an Inclusive Education Project from 1993–2009. The project resulted in a centralized, national approach to the development of policy and practice in inclusive education. Services began in 1993, when a pilot school opened in the capital, Vientiane. There are now 539 schools across 141 districts providing inclusive education and specialized support for more than 3000 children with disabilities (*102*).

While the costs of special schools and inclusive schools are difficult to determine it is generally agreed that inclusive settings are more cost-effective (*33*). Inclusion has the best chance of success when school funding is decentralized, budgets are delegated to the local level, and funds are based on total enrolment and other indicators. Access to small amounts of flexible funds can promote new approaches (*103*).

School interventions

Recognizing and addressing individual differences

Education systems need to move away from more traditional pedagogies and adopt more learner-centred approaches which recognize that each individual has an ability to learn and a specific way of learning. The curricula, teaching methods and materials, assessment and examination systems, and the management of classes all need to be accessible and flexible to support differences in learning patterns (*19, 69*).

Assessment practices can facilitate or hinder inclusion (*103*). The need to attain academic excellence often pervades school cultures, so policies on inclusion need to ensure that all children reach their potential (*104*). Streaming

into ability groups is often an obstacle to inclusion whereas mixed-ability, mixed-age classrooms can be a way forward (*17, 69*). In 2005 the European Agency for Development in Special Needs Education studied forms of assessment that support inclusion in mainstream settings (*105*). Involving 50 assessment experts in 23 countries, the study addressed how to move from a deficit – mainly medically-based – approach to an educational or interactive approach. The following principles were proposed:

- Assessment procedures should promote learning for all students.
- All students should be entitled to be part of all assessment procedures.
- The needs of students with disabilities should be considered within all general assessment policies as well as within policies on disability-specific assessment.
- The assessment procedures should complement each other.
- The assessment procedures should aim to promote diversity by identifying and valuing the progress and achievements of each student.
- Inclusive assessment procedures should explicitly aim to prevent segregation by avoiding – as far as possible – forms of labelling. Instead, assessments should focus on learning and teaching practices that lead to more inclusion in a mainstream setting.

Individualized education plans are a useful tool for children with special educational needs to help them to learn effectively in the least restrictive environments. Developed through a multidisciplinary process, they identify needs, learning goals and objectives, appropriate teaching strategies, and required accommodations and supports. Many countries such as Australia, Canada, New Zealand, the United Kingdom and the United States have policies and documented processes for such plans (*106*).

Creating an optimum learning environment will assist children in learning and achieving their potential (*107*). Information and communication technologies, including assistive technologies, should be used whenever possible (*69, 108*). Some students with disabilities might require accommodations such as large print, screen readers, Braille and sign language, and specialized software. Alternative formats of examination may also be needed, such as oral examinations for non-readers. Learners with difficulty in understanding as a result of intellectual impairments may need adapted teaching styles and methods. The choices regarding reasonable accommodations will depend on the available resources (*71*).

Providing additional supports

To ensure the success of inclusive education policies some children with disabilities will require access to additional support services (*5*). The additional costs associated with these is likely to be offset in part by savings from students in specialized institutions transferring to mainstream schools.

Schools should have access to specialist education teachers where required. In Finland the majority of schools are supported by at least one permanent special education teacher. These teachers provide assessments, develop individualized education plans, coordinate services, and provide guidance for mainstream teachers (*109*). In El Salvador "support rooms" have been set-up in mainstream primary schools to provide services to students with special education needs, including those with disabilities. The services include assessments of students, instruction on an individual basis or in small groups, support for general education teachers, and speech and language therapy and similar services. Support room teachers work closely with parents, and receive a budget from the Ministry of Education for training and salaries. In 2005 about 10% of the schools nationwide had support rooms (*68*).

Teaching assistants – also known as learning support assistants, or special needs assistants – are increasingly used in mainstream classrooms. Their role varies in different settings, but their main function is to support children with disabilities to participate in mainstream classrooms – they should not be regarded as substitute teachers. Their successful deployment requires effective communication and planning with the classroom teacher, a shared understanding of their role and responsibilities, and ongoing monitoring of the way support is provided (*110, 111*). There is a danger that extensive use of teaching assistants may discourage more flexible approaches and sideline disabled children in class (*93*). Special needs assistants should not hinder children with disabilities from interacting with non-disabled children or from engaging in age-appropriate activities (*88*).

Early identification and intervention can reduce the level of educational support children with disabilities may require throughout their schooling and ensure they reach their full potential (*107*). Children with disabilities may require access to specialist health and education professionals such as occupational therapists, physiotherapists, speech therapists, and educational psychologists to support their learning (*107*). A review of early childhood interventions in Europe stressed the need for proper coordination among health, education, and social services (*112*).

Making better use of existing resources to support learning is also important, particularly in poorer settings. For example, while schools in poor rural environments may have large class sizes and fewer material resources, stronger community involvement and positive attitudes can overcome these barriers (*65*). Many teaching materials that significantly enhance learning processes can be locally made (*103*). Special schools, where they exist, can be valuable for disability expertise (early identification and intervention) and as training and resource centres (*5*). In low-income settings itinerant teachers can be a cost-effective means of addressing teacher shortages, assisting children with disabilities to develop skills – such as Braille literacy, orientation and mobility – and developing teaching materials (*113*).

Box 7.4. Teacher education in Ethiopia

Teacher training on special educational needs has been conducted in Ethiopia since the 1990s, a focus for much international support. Until the early 1990s, teacher education on special educational needs was primarily through short nongovernmental organization-funded workshops. This approach did not produce lasting changes in teaching and learning processes. Nor did it enable the government to be self-reliant in training special education staff.

Starting in 1992, with support from the Finnish government, a six-month training course was launched at a teacher training institute (*114*). This was part of a drive to support existing special schools, introduce more special classes, and increase the number of learners within mainstream classes with support from itinerant teachers. Fifty teachers received university education from Finnish universities – 6 in Finland itself, 44 through distance learning, which cost around 10% of the direct education.

Short support courses were developed at Addis Ababa University, and a special centre, the Sebeta Teacher Training Institute, was created as part of Sebeta School for the Blind. Between 1994 and 1998, 115 people graduated as special education teachers, and thousands of mainstream teachers received in-service training. But the facilities do not train enough teachers to meet the full demand for inclusive education (*115*).

Other regular colleges and universities in Ethiopia now offer special needs education courses to all students, and Sebeta continues to offer a 10-month course to qualified teachers. As a result of Sebeta's training programme, there has been an expansion in the numbers of special classes and disabled children attending school. But using Ministry of Education statistics, it is estimated that only 6000 identified disabled children have access to education of a primary school population of nearly 15 million (*64*).

Building teacher capacity

The appropriate training of mainstream teachers is crucial if they are to be confident and competent in teaching children with diverse educational needs. The principles of inclusion should be built into teacher training programmes, which should be about attitudes and values not just knowledge and skills (*103*). Post-qualification training, such as that offered at Ethiopia's Sebeta Teacher Training Institute, can improve provision and – ultimately – the rate of enrolment of students with disabilities (see Box 7.4).

Teachers with disabilities should be encouraged as role models. In Mozambique a collaboration between a teacher training college and a national disabled people's organization, ADEMO, trains teachers to work with learners with disabilities and also provides scholarships for students with disabilities to train as teachers (*116*).

Several resources can assist teachers to work towards inclusive approaches for students with disabilities such as:

- *Embracing diversity: Toolkit for creating inclusive, learning friendly environments* contains nine self-study booklets to assist teachers to improve their skills in diverse classroom settings (*107*).

- *Module 4: Using ICTs to promote education and job training for persons with disabilities* in *Toolkit of best practices and policy advice* provides information on how information and communication technologies can facilitate access to education for people with disabilities (*108*).

- *Education in emergencies: Including everyone: INEE pocket guide to inclusive education* provides support for educators working in emergency and conflict situations (*117*).

Teacher training should also be supported by other initiatives that provide teachers with opportunities to share expertise and experiences about inclusive education and to adapt and experiment with their own teaching methods in supportive environments (*69, 102*).

Where segregated schools feature prominently, enabling special education teachers to make the transition to working in an inclusive system should be a priority. In extending inclusive education, special schools and mainstream schools have to collaborate (*62*). In the Republic of Korea at least one special school in each district is selected by the government to work closely with a partner mainstream school, to encourage inclusion of disabled children through various initiatives such as peer support and group work (*76*).

Removing physical barriers

Principles of universal design should underlie policies of access to education. Many physical barriers are relatively straightforward to overcome: changing physical layout of classrooms can make a major difference (*118*). Incorporating universal design into new building plans is cheaper than making the necessary changes to an old building and adds only around 1% to the total construction cost (*119*).

Overcoming negative attitudes

The physical presence of children with disabilities in schools does not automatically ensure their participation. For participation to be meaningful and produce good learning outcomes, the ethos of the school – valuing diversity and providing a safe and supportive environment – is critical.

The attitudes of teachers are critical in ensuring that children with disabilities stay in school and are included in classroom activities. A study carried out to compare the attitudes of teachers towards students with disabilities in Haiti and the United States showed that teachers are more likely to change their attitudes towards inclusion if other teachers demonstrate positive attitudes and a supportive school culture exists (*36*). Fear and a lack of confidence among teachers regarding the education of students with disabilities can be overcome:

- In Zambia teachers in primary and basic schools had expressed interest in including children with disabilities, but believed that this was reserved for specialists. Many had fears that such conditions as albinism were contagious. They were encouraged to discuss their negative beliefs and to write about them reflectively (*120*).

- In Uganda teachers' attitudes improved simply by having regular contact with children with disabilities (*56*).
- In Mongolia a training programme on inclusive education was run for teachers and parents with the support of specialist teachers. The 1600 teachers trained had highly positive attitudes towards the inclusion of children with disabilities and towards working with the parents: the enrolment of children with disabilities in preschool facilities and primary schools increased from 22% to 44% (*121*).

The role of communities, families, disabled people, and children with disabilities

Communities

Approaches involving the whole community reflect the fact that the child is an integral member of the community and make it more likely that sustainable inclusive education for the child can be attained (see Box 7.5).

Community-based rehabilitation (CBR) projects have often included educational activities for children with disabilities and share the goal of inclusion (*5, 125*). CBR-related activities that support inclusive education include referring children with disabilities to appropriate schools, lobbying schools to accept children with disabilities, assisting teachers to support children with disabilities, and creating links between families and communities (*59*).

CBR workers can also be a useful resource to teachers in providing assistive devices, securing medical treatment, making the school environment accessible, establishing links to disabled people's organizations, and finding employment or vocational training placements for children at the end of their school education.

Examples of innovative practices that link CBR to inclusive education can be found in many low-income countries:

- In the Karamoja region of Uganda, where most people are nomads and only 11.5% of the population are literate, children's

Box 7.5. Sport for children with disabilities in Fiji

Since March 2005 the Fiji Paralympic Committee (FPC) and the Australian Sports Commission have worked together to provide inclusive sport activities for children with disabilities in Fiji's 17 special education centres. These activities are part of the Australian Sports Outreach Program, an Australian government initiative that seeks to help individuals and organizations deliver high-quality, inclusive sport-based programmes that contribute to social development.

FPC's grassroots programmes are designed to increase the variety and quality of sport choices available for children in Fijian schools. Its activities include:

- Pacific Junior Sport – a games-based programme that provides opportunities for children to participate and develop their skills;
- *qito lai lai* ("children's games") for smaller children;
- arranging for sport federations – such as those of golf, table tennis, tennis, and archery – to run sessions in schools;
- supporting schools so that students can play popular sports, such as football, volleyball, and netball, and paralympic sports such as boccia, goalball, and sitting volleyball;
- managing regional and national sport tournaments, as well as festivals in which students test their skills in football, netball, and volleyball against children from mainstream schools;
- providing role models through the athlete ambassador programme, in which athletes with a disability regularly visit schools, including mainstream schools.

Sport can improve the inclusion and well-being of people with a disability:

- by changing what communities think and feel about people with a disability – and in that way reducing stigma and discrimination;
- by changing what people with a disability think and feel about themselves – and in that way empowering them to recognize their own potential;
- by reducing their isolation and helping them integrate more fully into community life;
- by providing opportunities which assists young people to develop healthy body systems (musculoskeletal, cardiovascular) and improve coordination.

As a result of FPC's work, each Friday afternoon across the country more than 1000 children with a disability are playing a sport. As the FPC's sport development officer points out, "when people see children with a disability playing sport, they know that they are capable of doing many different things".

Source (*122–124*).

domestic duties are essential to the survival of their families. In this region a project called Alternative Basic Education for Karamoja has been set up. This community-based project has pushed for inclusion in education (*126*). It encourages the participation of children with disabilities and school instruction in the local language. The curriculum is relevant to the community's livelihood, containing instruction on such topics as livestock and crop production.

- The Oriang project in western Kenya has introduced inclusive education in five primary schools. Technical and financial assistance is provided by Leonard Cheshire Disability (*60*). The support includes training new teachers and working with students, parents, teachers, and the wider community to change attitudes and build the right structures for delivering inclusive education. The project benefits 2568 children, of whom 282 have a mild to severe disability (*127*).

Parents

Parents should be involved in all aspects of learning (*128*). The family is the first source of education for a child, and most learning occurs at home. Parents are frequently active in creating educational opportunities for their children, and they need to be brought on board to facilitate the process of inclusion. In several countries individual parents, often with the support of parents' associations, have taken their governments to court, setting precedents that opened regular schools to children with disabilities. Inclusion Panama pressured the Panamanian government to change the law requiring children with disabilities to be educated in a separate system. In 2003, as a result of its campaign, the government introduced a policy to make all schools inclusive. NFU, a parents' organization in Norway, has lent support to parents in Zanzibar to collaborate with the education ministry in introducing inclusive education. In 2009 a parents' organization in Lebanon persuaded a teachers' training college to conduct its practical training for teachers in the community instead of in institutions.

Disabled people's organizations

Disabled people's organizations also have a role in promoting the education of disabled children – for example, working with young disabled people, providing role models, encouraging parents to send their children to school and become involved in their children's education, and campaigning for inclusive education. The Southern Africa Federation of the Disabled, for instance, has set up a range of programmes involving people with disabilities, including its children and youth programme, running for the past 15 years. The programme focuses on all aspects of discrimination and abuse of children with disabilities and their exclusion from education and other social activities. However such organizations frequently lack the resources and capacity to develop their role in education.

Children with disabilities

The voices of children with disabilities themselves must be heard, though they frequently are not. In recent years children have been more involved in studies of their experiences of education. The results of such child-informed research are of great benefit for educational planners and policy-makers and can be a source of evidence as educational systems become more inclusive. Child-to-child cooperation should be better used to promote inclusion (94).

Audiovisual methods have been particularly effective in bringing out the views of children in a range of socioeconomic settings (129, 130).

- Young people in nine Commonwealth countries were consulted about their views on the CRPD through a series of focus groups. The right to education featured in the top three issues in three quarters of these groups (131).
- In a refugee programme in Jhapa, Nepal, children with disabilities were found to be a neglected and vulnerable group (132). A full-time disability coordinator for the programme was therefore appointed to undertake participatory action research. Disabled children talked about their family lives and described how they were taunted if they left their homes. Both children and parents listed education as the top priority. After 18 months more than 700 children had been integrated into schools, and sign-language training had been introduced in all refugee camps, for Deaf and non-deaf children.
- In September 2007 the Portuguese Ministry of Education organized a Europe-wide consultation in collaboration with the European Agency for Development in Special Needs Education (133). The young people consulted favoured inclusive education, but insisted that each person should be able to choose where to be educated. Acknowledging that they gained social skills and experience of the real world in inclusive schools, they also said that individualized specialist support had helped them to prepare for higher education.

Conclusion and recommendations

Children with disabilities are less likely than children without disabilities to start school and have lower rates of staying and being promoted in school. Children with disabilities should have equal access to quality education, because this is key to human capital formation and their participation in social and economic life.

While children with disabilities have historically been educated in separate special schools, inclusive mainstream schools in both urban and rural areas provide a cost-effective way forward. Inclusive education is better able to reach the majority and avoids isolating children with disabilities from their families and communities.

A range of barriers within education policies, systems and services limit disabled children's mainstream educational opportunities. Systemic and school-level change to remove physical and attitudinal barriers and provide reasonable accommodation and support services is required to ensure that children with disabilities have equal access to education.

A broad range of stakeholders – policy-makers, school administrators, teachers, families, and children with and without disabilities – can contribute to improving educational opportunities and outcomes for children with disabilities, as outlined in the following recommendations.

Formulate clear policies and improve data and information

- Develop a clear national policy on the inclusion of children with disabilities in education supported by the necessary legal framework, institutions, and adequate resources. Definitions need to be agreed on what constitutes "inclusive education" and "special educational needs", to help policy-makers develop an equitable education system that includes children with disabilities.
- Identify, through surveys, the level and nature of need, so that the correct support and accommodations can be introduced. Some students may require only modifications to the physical environment to gain access, while others will require intensive instructional support.

- Establish monitoring and evaluation systems. Data on the numbers of learners with disabilities and their educational needs, both in special schools and in mainstream schools, can often be collected through existing service providers. Research is needed on the cost–effectiveness and efficiency of inclusive education.
- Share knowledge about how to achieve educational inclusion among policy-makers, educators, and families. For developing countries the experience of other countries that have already moved towards inclusion can be useful. Model projects of inclusive education could be scaled up through local-to-regional-to-global networks of good practice.

Adopt strategies to promote inclusion

- Focus on educating children as close to the mainstream as possible. This includes, if necessary, establishing links between special education facilities and mainstream schools.
- Do not build a new special school if no special schools exist. Instead, use the resources to provide additional support for children with disabilities in mainstream schools.
- Ensure an inclusive educational infrastructure – for example, by mandating minimum standards of environmental accessibility to enable access to school for children with disabilities. Accessible transport is also vital.
- Make teachers aware of their responsibilities towards all children and build and improve their skills for teaching children with disabilities. Educating teachers about including children with disabilities should ideally take place in both pre-service and in-service teacher education. It should have a special emphasis on teachers in rural areas, where there are fewer services for children with disabilities.
- Support teachers and schools to move away from a one-size-fits-all model towards flexible approaches that can cope with

diverse needs of learners – for example, individualized education plans can ensure the individual needs of students with disabilities are met.

- Provide technical guidance to teachers that can explain how to group students, differentiate instruction, use peers to provide assistance, and adopt other low-cost interventions to support students having learning difficulties.

- Clarify and reconsider policies on the assessment, classification, and placement of students so that they take into consideration the interactional nature of disability, do not stigmatize children, and benefit the individuals with disabilities.

- Promote Deaf children's right to education by recognizing linguistic rights. Deaf children should have early exposure to sign language and be educated as multilinguals in reading and writing. Train teachers in sign language and provide accessible educational material.

Provide specialist services, where necessary

- Increase investment in school infrastructure and personnel so that children with disabilities that are identified as having special educational needs obtain the needed support, and continue to receive that support during their education.

- Make available speech and language therapy, occupational therapy, and physiotherapy to learners with moderate or significant disabilities. In the absence of specialist providers, use existing community-based rehabilitation services to support children in educational settings. If these resources are absent, an attempt should be made to develop these services gradually.

- Consider introducing teaching assistants to provide special support to children with disabilities, while ensuring that this does not isolate them from other students.

Support participation

- Involve parents and family members. Parents and teachers should jointly decide on the educational needs of a child. Children do better when families get involved, and this costs very little.

- Involve the broader community in activities related to the education of children with disabilities. This is likely to be more successful than policy decisions handed down from above.

- Develop links between educational services and community-based rehabilitation – and other rehabilitation services, where they exist. In this way, scarce resources can be used more efficiently, and education, health care, and social services can be properly integrated.

- Encourage adults with disabilities and disabled people's organizations to become more involved in promoting access to education for children with disabilities.

- Consult and involve children in decisions about their education.

References

1. *Global burden of disease: 2004 update*. Geneva, World Health Organization, 2008.
2. *World population prospects: the 2008 revision population database*: *highlights*. United Nations, Department of Economic and Social Affairs, 2009 (http://www.un.org/esa/population/publications/wpp2008/wpp2008_highlights.pdf, accessed 12 January 2011).
3. *The State of the World's Children 2006: excluded and invisible*. New York, United Nations Children's Fund, 2005.
4. *The present situation of special education*. Paris, United Nations Educational, Scientific and Cultural Organization, 1988.
5. *Education for All. Salamanca framework for action*. Washington, United Nations Educational, Scientific and Cultural Organization, 1994.
6. *The Dakar framework for action: Education for All: meeting our collective commitments*. Adopted by the World Education Forum, Dakar, United Nations Educational, Scientific and Cultural Organization, 26–28 April 2000. Paris, 2000a.

7. *Convention on the Rights of Persons with Disabilities*. New York, United Nations, 2006.

8. Filmer D. Disability, poverty, and schooling in developing countries: results from 14 household surveys. *The World Bank Economic Review*, 2008,22:141-163. doi:10.1093/wber/lhm021

9. *Education for All Global Monitoring Report*. Paris, United Nations Educational, Scientific and Cultural Organization, 2009.

10. Nott J. *Impaired identities? Disability and personhood in Uganda and implications for an international policy on disability*. Oslo, Department of Social Anthropology, University of Oslo, 1998.

11. *People with disabilities in India: from commitments to outcomes*. Washington, Human Development Unit, South Asia Region, World Bank, 2009.

12. *World Health Survey*. Geneva, World Health Organization, 2002–2004 (http://www.who.int/healthinfo/survey/en/, accessed 20 August 2009).

13. Loeb ME, Eide AH, eds. *Living conditions among people with activity limitations in Malawi: a national representative study*. Oslo, SINTEF, 2004.

14. Eide AH, van Rooy G, Loeb ME. *Living conditions among people with disabilities in Namibia: a national, representative study*. Oslo, SINTEF, 2003.

15. Eide AH, Loeb ME, eds. *Living conditions among people with activity limitations in Zambia*. Oslo, SINTEF, 2006.

16. Eide AH et al. *Living conditions among people with disabilities in Zimbabwe: a representative, regional study*. Oslo, SINTEF, 2003.

17. *Reaching the marginalized EFA Global Monitoring Report 2010*. Paris, United Nations Educational, Scientific and Cultural Organization, 2010.

18. Karangwa E, Kobusingye M. *Consultation report on education of the Deaf in Rwanda*. Kigali, Ministry of Education, 2007.

19. Porter GL. *Disability and inclusive education*. Paper prepared for the InterAmerican Development Bank seminar, Inclusion and Disability, Santiago, 2001 (http://www.disabilityworld.org/05-06_01/children/inclusiveed.shtml, accessed 1 May 2009).

20. *Summary report. Violence against children. UN Secretary-General's report on violence against children. Thematic group on violence against children. Findings and recommendations*. New York, United Nations Children's Fund, 2005.

21. Singal N. Inclusive education in India: international concept, national interpretation. *International Journal of Disability Development and Education*, 2006,53:351-369. doi:10.1080/10349120600847797

22. *Education for All global monitoring report 2009. Regional overview: sub-Saharan Africa*. Paris, United Nations Educational, Scientific and Cultural Organization, 2009 (http://unesdoc.unesco.org/images/0017/001784/178418e.pdf, accessed 20 August 2009).

23. Tirussew T. Overview of the development of inclusive education in the last fifteen years in Ethiopia. In: Savolainen H, Matero M, Kokkala H, eds. *When all means all: experiences in three African countries with EFA and children with disabilities*. Helsinki, Ministry for Foreign Affairs, 2006.

24. Kett M, Geiger M, Boersma M. Community-based rehabilitation and families in crisis. In: Hartley S, Okune J. *CBR: inclusive policy development and implementation*. Norwich, University of East Anglia, 2008.

25. Lewis I. *Education for disabled people in Ethiopia and Rwanda*. Manchester, Enabling Education Network, 2009.

26. Mete C, ed. *Economic implications of chronic illness and disability in Eastern Europe and the former Soviet Union*. Washington, World Bank, 2008.

27. *Project appraisal document on a proposed credit to the People's Republic of Bangladesh for a disability and children-at-risk project project*. Washington, World Bank, 2008 (http://tinyurl.com/yhuqa6u, accessed 19 October 2009).

28. *SNE country data 2010: background information*. Odense, European Agency for Development in Special Needs Education, 2010. Unpublished.

29. Florian L et al. Cross-cultural perspectives on the classification of children with disabilities: Part 1 issues in the classification of children with disabilities *The Journal of Special Education*, 2006,40:36-45. doi:10.1177/00224669060400010401

30. Educational Quality Improvement Program. *Issues brief: educating children with disabilities: Who are the children with disabilities?* Washington, United States Agency for International Development, 2005 (http://www.equip123.net/webarticles/anmviewer.asp?a=359&z=92, 12 January 2011).

31. *Students with disabilities, learning difficulties and disadvantages: policies, statistics and indicators*. Paris, Organisation for Economic Co-operation and Development, 2007.

32. Naidhu A. Collaboration in the era of inclusion. In: Forlin C, Lian M-GJ, eds. *Reform, inclusion and teacher education: toward a new era of special education in the Asia Pacific Region*. London, Routledge, 2008.

33. *Inclusive education at work: students with disabilities in mainstream schools*. Paris, Organisation for Economic Co-operation and Development, 1999.

34. *Special needs education: country data 2010*. Odense, European Agency for Development in Special Needs Education, 2010.

35. *Understanding and responding to children's needs in inclusive classrooms*. Paris, United Nations Educational, Scientific and Cultural Organization, 2001 (http://unesdoc.unesco.org/images/0012/001243/124394e.pdf, accessed 13 August 2009).

36. Dupoux E, Wolman C, Estrada E. Teachers' attitudes toward integration of students with disabilities in Haiti and the United States. *International Journal of Disability Development and Education*, 2005,52:43-58. doi:10.1080/10349120500071894

37. Silverstein J. *Framework for understanding IDEA in general and the discipline provisions in particular.* Washington, Center for Study and Advancement of Disability Policy, 2002.

38. Farrell P et al. SEN inclusion and pupil achievement in English schools. *Journal of Research in Special Educational Needs*, 2007,7:172-178. doi:10.1111/j.1471-3802.2007.00094.x

39. Norwich B. Education, inclusion and individual differences: recognising and resolving dilemmas. *British Journal of Educational Studies*, 2002,50:482-502. doi:10.1111/1467-8527.t01-1-00215

40. Pitt V, Curtin M. Integration versus segregation: the experiences of a group of disabled students moving from mainstream school into special needs further education. *Disability & Society*, 2004,19:387-401. doi:10.1080/09687590410001689485

41. Foster S, Emerton G. Mainstreaming the Deaf student: A blessing or a curse? *Journal of Disability Policy Studies*, 1991,2:61-76. doi:10.1177/104420739100200205

42. Fuchs D, Fuchs LS. Sometimes separate is better (education for learning disabled children). *Educational Leadership*, 1994,54:22-27.

43. Hocutt AM. Effectiveness of special education: is placement the critical factor? *The Future of children / Center for the Future of Children, the David and Lucile Packard Foundation*, 1996,6:77-102. PMID:8689263

44. McLaughlin MJ et al. *The education of children with disabilities and interpretations of equity: a review of policy and research.* New York, Teachers College, Columbia University, 2008.

45. Fisher M, Meyer LH. Development and social competence after two years for students who enrolled in inclusive and self-contained educational programs. *Research and Practice for Persons with Severe Disabilities*, 2002,27:165-174. doi:10.2511/rpsd.27.3.165

46. Kishi GS, Meyer LH. What children report and remember: A six-year follow-up of the effects of social contact between peers with and without severe disabilities. *The Journal of the Association for Persons with Severe Handicaps*, 1994,19:277-289.

47. Helmstetter E et al. Comparison of general and special education classrooms of students with severe disabilities. *Education and Training in Mental Retardation and Developmental Disabilities*, 1998,33:216-227.

48. Peck CA, Donaldson J, Pezzoli M. Some benefits nonhandicapped adolescents perceive for themselves from their social relationships with peers who have severe handicaps. *The Journal of the Association for Persons with Severe Handicaps*, 1990,15:241-249.

49. Baker ET, Wang MC, Walberg HJ. The effects of inclusion on learning. *Educational Leadership*, 1994–1995,52:33-35.

50. Baines L, Baines C, Masterson C. Mainstreaming: one school's reality. *Phi Delta Kappan*, 1994,76:39-40.

51. Zigmond N, Baker JM. An exploration of the meaning and practice of special education in the context of full inclusion of students with learning disabilities. *The Journal of Special Education*, 1995,29:109-115. doi:10.1177/002246699502900201

52. Salend SJ, Duhaney LMG. The impact of inclusion on students with and without disabilities and their educators. *Remedial and Special Education*, 1999,20:114-126. doi:10.1177/074193259902000209

53. Kalambouka A et al. The impact of population inclusivity in schools on student outcomes. In: *Research evidence in education library*. London, EPPI-Centre, Social Science Research Unit, Institute of Education, University of London, 2005.

54. Dyson A et al. *Inclusion and pupil achievement.* London, Department for Education and Skills, 2004.

55. Schneider M et al. *We also count! The extent of moderate and severe reported disability and the nature of the disability experience in South Africa.* Pretoria, Department of Health and CASE, 1999.

56. Afako R et al. *Implementation of inclusive education policies in Uganda.* Collaborative research between the Centre of International Child Health and the Uganda National Institute of Special Education. Paris, United Nations Educational, Scientific and Cultural Organization, 2002.

57. *Table 4–3. Students with disabilities served under IDEA, Part B, in the U.S. and outlying areas who exited school, by exit reason, reporting year, and student's age: 1995–96 through 2004–05.* Rockville, Data Accountability Centre, 2009 (https://www.ideadata.org/tables30th/ar_4-3.xls, accessed 16 October 2009).

58. Newman L et al. *The post-high school outcomes of youth with disabilities up to 4 years after high school: a report of findings from the National Longitudinal Transition Study-2 (NLTS2) (NCSER 2009–3017).* Menlo Park, SRI International, 2009 (www.nlts2.org/reports/2009_04/nlts2_report_2009_04_complete.pdf, accessed 22 October 2009).

59. Ogot O, McKenzie J, Dube S. Inclusive Education (IE) and community-based rehabilitation. In: Hartley S, Okune J, eds. *CBR: inclusive policy development and implementation.* Norwich, University of East Anglia, 2008.

60. *Report to Comic Relief on Oriang Cheshire inclusive education project.* London, Leonard Cheshire Disability, 2006.

61. Barton L, Armstrong F. *Policy, experience and change: cross-cultural reflections on inclusive education.* Dordrecht, Springer, 2007.

62. Forlin C, Lian MGJ, eds. *Reform, inclusion and teacher education: toward a new era of special education in the Asia Pacific Region.* London, Routledge, 2008.

63. *Education access and retention for educationally marginalised children: innovations in social protection*. KwaZulu-Natal, Mobile Task Team, Health Economics & HIV and AIDS Research Division, University of KwaZulu-Natal, 2005. (http://www.schoolsandhealth.org/sites/ffe/Key%20Information/Education%20Access%20and%20Retention%20for%20Educationally%20Marginalised%20Children.pdf, accessed 12 January 2011).

64. Bines H, Lei P, eds. *Education's missing millions: including disabled children in education through EFA FTI processes and national sector plans*. Milton Keynes, World Vision UK, 2007 (http://www.worldvision.org.uk/upload/pdf/Education%27s_Missing_Millions_-Main_Report.pdf, accessed 22 October 2009).

65. Stubbs S. *Inclusive education: where there are few resources*. Oslo, Atlas Alliance, 2008 (http://www.eenet.org.uk/theory_practice/IE%20few%20resources%202008.pdf, accessed 20 July 2009).

66. Chambers J, Shkolnik J, Pérez M. *Total expenditures for students with disabilities, 1999–2000: spending variation by disability*. Palo Alto, American Institutes for Research, Center for Special Education Finance, 2003 (No. ED481398).

67. *Education for all: global synthesis*. Paris, United Nations Educational, Scientific and Cultural Organization, 2000.

68. Hernandez G. *Assessing El Salvador's capacity for creating inclusive educational opportunities for students with disabilities using a capacity assessment framework*. College Park, University of Maryland, 2006.

69. *Policy Guidelines on Inclusion in Education*, Paris, United Nations Educational, Scientific and Cultural Organization, 2009.

70. Wright SL, Sigafoos J. Teachers and students without disabilities comment on the placement of students with special needs in regular classrooms at an Australian primary school. *Australasian Journal of Special Education*, 1997,21:67-80. doi:10.1080/1030011970210203

71. Chimedza R, Peters S. *Disability and special educational needs in an African context*. Harare, College Press, 2001.

72. *Proposal for a national plan for special needs education and related services in Rwanda*. Kigali, Government of the Republic of Rwanda, 2005 (http://payson.tulane.edu/gsdl-2.73//collect/mohnonve/index/assoc/HASH2410. dir/doc.pdf, accessed 18 August 2009).

73. Haualand H, Allen C. *Deaf people and human rights*. Helsinki, World Federation of the Deaf and Swedish National Association of the Deaf, 2009.

74. *Researching our experience: a collection of writings by Zambian teachers*. Mpika and Manchester, Enabling Education Network, 2003.

75. Macdonald SJ. *Toward a sociology of dyslexia: exploring links between dyslexia, disability and social class*. Saarbrücken, VDM Publishing House, 2009.

76. Kwon H. Inclusion in South Korea: the current situation and future directions. *International Journal of Disability Development and Education*, 2005,52:59-68. doi:10.1080/10349120500071910

77. Huang HH, Diamond KE. Early childhood teachers' ideas about including children with disabilities in programs designed for typically developing children. *International Journal of Disability Development and Education*, 2009,56:169-182. doi:10.1080/10349120902868632

78. Price P. Education for All (EFA): an elusive goal for children with disabilities in developing countries in the Asian Pacific Region. *Asia Pacific Disability Rehabilitation Journal*, 2003,14:3-9.

79. Inclusion International. *Better education for all: when we're included too*. Salamanca, Instituto Universitario de Integracion en la Comunidad, 2009.

80. Ingstad B, Whyte SR, eds. *Disability and culture*. Berkley, University of California Press, 2005.

81. O'Sullivan C, MacLachlan M. Childhood disability in Burkina Faso and Sierra Leone: an exploratory analysis. In: M.Machlan, L.Swartz, eds. *Disability and international development: towards inclusive global health*. Dordrecht, Springer, 2009.

82. Karangwa E. *Grassroots community-based inclusive education: exploring educational prospects for young people with disabilities in the post-conflict Rwandan communities*. Louvain, Centre for Disability, Special Needs Education and Child Care, 2006 (https://repository.libis.kuleuven.be/dspace/handle/1979/424, accessed 1 July 2008).

83. Karangwa E, Ghesquière P, Devlieger P. The grassroots community in the vanguard of inclusion: the Rwandan perspective. *International Journal of Inclusive Education*, 2007,11:607-626.

84. Kvam MH, Braathen SH. *Violence and abuse against women with disabilities in Malawi*. Oslo, SINTEF, 2006.

85. Howell C. Changing public and professional discourse. In: Engelbrecht P, Green L, eds. *Responding to the challenges of inclusive education in Southern Africa*. Pretoria, Van Schaik Publishers, 2006:89–100.

86. Boersma FJ, Chapman JW. Teachers' and mothers' academic achievement expectations for learning disabled children. *Journal of School Psychology*, 1982,20:216-221. doi:10.1016/0022-4405(82)90051-6

87. McGrew KS, Evans J. *Expectations for students with cognitive disabilities: Is the cup half empty or half full? Can the cup flow over?* Minneapolis, National Center on Educational Outcomes, University of Minnesota, 2003 (http://education.umn.edu/NCEO/OnlinePubs/Synthesis55.html, accessed 9 August 2010).

88. Watson N et al. *Life as a disabled child: research report*. Edinburgh, University of Edinburgh, 1998.

89. McGregor G, Vogelsberg RT. *Inclusive schooling practices: pedagogical and research foundations. A synthesis of the literature that informs best practices about inclusive schooling*. Baltimore, Paul H Brookes, 1998.

90. Villa RA et al. Inclusion in Viet Nam: more than a decade of implementation. *Research and Practice for Persons with Severe Disabilities*, 2003,28:23-32. doi:10.2511/rpsd.28.1.23

91. Begeny JC, Martens BK. Inclusionary education in Italy: a literature review and call for more empirical research. *Remedial and Special Education*, 2007,28:80-94. doi:10.1177/07419325070280020701

92. Cornoldi C et al. Teacher attitudes in Italy after twenty years of inclusion. *Remedial and Special Education*, 1998,19:350-356. doi:10.1177/074193259801900605

93. *Disabled children's right to education.* Auckland, New Zealand Human Rights Commission, 2009.

94. *Open file on inclusive education: support materials for managers and administrators.* Paris, United Nations Educational, Scientific and Cultural Organization, 2003 (http://unesdoc.unesco.org/images/0013/001321/132164e.pdf, accessed 13 August 2009).

95. Khatleli P et al. Schools for all: national planning in Lesotho. In: O'Toole B, McConkey R, eds. *Innovations in developing countries for people with disabilities.* Chorley, Lisieux Publications, 1995.

96. Johnstone CJ, Chapman D. Contributions and constraints to the implementation of inclusive education in Lesotho. *International Journal of Disability Development and Education*, 2009,56:131-148. doi:10.1080/10349120902868582

97. *Annual report of the United Nations High Commissioner for Human Rights and reports of the office of the High Commissioner and the Secretary-General: thematic study by the office of the United Nations High Commissioner for Human Rights on enhancing awareness and understanding of the convention on the rights of persons with disabilities.* Geneva, Office of the High Commissioner on Human Rights, 2009 (http://www.un.org/disabilities/documents/reports/ohchr/A.HRC.10.48AEV.pdf, accessed 12 January 2011).

98. Hartman WT. State funding models for special education. *Remedial and Special Education*, 1992,13:47-58. doi:10.1177/074193259201300610

99. Parrish TB. *Fiscal policies in special education: removing incentives for restrict placements.* Palo Alto, Center for Special Education Finance, American Institutes for Research, 1994 (Policy Paper No. 4).

100. *Student with disabilities, learning difficulties and disadvantages: statistics and indicators.* Paris, Organisation for Economic Co-operation and Development, 2005.

101. *Students with disabilities, learning difficulties and disadvantages: statistics and indicators for curriculum access and equity (special educational needs) in the countries of the organisation of American States (OAS) – outputs.* Paris, Organisation for Economic Co-operation and Development, 2007b.

102. Grimes PA. *Quality education for all: a history of the Lao PDR inclusive education project 1993–2009.* Vientiane, Save the Children Norway, 2009.

103. *Overcoming Exclusion through Inclusive Approaches in Education: a challenge and a vision*, Paris, United Nations Educational, Scientific and Cultural Organization, 2003.

104. Slee R. Teacher education, government and inclusive schooling. In: Allen J, ed. *Inclusion, participation and democracy.* Dordrecht, Kluwer Publishers, 2003.

105. *Assessment in inclusive settings: key issues for policy and practice.* Odense, Denmark, European Agency for Development in Special Needs Education, 2007.

106. McCausland D. *International experience in the provision of individual education plans for children with disabilities.* Dublin, National Disability Authority, 2005.

107. *Embracing diversity: toolkit for creating inclusive, learning-friendly environments.* Bangkok, Thailand, United Nations Educational, Scientific and Cultural Organization, 2009 (http://www2.unescobkk.org/elib/publications/032revised/index.htm, accessed 12 January 2011).

108. *Toolkit of best practices and policy advice.* Geneva, International Telecommunication Union, 2009 (http://www.connec-taschool.org/itu-module-list, accessed 12 January 2011).

109. Takala M, Pirttimaa R, Törmänen M. Inclusive special education: the role of special education teachers in Finland. *British Journal of Special Education*, 2009,36:162-172. doi:10.1111/j.1467-8578.2009.00432.x

110. Jerwood L. Focus on practice: using special needs assistants effectively. *British Journal of Special Education*, 1999,26:127-129. doi:10.1111/1467-8527.t01-1-00123

111. Logan A. The role of the special needs assistant supporting pupils with special educational needs in Irish mainstream primary schools. *Support for Learning*, 2006,21:92-99. doi:10.1111/j.1467-9604.2006.00410.x

112. *Early childhood intervention: analysis of situations in Europe.* Middlefart, Denmark, European Agency for Development in Special Needs Education, 2005.

113. Education for children with disabilities: improving access and quality. London, UK Department for International Development, 2010 (http://www.dfid.gov.uk/Media-Room/News-Stories/2010/Education-for-children-with-disabilities/, accessed 12 January 2011).

114. Lasonen J, Kemppainen R, Raheem K. *Education and training in Ethiopia: an evaluation of approaching EFA goals*. Jyväskylä, Finland, Institute for Educational Research, University of Jyväskylä, 2005 (http://ktl.jyu.fi/arkisto/verkkojulkaisuja/TP_23_Lasonen.pdf, accessed 30 September 2009).

115. *Putting children at the centre of education: how VSO supports practice and policy in primary schools*. Addis Ababa, VSO Ethiopia, 2008.

116. Schurmann E. *Training disabled teachers in Mozambique*. Manchester, Enabling Education, 2006 (Newsletter 10) (http://www.eenet.org.uk/resources/eenet_newsletter/news10/page15.php, accessed 30 September 2009).

117. *Education in emergencies: including everyone. INEE pocket guide to inclusive education*. Geneva, Inter-Agency Network on Education in Emergencies, 2009.

118. Ferguson DL. International trends in inclusive education: the continuing challenge to teach one and everyone. *European Journal of Special Needs Education*, 2008,23:109-120. doi:10.1080/08856250801946236

119. *Accessibility program and school restoration in Lisbon*. Paris, Organisation for Economic Co-operation and Development, 2006.

120. Miles S. Engaging with teachers' knowledge: promoting inclusion in Zambian schools. *Disability & Society*, 2009,24:611-624. doi:10.1080/09687590903010990

121. *Making schools inclusive: how change can happen: Save the Children's experiences*. London, Save the Children, 2008.

122. *Development for all: towards a disability-inclusive Australian aid program 2009–2014*. Canberra, Australian Agency for International Development, 2008a.

123. . Australian Agency for International DevelopmentSport and Development. *Focus Magazine*, 2008,b23:2-22.

124. Sport for Development and Peace International Working Group. *Harnessing the power of sport for development and peace: recommendations to governments*. Toronto, Right to Play, 2008.

125. International Labour Organization, United Nations Educational, Scientific and Cultural Organization, World Health Organization. *CBR: A strategy for rehabilitation, equalization of opportunities, poverty reduction and social inclusion of people with disabilities*. Geneva, World Health Organization, 2004.

126. Focas-Licht M. Alternative basic education for Karamoja, Uganda. *Enabling Education*, 2000, 4.

127. Chavuta AHP, Kimuli E, Ogot O. Community-based rehabilitation as part of inclusive education and development. In: Hartley S, ed. *CBR as part of community development: a poverty reduction strategy*. London, University College London, Centre for International Child Health, 2006:54–63 (http://www.afri-can.org/cbr_book.php, accessed 21 September 2009).

128. Brady JP et al. *Evaluation of the Step By Step Program: executive summary*. Arlington, VA, Improving Educational Quality and Children's Resources International, 1999 (http://www.childrensresources.org/stepbystep.pdf, accessed 7 September 2009).

129. Carrington S, Allen K, Osmolowski D. Visual narrative: a technique to enhance secondary students' contribution to the development of inclusive, socially just school environments. Lessons from a box of crayons. *Journal of Research in Special Educational Needs*, 2007,7:8-15. doi:10.1111/j.1471-3802.2007.00076.x

130. Kaplan I, Lewis I, Mumba P. Picturing global educational inclusion? Looking and thinking across students' photographs from the UK, Zambia and Indonesia. *Journal of Research in Special Educational Needs*, 2007,7:23-35. doi:10.1111/j.1471-3802.2007.00078.x

131. Rieser R. *Implementing inclusive education: a Commonwealth guide to implementing Article 24 of the UN Convention on the Rights of Persons with Disabilities*. London, Commonwealth Secretariat, 2008.

132. *Schools for all: including disabled children in education*. London, Save the Children UK, 2002.

133. *Young people's views on inclusive education: Lisbon declaration*. Odense, Denmark, European Agency for Development in Special Needs Education, 2007.

Chapter 8

Work and employment

"My disabilities deprived me of the chance to participate in farming; nevertheless I didn't give up. I raised ducks, sold aqua-cultural products, and traded waste materials. Although social discrimination and physical disability caused lots of difficulties, I never yielded. However, due to the hardship of the work, the ulcer on my right foot deteriorated, finally I had to have an amputation. Luckily with the help of friends and neighbours, I was successfully fitted with a prosthesis and restarted my career to seek a meaningful and independent life. From scratch, I began to raise cattle. I set up the Centre of Cattle Trading. It not only provides me a sufficient life, but also enables me to help many others who are also facing the challenges of leprosy."

Tiexi

"A lot of people, when I tried to get into university and when I applied for jobs, they struggled to see past the disability. People just assumed because I had a disability, that I couldn't perform even the simplest of tasks, even as much as operating a fire extinguisher… I think the main reason I was treated differently, since I set out to become a nurse, was probably because people were scared, because they've never been faced with anyone like me before."

Rachael

"I work at the catering unit of an NGO, supplying meals to 25 people who work there and sewing dolls when I am not cooking. The products are made for shops who buy because of the good quality, not because the things are made by people with disabilities. I have many friends at work. We all have intellectual disabilities. I do not have any other job choices because no one else would hire someone like me. It is hard to think what I would do if I had more choices, but maybe I would like to sing and dance and make music."

Debani

"Before the earthquake we were a big family with seven children all with our wishes and dreams. But only three of us survived in the ruined blocks of the buildings. The US doctors managed to save only one of my legs. With prosthesis I restarted attending school. I was living with memories of past, which were only a few pictures left. Even though I acknowledged the need to further my education I had no wish to do it. The turning point in my life was an offer to work in the local TV channel as a starting journalist. At first I had the anticipation that disability could be a hindrance upon becoming a professional journalist. But I had a very warm welcome; I was encouraged and had an on-job training for becoming a journalist. Very soon I felt comfortable in my new environment and position, was given equal number of responsibilities as others had and was not given any privilege."

Ani

8

Work and employment

Across the world, people with disabilities are entrepreneurs and self-employed workers, farmers and factory workers, doctors and teachers, shop assistants and bus drivers, artists, and computer technicians (*1*). Almost all jobs can be performed by someone with a disability, and given the right environment, most people with disabilities can be productive. But as documented by several studies, both in developed and developing countries, working age persons with disabilities experience significantly lower employment rates and much higher unemployment rates than persons without disabilities (*2–9*). Lower rates of labour market participation are one of the important pathways through which disability may lead to poverty (*10–15*).

In Article 27 the United Nations *Convention on the Rights of Persons with Disabilities* (CRPD) "recognizes the right of persons with disabilities to work, on an equal basis with others; this includes the opportunity to gain a living by work freely chosen or accepted in a labour market and work environment that is open, inclusive and accessible to persons with disabilities" (*16*). Furthermore, the CRPD prohibits all forms of employment discrimination, promotes access to vocational training, promotes opportunities for self-employment, and calls for reasonable accommodation in the workplace, among other provisions.

A number of factors impact labour market outcomes for persons with disabilities including; productivity differentials; labour market imperfections related to discrimination and prejudice, and disincentives created by disability benefit systems (*2, 17–19*). To address labour market imperfections and encourage the employment of people with disabilities, many countries have laws prohibiting discrimination on the basis of disability. Enforcing antidiscrimination laws is expected to improve access to the formal economy and have wider social benefits. Many countries also have specific measures, for example quotas, aiming to increase employment opportunities for people with disabilities (*20*). Vocational rehabilitation and employment services – job training, counselling, job search assistance, and placement – can develop or restore the capabilities of people with disabilities to compete in the labour market and facilitate their inclusion in the labour market. At the heart of all this is changing attitudes in the workplace (see Box 8.1).

> **Box 8.1. Key concepts**
>
> The term "work" is broad and includes unpaid work in the home or in a family enterprise, paid work for another person or organization in the formal or informal economy, and self-employment.
>
> Livelihood is "the means by which an individual secures the necessities of life" (*21*). It may involve work at home or in the community, work alone or in a group, or for an organization, a government body, or a business. It may be work that is remunerated in kind, in cash, or by a daily wage or a salary (*21*). In many countries, people with disabilities are found predominantly in non-wage or non-salary forms of work (*22*).
>
> The "formal economy" is regulated by the government and includes employment in the public and private sectors where workers are hired on contracts, and with a salary and benefits, such as pension schemes and health insurance. The "informal economy" is the unregulated part of a country's economy. It includes small-scale agriculture, petty trading, home-based enterprises, small businesses employing a few workers, and other similar activities (*22*).
>
> The term "labour force" refers to all adults of working age who are available, capable, and working or wanting to work (*23*). The "unemployed" includes people who are not employed but are available and searching for work. There are different indicators for measuring the work status of people with disabilities:
>
> - the **unemployment rate** is the number of unemployed people expressed as a percentage of the labour force;
> - the **employment rate** is the share of the working age population which works for pay;
> - the **labour force participation rate** is the proportion of the adult population which is economically active, whether employed or unemployed (*22*).
> - the **employment ratio** is the ratio of the employment rate of people with disabilities compared to the employment rate of the general population.

Understanding labour markets

Participation in the labour market

If people with disabilities and their households are to overcome exclusion, they must have access to work or livelihoods, breaking some of the circular links between disability and poverty (*14, 24–26*). Some employers continue to fear that people with disabilities are unqualified and not productive (*27, 28*). But people with disabilities often have appropriate skills, strong loyalty and low rates of absenteeism, and growing numbers of companies find it efficient and profitable to hire people with disabilities (*29, 30*).

The participation of people with disabilities in the labour force is important for other reasons:

- **Maximizing human resources.** Productive engagement of persons with disabilities increases individual well-being and contributes to the national output (*31, 32*).
- **Promoting human dignity and social cohesion.** Apart from income, employment brings personal and social benefits, adding to a sense of human dignity and social cohesion (*33*). All individuals should be able to freely choose the direction of their personal lives, to develop their talents and capabilities to the full (*16*).
- **Accommodating the increasing numbers of people with disabilities in the working age population.** The prevalence of disability is expected to increase in the coming decades because of a rise in chronic conditions together with improved health and medical rehabilitation services that preserve and prolong life. The ageing of the world's population is also expected to increase the prevalence of disability. In all world regions the proportion of people over the age of 60 is predicted to rise over the next few decades (*17, 18*).

Labour market theory suggests, for reasons of both supply and demand, that the employment rate of people with disabilities will be lower than that of people without disabilities.

On the supply side, people with disabilities will experience a higher cost of working, because more effort may be required to reach the workplace and to perform the work, and in countries with more generous disability allowances, employment may result in a loss of benefits and health care coverage, whose value is greater than the wages that could be earned (*34*). So the "reservation wage" of a person with disability – the lowest wage a person is willing to work for – is likely to be higher than that of a person without a disability. The resulting "benefit trap" is a source of concern in many high-income countries (*2, 35*).

On the demand side, a health condition may make a person less productive, especially if the workplace environment does not accommodate people with disabilities. In such circumstances, the person would be expected to be offered a lower market wage. The effects of a disability on productivity are hard to calculate, because they depend on the nature of impairment, the working environment, and the tasks required in the job. A blind person, for example, might find it difficult to operate a crane but face no impediment to productivity as a telephone operator (*36*). In an agrarian economy most jobs are in the primary sector and involve heavy manual labour, which those with limited walking or carrying abilities may not be able to perform. In addition, a person with a disability may be offered a lower wage purely as a result of discrimination.

A higher reservation wage and a lower market wage thus make a person with disability less likely to be employed than one without disability.

Employment rates

In many countries data on the employment of people with disabilities are not systematically available. Responses to an International Labour Organization (ILO) survey in 2003 showed that 16 of the 111 countries and territories responding had no data at all on employment in relation to disability (*22*). In low-income and middle-income countries, the availability of data continues to be limited, despite recent improvements (*37*). And in many of these countries, a significant proportion of people work in the informal economy, and so do not appear in all labour market statistics. Nor are they covered by employment legislation.

Data from several countries show that employment rates for people with disabilities are below that of the overall population (see Table 8.1 and see Table 8.2) with the employment ratio varying from lows of 30% in South Africa and 38% in Japan to highs of 81% in Switzerland and 92% in Malawi.

Because non-working people with disabilities often do not look for jobs and are thus not counted as part of the labour force, the unemployment rate may not give the full picture of their status in the labour market. Instead, the employment rate is more commonly used as an indicator of the labour market status of people with disabilities.

Analysis of the World Health Survey results for 51 countries gives employment rates of 52.8% for men with disability and 19.6% for women with disability, compared with 64.9% for non-disabled men, and 29.9% for non-disabled women. A recent study from the Organization for Economic Co-operation and Development (OECD) (*2*) showed that in 27 countries working-age persons with disabilities experienced significant labour market disadvantage and worse labour market outcomes than working-age persons without disabilities. On average, their employment rate, at 44%, was over half that for persons without disability (75%). The inactivity rate was about 2.5 times higher among persons without disability (49% and 20%, respectively).

The employment rate varies considerably for people with different disabilities with individuals with mental health difficulties or intellectual impairments (*28, 44*) experiencing the lowest employment rates. A British analysis found that people with mental health difficulties faced greater difficulties in gaining entry into the labour market and in obtaining

Table 8.1. Employment rates and ratios in selected countries

Country	Year	Employment rate of people with disabilities (%)	Employment rate of overall population (%)	Employment ratio
Australia[a]	2003	41.9	72.1	0.58
Austria[a]	2003	43.4	68.1	0.64
Canada[a]	2003	56.3	74.9	0.75
Germany[a]	2003	46.1	64.8	0.71
India[b]	2002	37.6	62.5	0.61
Japan[a]	2003	22.7	59.4	0.38
Malawi[f]	2003	42.3	46.2	0.92
Mexico[a]	2003	47.2	60.1	0.79
Netherlands[a]	2003	39.9	61.9	0.64
Norway[a]	2003	61.7	81.4	0.76
Peru[c]	2003	23.8	64.1	0.37
Poland[a]	2003	20.8	63.9	0.33
South Africa[d]	2006	12.4	41.1	0.30
Spain[a]	2003	22.1	50.5	0.44
Switzerland[a]	2003	62.2	76.6	0.81
United Kingdom[a]	2003	38.9	68.6	0.57
USA[e]	2005	38.1	73.2	0.52
Zambia[g]	2005	45.5	56.5	0.81

Note: The employment rate is the proportion of the working age population (with or without disabilities) in employment. Definitions of working age differ across countries.
Sources: a (*38*); b (*8*); c (*39*); d (*7*); e (*40*); f (*41*); g (*42*).

Table 8.2. Employment rates, proportion of disabled and not disabled respondents

Individuals	Percent					
	Low-income countries		High-income countries		All countries	
	Not disabled	Disabled	Not disabled	Disabled	Not disabled	Disabled
Male	71.2	58.6*	53.7	36.4*	64.9	52.8*
Female	31.5	20.1*	28.4	19.6*	29.9	19.6*
18–49	58.8	42.9*	54.7	35.2*	57.6	41.2*
50–59	62.9	43.5*	57.0	32.7*	60.9	40.2*
60 and over	38.1	15.1*	11.2	3.9*	26.8	10.4*

Note: Estimates are weighted using WHS post-stratified weights, when available (probability weights otherwise), and age-standardized. * *t*-test suggests significant difference from "Not disabled" at 5%.
Source (*43*).

earnings compared with other workers (*45*). Another study found that people with intellectual impairments were three to four times less likely to be employed than people without disabilities – and more likely to have more frequent and longer periods of unemployment. They were less likely to be competitively employed and more likely to be employed in segregated settings (*46*).

Types of employment

In many countries, labour markets are largely informal, with many self-employed workers. In

India, for example, 87% of people with disabilities who work are in the informal sector (*47*).

People with disabilities may need flexibility in the scheduling and other aspects of their work – to give them proper time to prepare for work, to travel to and from work, and to deal with health concerns. Contingent and part-time work arrangements, which often provide flexibility, may therefore be attractive to them. But such jobs may provide lower pay and fewer benefits. Research in the United States of America has shown that 44% of workers with disabilities are in some contingent or part-time employment arrangement, compared with 22% of those without disabilities (*48*). Health issues were the most important factor explaining the high prevalence of contingent or part-time work.

Wages

If people with disabilities are employed, they commonly earn less than their counterparts without disabilities; women with disabilities commonly earn less than men with disabilities. The wage gaps between men and women with and without disabilities are thus as important as the difference in employment rates (*45, 49*). In the United Kingdom of Great Britain and Northern Ireland only half of the substantial difference in wages and participation rates between disabled and non-disabled male workers was attributable to differences in productivity (*19*). Empirical research in the United States found that discrimination reduced wages and opportunities for employment. While prejudice had a strong effect for a relatively small minority of men with disabilities, it appeared relatively unimportant in determining wage differentials for a much larger group (*36*).

It is unclear whether the wage gap is as marked in developing countries. Recent studies in India have produced mixed results, with a significant wage gap found for males in rural labour markets in Uttar Pradesh but not for similar workers in Tamil Nadu (*50, 51*). Further research is needed in this area, based on nationally representative data.

Barriers to entering the labour market

People with disabilities are disadvantaged in the labour market. For example, their lack of access to education and training or to financial resources may be responsible for their exclusion from the labour market – but it could also be the nature of the workplace or employers' perceptions of disability and disabled people. Social protection systems may create incentives for people with disabilities to exit employment onto disability benefits (*2*). More research is needed on factors that influence labour market outcomes for persons with disabilities.

Lack of access

Education and training are central to good and productive work for a reasonable income (*52–54*). But young people with disabilities often lack access to formal education or to opportunities to develop their skills – particularly in the increasingly important field of information technology (*55–57*). The gap in educational attainment between those with a disability and those without is thus an ever-increasing obstacle (*9*).

People with disabilities experience environmental obstacles that make physical access to employment difficult. Some may not be able to afford the daily travel costs to and from work (*58, 59*). There may also be physical barriers to job interviews, to the actual work setting, and to attending social events with fellow employees (*54*). Access to information can be a further barrier for people with visual impairments (*60*).

A lack of access to funding is a major obstacle for anyone wanting to set up a business. For a person with a disability, particularly a disabled woman, it is usually even more difficult, given the frequent lack of collateral. Many potential lenders – wrongly – perceive people with disabilities to be high risks for loans. So credit markets can prevent people with disabilities from obtaining funds for investment (*49*).

assumption that quotas correct labour market imperfections to the benefit of persons with disabilities is yet to be documented empirically, as no thorough impact evaluation of quotas on employment of persons with disabilities has been performed.

Germany has a quota of 5% for the employment of severely disabled employees in firms employing more than 20 people. In 2002 the figure for private firms was 3.4%, and in 2003 7.1% for government employment (80). In South Africa government departments and state bodies are bound by statutory provisions stipulating that at least 2% of their workforce must consist of people with disabilities. But the quota in the state sector has not been met (81). Turkey has a 3% quota for firms with more than 50 workers, with the state paying all the employers' social security contributions for disabled workers up to the limit of the quota, and half the contributions for disabled workers above the quota.

In many cases fines are imposed on employers who fail to meet their quotas. Such fines can be used to support initiatives to boost disability employment. In China companies that fail to meet the 1.5% quota pay a fee to the Disabled Persons Employment Security Fund, which supports training and job placement services for people with disabilities (82).

During the transition to free market economies, several countries in Eastern Europe and the former Soviet Union introduced quotas to replace the former system where jobs were set aside in specific industries for workers with disabilities. Fines for not meeting quotas paid for vocational rehabilitation and job training programmes.

In most Organisation for Economic Co-operation and Development (OECD) countries the rate of filling quotas ranges from 50% to 70% (73, 83). Quotas attract controversy. They can be unpopular with employers, who would often rather pay a fine than attempt to fill their statutory quotas. Among disabled people's organizations, they are sometimes regarded as diminishing the potential value of workers with disabilities (84).

Incentives to employers

If employers bear the cost of providing reasonable accommodations, they may be less likely to hire people with disabilities – to avoid additional costs of labour. If employees bear the cost, their mobility in the market may be reduced because of the risk of incurring further accommodation-related expenses in a new job. To counter these obstacles, various financial incentives can be offered:

- Tax incentives are often offered to employers, especially smaller employers (85).
- Government employment agencies can provide advice and funding for employment-related accommodations, as with one state's vocational rehabilitation agency in the United States (86).
- Workplace modifications can be supported. In Australia the Department of Employment and Workplace Relations funds the Workplace Modifications Scheme, which provides up to A$ 10 000 for modifications to accommodate new employees with disabilities (87).

Supported employment

Special employment programmes can make an important contribution to the employment of people with severe disabilities, particularly those with intellectual impairments and mental health conditions (38).

Supported employment can integrate people with disabilities into the competitive labour market. It provides employment coaching, specialized job training, individually tailored supervision, transportation, and assistive technology, all to enable disabled people to learn and perform better in their jobs (88). Its success has been documented for people with severe disabilities, including those with psychiatric or intellectual impairment, learning disabilities, and traumatic brain injury (89–92).

Social firms and other social enterprises work in the open market, but have the social objective of employing people experiencing the greatest disadvantage in the labour market. Often such enterprises seek to give employment opportunities for persons with disabilities, particularly those with intellectual impairments and mental health conditions, alongside non-disabled people (*93, 94*). Recent estimates suggest there are around 3800 social firms in Europe, predominantly in Germany and Italy, employing around 43 000 people with disabilities (*95*). The evidence base for social firms is currently weak. Where successful, it is argued that enterprises can result in savings for health and social care budgets, as well as social returns on investment, in the form of well-being and independence. For example, analysis of the Six Mary's Place guesthouse project in Edinburgh (*96*) suggested that for every £1 invested, £5.87 was returned in the form of savings in mental health and welfare benefits, new tax income, and increased personal income. Cost–benefit assessments of social firms and supported employment also need to include the wider health, social, and personal benefits (*97*).

Sheltered employment

Sheltered work provides employment in separate facilities, either in a sheltered business or in a segregated part of a regular enterprise (*73*), and is intended for those who are perceived as unable to compete in the open labour market. For example, in Switzerland, a country with one of the highest employment rates for people with disabilities, much of the employment is in segregated settings (*38*). In France sheltered employment offers regular pay and full social security coverage for people with one third or less work capacity loss and merely symbolic remuneration for those with more than two thirds of work-capacity loss (*38*). Sheltered workshops are controversial, because they segregate people with disabilities and are associated with the charity ethos.

The CRPD promotes the opportunity for people with disabilities to work in an open labour market (*16*). However, there may be a disincentive for sheltered workshops to move disabled people onto the open labour market because they may then lose their "best workers" (*98*). In New Zealand there have been attempts to make sheltered employment more professional and competitive and to ease the transition to the open market (see Box 8.2) (*38*). A recent European trend has been for sheltered workshops to transition to become social firms.

Employment agencies

General employment agencies have been encouraged – and in some cases required by law – to serve job seekers with disabilities in the same setting as other job seekers, rather than referring people with disabilities to special placement services. In the United States the Workforce Investment Act of 1998 brought together a wide range of job placement programmes into the "One Stop Centers". Countries such as Austria, Belgium, Denmark, and Finland include people with disabilities in services offered by mainstream employment agencies (*101*). Other countries have targeted services, such as BizLink, Singapore (*102*). More than 3000 employment service agencies for people with disabilities operate in China (*103*), where the Chinese Disabled Persons' Federation has a leading role in fostering employment.

Thinking behind the provision of employment services for people with disabilities is changing:

- There has been a move from a model of job placement that tried to fit people into available job openings to a "person-centred" model involving the interests and skills of the individual. The aim is to find a match that will lead to viable longer term employment and a life-long career (*104*).
- There has been a shift from using sheltered employment towards supported employment – that is, from "train and place" to "place and train". The idea is to employ people first, before they are trained, to help dispel beliefs that disabled people cannot perform a particular job (*105–107*).

Box 8.2. Improving vocational services for people with disabilities in New Zealand

In 2001 the New Zealand government launched Pathways to Inclusion to increase the participation of people with disabilities both in the workforce and in communities (*99*).

People with disabilities working in sheltered workshops had been paid less than the minimum wage, regardless of their skills or abilities.

Providers of sheltered employment, with advice and government funding, shifted their operations to include supported employment and community participation services. Although sheltered work is still part of a range of vocational services funded through the Ministry of Social Development, supported employment services have now largely replaced it.

An evaluation of the Pathways to Inclusion programme since its inception found the following (*100*):

- the number of people participating in vocational services increased from 10 577 in 2003 to 16 130 in 2007;
- employment outcomes have improved, with more participants either moving off benefits or declaring earnings while remaining on benefits;
- the number of providers of vocational services that aim to achieve paid employment increased from 44% to 76% over three years;
- the proportion of services providing segregated employment that paid at least the minimum wage all or most of the time increased from 10% in 2004 to 60% in 2007;
- the number of service users moving off benefits or declaring earnings within 12 to 24 months of starting the service has increased – an indication of the long-term effectiveness of the services.

Several successful user-controlled disability employment services have been launched in recent years:

- In Rio de Janeiro, Brazil, the Centro de Vida Independiente serves as an employment broker and ongoing support agency for disabled people (*108*).
- In Spain Fundación ONCE was founded in 1988 to promote training and employment and accessibility, funded by the national lottery – which is operated by ONCE, the association of blind people (*109*).
- In Manchester, United Kingdom, "Breakthrough" is an innovative user-controlled employment service that works with disabled people and employers, helping to find and sustain employment and to find training for work (*110*).
- In South Africa, Disability Employment Concerns was established in 1996 with the aim of emulating the ONCE model. Owned by disabled people's organizations, it invests in and supports companies to promote disability employment equity targets (*111, 112*).

- In India the National Centre for Promotion of Employment for Disabled People (*113*) sensitizes the corporate world, campaigns for access, promotes education, and raises awareness.

These programmes suggest that disabled people's organizations could expand their range of activities for improving disability employment – such as job search and job matching, training in technology and other job skills, and in interview skills.

Disability management

Disability management refers to interventions applied to individuals in employment who develop a health condition or disability. The main elements of disability management are generally effective case management, education of supervisors, workplace accommodation, and an early return to work with appropriate supports (*114*). The Canadian National Institute of Disability Management and Research (*115*) is an international resource that promotes education, training, and research on workplace-based reintegration – the process that maintains workers' abilities while reducing costs of disability for employers and governments.

In the United Kingdom the Pathways to Work programme is an initiative providing support in the fields of employment and health for people claiming the Employment and Support Allowance. It consists of mandatory work-related interviews and a range of services to help disabled people and those with health conditions move into work. Personal advisers offer help in finding jobs, work-related training, and assistance in managing disabilities or health conditions. Early research with a sample of beneficiaries found that the programme increased the probability of being employed by 7.4% (*116*).

People with disabilities are not a homogeneous group, and some subgroups require tailored approaches. The problems of impaired hearing, for instance, will differ from those of being blind (*117, 118*). Particular issues arise for people who have intermittent or episodic problems, such those with mental health difficulties.

Research has found considerable differences between countries in the proportion of people who return to work after the onset of disability, with figures in one study ranging from 40% to 70% (*119*). Organizations with established disability management programmes have improved the rates of return to work (see Box 8.3) (*120*).

Vocational rehabilitation and training

Vocational rehabilitation services develop or restore the capabilities of people with disabilities so they can participate in the competitive labour market. The services usually relate to job training, counselling, and placement. For example, in Thailand the Redemptorist Vocational School for the Disabled offers job placement as well as training in computer skills and business management (*121*). Mainstream vocational guidance and training programmes are less segregating than dedicated vocational training programmes.

Traditional training and mainstream programmes

In OECD countries there is insufficient investment in rehabilitation and employment measures, and take-up is low (*122*). In developing countries, vocational services tend to consist of small rehabilitation and training programmes (*9, 123*). Because of their high costs, such programmes fail to reach a significant proportion of their target group (*124*). Furthermore, traditional training programmes – focused on a limited range of specialized technical skills and provided in segregated centres – have not put many people with disabilities into jobs (*38,*

Box 8.3. Returning to work in Malaysia

Social security programmes help people with disabilities engage in community and working life. Whether financed by social insurance or through tax-funded benefits, cash payments and in-kind benefits can provide a means of contributing to society. This, in turn, will create more positive attitudes towards people with disabilities and make society more "disability-inclusive".

In Malaysia, following a year-long pilot scheme in 2005, the Social Security Organization is extending its Return to Work programme throughout the country, combining financial support through social security payments with physical and vocational rehabilitation to help workers with employment-related injuries and diseases return to work. A pilot demonstrated that, with rehabilitation, 60% of those injured in the workplace can return to full employment.

The programme works with rehabilitation service providers and has established links with several large employers to provide work for participants. A case manager coordinates the rehabilitation with the injured person and his or her family, employer, and doctor – bringing in professionals from different disciplines as needed, such as physical therapy, occupational therapy, counselling, and pain management.

125). Such programmes are typically in urban areas, often distant from where people with disabilities live. The trades they teach – such as carpentry and shoemaking – are frequently not responsive to changes in the labour market. In addition, an underlying assumption of these programmes tends to be that people with disabilities are capable of only a limited number of occupations.

In South Africa, however, a mainstreaming approach, under the country's National Skills Strategy, Sectoral Education and Training Authorities requires the allocation of 4% of traineeships to people with disabilities (*111*).

Alternative forms of training

Apart from imparting technical skills, recent programmes have also concentrated on improving the self-confidence of trainees and raising awareness of the wider business environment. The Persons with Disabilities' Self-Initiative to Development programme in Bangladesh helps people with disabilities form self-help organizations within the community (*126*). In Soweto, South Africa, training in competencies forms part of an entrepreneurship training programme, and the survival rate of businesses has been high (*127*).

Recent initiatives to provide alternative forms of training show promise:

- **Community-based vocational rehabilitation.** Trainers are local artisans who provide trainees with the skills to become self-reliant in the community. In Nigeria participants are given training as well as help with microfinance, so that they can be self-employed when they have finished the programme (*125*).
- **Peer training.** In Cambodia a successful home-based peer-training programme encourages village entrepreneurs in rural villages to teach technical and business skills to people with disabilities (*128*).
- **Early interventions.** In Australia a project providing computer training to people with recent spinal cord injuries – while still in hospital – has increased the rates of return to further education and training or work (*129*).
- **Mentoring.** In the United States collaboration between the government and private enterprise provides summer internships to hundreds of young people with disabilities. This mentoring project – raising career awareness and building skills – has in many cases led to permanent placements at the employers offering the internships (*130*).
- **Continuity of training.** Being able to keep in touch with rehabilitation centres, and to build on earlier training, is important. The Leprosy Mission in India sponsors associations of alumni from its vocational rehabilitation centres, enabling those trained to keep in touch with other graduates and with the training centres (see Box 8.4).

Promoting employment and the development of livelihoods is often undertaken through community-based rehabilitation (CBR), discussed throughout this Report. Interventions typically aim to:

- teach skills for developing income-generating opportunities and for being employed;
- impart knowledge about the labour market;
- shape appropriate attitudes to work;
- provide guidance on developing relationships with employers to find a job or receive in-job training.

CBR also seeks to create support in the community for including people with disabilities. A resource from the ILO offers examples of good practices on CBR and employment, together with practical suggestions for skills development, self-employment, and access to the job market (*52*).

Despite these promising initiatives, the evaluation of vocational rehabilitation is difficult and, in general, its effects are still largely unknown. The evaluation is made more difficult by the fact that disability benefits often act as disincentives to work, and by the wide range of different services provided to individuals (*75*).

Box 8.4. Vocational training at the Leprosy Mission

The Leprosy Mission in India runs vocational training centres for young people affected by leprosy. Students are taught a wide range of technical skills – including car repairing, tailoring, welding, electronics, radio and television repairing, stenography, silk production, offset printing, and computing. The qualifications obtained by those graduating are officially recognized by the government. The schools also teach other types of skills, such as business management and core life skills.

Core life skills are taught through the timetable and activities of the centres, nurtured through the examples of the staff.

The aims are to develop:

- personal skills – including those related to self-esteem, positive thinking, motivation, goal setting, problem solving, decision-making, time management, and stress management;
- coping mechanisms – including how to deal with one's sexuality, shyness, loneliness, depression, fear, anger, alcoholism, failure, criticism, and conflict;
- fitness for a job – including leadership skills, team work skills, and career planning.

In interviews and focus group discussions, former students were asked to name the most important thing they had learned from their training. No one mentioned technical skills. Instead, they mentioned discipline, punctuality, obedience, personality development, self-confidence, responsibility, and communication skills.

The Leprosy Mission's training centres have a job placement rate of more than 95%.

Among the reasons for the success are that the Mission has active job placement officers with good relations with local employers, who know that graduates from the Mission's training centres will be of a high standard, and the training centres have a strong alumni association that keeps graduates in touch with each other and with their training centre.

Self-employment and microfinance

Funding to help start small businesses can provide an alternative to scarce formal employment (*131, 132*). For self-employment programmes for people with disabilities to succeed, however, marketing skills, access to credit, and long-term support and follow-up are needed (*133*). The International Study on Income Generation Strategies analysed 81 self-directed employment projects and highlighted four success factors:

- a self-directed identity (self-confidence, energy, risk-taking);
- relevant knowledge (literacy and numeracy, technical skills, business skills);
- availability of resources (advice, capital, marketing assistance);
- an enabling social and policy environment (political support, community development, disability rights).

It identified successful examples of income generation schemes from Jamaica, the Philippines, and Thailand (*134*).

Many people with disabilities have few assets to secure loans, and may have lived in poverty for years. Microfinance programmes are in principle open to all, including disabled people. But anecdotal evidence suggests that few people with disabilities benefit from such schemes. Some microfinance programmes have been set up by disability NGOs and others target people with disabilities, but more evidence is needed on their effectiveness.

- a targeted microfinance programme in Ethiopia had a positive impact on the lives of women who became disabled during war (*135*);
- Handicap International evaluated 43 projects and found that targeted microfinance schemes were beneficial and that almost two thirds of them were sustainable (*132*);
- a disability organization typically faces difficulties in developing and administering

microfinance programmes, and targeted microfinance programmes set up by a disability organization can reach only a small number of people with disabilities (*136*).

A review of the literature found obstacles in mainstream microfinance, so provisional schemes run by NGOs and disabled people's organizations can help, because they give rise to social inclusion, participation, and empowerment. But both approaches are needed to achieve wider coverage and sustainability, given that microfinance has great social and economic impact for persons with disabilities (*137*).

Social protection

Long-term disability benefits can provide disincentives for people to seek employment and return to work (*2, 138, 139*). This is especially the case for those who are less skilled or whose jobs, if they were seeking them, would be lower paying. One reason is that the benefit provides a regular income – even though small – that the person can rely on. Loss of this regular payment and reliance on menial, low-paid work may result in no regular income and little sense of security (*34*).

But social assistance benefits can also have positive effects on employment for people with disabilities. Returning to work after disability may involve a period of unemployment and income insecurity. Social assistance programmes therefore need to take this into account when planning the transitional phases away from and back onto benefits. Such transitions should be factored into the benefit programmes so that people feel an incentive to work, while at the same time being secure in the knowledge that a benefit is still available should they not succeed (*73*).

The growth in disability benefit costs and the low employment rates for people with disabilities are concerns for policy-makers in developing countries (*2, 7, 35, 140*). In OECD countries there has been substantial growth in disability

beneficiary rates over the past decade, which now represents around 6% of working age population (*2, 141*). Disability benefits have become a benefit of last resort because: unemployment benefits are harder to access, early retirement schemes have been phased out, and low-skilled workers face labour market disadvantages (*2*). Spending on disability benefits is an increasing burden on public finances, rising to as much as 4–5% of GDP in countries such as the Netherlands, Norway, and Sweden. People with mental health difficulties make up the majority of claims in most countries. People almost never leave disability benefits for a job (*2*).

System reform to replace passive benefits with active labour market programmes can make a difference. Evidence from Hungary, Italy, the Netherlands, and Poland suggests that tighter obligations for employers to provide occupational health services and to support reintegration, together with stronger work incentives for workers and better employment supports, can help disability beneficiaries into work (*2*).

The work disincentives of benefit programmes, together with the common perception that disability is necessarily an obstacle to work, can be significant social problems (*38*). So the status of disability should be independent of the work and income situation. Disability should be recognized as a health condition, interacting with contextual factors, and should be distinct from eligibility for and receipt of benefits, just as it should not automatically be treated as an obstacle to work (*38, 142*). Assessment should focus on the capacity for work, not disability. Guidance for doctors should emphasize the value and possibility of work and keep sickness absence as short as possible (*2*).

To ensure that social protection for people with disabilities does not operate as a disincentive to seeking employment, one policy option is to separate the income support element from the element to compensate for the extra costs incurred by people with disabilities. Temporary entitlements plus cost of disability components irrespective of work status, more flexible in-work payments, and options for putting benefits on hold while trying work are preferred options (*122, 141*).

Time-limited disability benefits may be another way to increase employment for disabled people, with particular importance for younger people (*2*). Germany, the Netherlands, and Norway recently adopted such programmes to encourage the return to work (*143*). These schemes accept the fact that some people have severe disabilities that will last for a longer period, but recognize that, with intervention, returning to work is possible. The limited duration of the benefit is in itself an incentive for people to return to work by the time benefits end. A critical factor in making the limited duration of the benefit an incentive to return to work, however, is the way in which the time-limited programme is linked to the permanent programme. If the transition to the permanent programme is smooth and expected by recipients, the incentive to return to the labour force is reduced. But there is no firm evidence on the effectiveness of time-limited benefits in encouraging the return to work.

Another priority is making sure it pays to be in work (*2*). The United Kingdom has recently been experimenting with ways outside the traditional disability benefit system to encourage people with disabilities to work (*139*). A Working Tax Credit is paid to a range of lower income employed and self-employed people, administered by the taxation authorities. A person qualifies for the disability element of the Working Tax Credit if he or she works at least 16 hours a week, has a disability that puts them at a disadvantage of finding a job, or receives a qualifying benefit such as the long-term disability pension. The idea is to encourage work among low-income households with a member with disabilities. The credit, introduced in April 2003, has proved complex to administer. But an early evaluation suggests that it is encouraging people to enter work and reducing previous disincentives for young people to seek work (*144*).

Working to change attitudes

Many disabled people's organizations already attempt to change perceptions on disability at the community level. Anecdotal evidence suggests that employing a disabled person in itself changes attitudes within that workplace (*54, 145*). In the United States, companies already employing a disabled person are more likely to employ other disabled people (*1*).

Many awareness campaigns have targeted specific conditions:
- the BBC World Service Trust has conducted a large-scale awareness campaign in India to counter misconceptions on leprosy;
- in New Zealand the organization Like Minds has worked to change public attitudes to people with mental health conditions (*146*);
- various initiatives have tackled the myths, ignorance, and fear often surrounding HIV/AIDS (*147*).

Light is a public electricity utility in Rio de Janeiro, Brazil, employing disabled people and generating positive publicity for its actions (*148*). On the reverse of the company's monthly electricity bill is a picture of a wheelchair, with the message:

> "At Light, the number of workers with disabilities is greater than that required by law. The reason is simple – for us, the most important thing is to have valuable people."

In the United Kingdom the Employers' Forum on Disability has developed innovative approaches for changing perceptions of disability (see Box 8.5). Similar initiatives have been developed in Australia, Germany, South Africa, Sri Lanka, and the United States. More data are needed to understand which interventions can shift embedded attitudes on disability and best promote positive attitudes about disability in the workplace.

- For larger businesses, aim to become model employers of people with disabilities.

Other organizations: NGOs including disabled people's organizations, microfinance institutions, and trade unions

- For organizations providing mainstream training opportunities, include people with disabilities.
- Provide targeted support when mainstream opportunities are not available.
- Support community-based rehabilitation, to enhance the development of skills and enable people with disabilities to make a decent living.
- Where the informal economy is predominant, promote micro-enterprises and self-employment for people with disabilities.
- For microfinance institutions, improve access to microfinance for persons with disabilities through better outreach, accessible information and customized credit conditions.
- Support the development of networks of people with disabilities that can campaign for the rights of people with disabilities.
- For labour unions, make disability issues, including accommodations, part of their bargaining agendas.

References

1. Domzal C, Houtenville A, Sharma R. *Survey of employer perspectives on the employment of people with disabilities*. McLean VA, CESSI, 2008.
2. *Sickness, disability and work: breaking the barriers. A synthesis of findings across OECD countries*. Paris, Organisation for Economic Co-operation and Development, 2010.
3. Houtenville AJ, et al., eds. *Counting working-age people with disabilities. What current data tell us and options for improvement*. Kalamazoo, W.E. Upjohn Institute for Employment Research, 2009.
4. Mitra S, Posarac A, Vick B. *Disability and poverty in developing countries: a snapshot from the World Health Survey*. forthcoming.
5. Contreras DG, et al.. *Socio-economic impact of disability in Latin America: Chile and Uruguay*. Santiago, Universidad de Chile, Departemento de Economia, 2006.
6. Mete C, ed. *Economic implications of chronic illness and disability in Eastern Europe and the Former Soviet Union*. Washington, World Bank, 2008.
7. Mitra S. The recent decline in the employment of persons with disabilities in South Africa, 1998–2006. *South African Journal of Economics*, 2008,76:480-492. doi:10.1111/j.1813-6982.2008.00196.x
8. Mitra S, Sambamoorthi U. Employment of persons with disabilities: evidence from the National Sample Survey. *Economic and Political Weekly*, 2006,a41:199-203.
9. *People with disabilities in India: from commitments to outcomes*. Washington, World Bank, 2009. (http://imagebank.world-bank.org/servlet/WDSContentServer/IW3P/IB/2009/09/02/000334955_20090902041543/Rendered/PDF/502090WP0Peopl1Box0342042B01PUBLIC1.pdf, accessed 2 February 2011).
10. Scott K, Mete C. Measurement of disability and linkages with welfare, employment, and schooling. In: Mete C, ed. *Economic implications of chronic illness and disability in Eastern Europe and the Former Soviet Union*. Washington, World Bank, 2008 (http://siteresources.worldbank.org/DISABILITY/Resources/Regions/ECA/EconomicImplicationsMete.pdf, accessed 2 February 2011).
11. Zaidi A, Burchardt T. Comparing incomes when needs differ: equivalization for the extra costs of disability in the UK. *Review of Income and Wealth*, 2005,51:89-114. doi:10.1111/j.1475-4991.2005.00146.x
12. Braitwaite J, Mont D. Disability and poverty: a survey of the World Bank poverty assessments and implications. *ALTER European Journal of Disability Research*, 2009,3:219-232.
13. Haveman R, Wolfe B. The economic well being of the disabled: 1962–1984. *The Journal of Human Resources*, 1990,25:32-54. doi:10.2307/145726
14. Hoogeveen JG. Measuring welfare for small but vulnerable groups: poverty and disability in Uganda. *Journal of African Economies*, 2005,14:603-631. doi:10.1093/jae/eji020
15. Peiyun . SLivermore G. Long-term poverty and disability among working age adults. *Journal of Disability Policy Studies*, 2008,19:244-256. doi:10.1177/1044207308314954

16.   *Convention on the Rights of Persons with Disabilities*. New York, United Nations, 2006.

17.   *Averting the Old Age Crisis: Policies to Protect the Old and Promote Growth. New York*. Washington, World Bank and Oxford University Press, 1994 (http://www-wds.worldbank.org/external/default/WDSContentServer/WDSP/IB/1994/09/01/0000 09265_3970311123336/Rendered/PDF/multi_page.pdf, accessed 2 February 2011).

18.   Kinsella K, Velkoff V. *An aging world* [United States Census Bureau, Series P95/01–1]. Washington, United States Government Printing Office, 2001.

19.   Kidd MP, Sloane PJ, Ferko I. Disability and the labour market: an analysis of British males. *Journal of Health Economics*, 2000,19:961-981. doi:10.1016/S0167-6296(00)00043-6 PMID:11186853

20.   Quinn G, Degener T. *The current use and future potential of the United Nations human rights instruments in the context of disability*. Geneva, United Nations, 2002 (http://www.ohchr.org/EN/PublicationsResources/Pages/SpecialIssues.aspx, accessed 2 July 2009).

21.   *CBR guidelines*. Geneva, World Health Organization, 2010.

22.   *The employment situation of people with disabilities: towards improved statistical information*. Geneva, International Labour Organization, 2007.

23.   Brandolini A, Cipollone P, Viviano E. *Does the ILO definition capture all employment?* [Temi de discussione del Servizio Studi No. 529]. Rome, Banca d'Italia, 2004 (http://www.bancaditalia.it/pubblicazioni/econo/temidi/td04/td529_04/td529/tema_529.pdf, accessed 18 March 2008).

24.   Yeo R, Moore K. Including disabled people in poverty reduction work: "nothing about us, without us" *World Development*, 2003,31:571-590. doi:10.1016/S0305-750X(02)00218-8

25.   Fujiura GT, Yamaki K, Czechowicz S. Disability among ethnic and racial minorities in the United States. *Journal of Disability Policy Studies*, 1998,9:111-130. doi:10.1177/104420739800900207

26.   Harriss-White B. On to a loser: disability in India. In: Harriss-White B, Subramanian S, eds. *Essays on India's social sector in honour of S. Guhan*. New Delhi, Sage Publications, 1999:135–163.

27.   Roberts S et al. *Disability in the workplace: employers' and service providers' responses to the Disability Discrimination Act in 2003 and preparation for 2004 changes*. London, Department of Work and Pensions Research Summary, 2004.

28.   *Ready, willing, and disabled: survey of UK employers*. London, Scope, 2003 (http://www.scope.org.uk/work/, accessed 17 March 2008).

29.   Bagshaw M. *Ignoring disability: a wasted opportunity*. Wellington, National Equal Opportunities Network, 2006 (http://www.neon.org.nz/newsarchive/bagshawplusfour/, accessed 18 June 2009).

30.   Unger D. Employers' attitudes toward persons with disabilities in the workforce: myths or realities? *Focus on Autism and Other Developmental Disabilities*, 2002,17:2-10. doi:10.1177/108835760201700101

31.   Buckup S. *The price of exclusion: the economic consequences of excluding people with disabilities from the world of work*. Geneva, International Labour Organization, 2009.

32.   McDaid D, Knapp M, Raja S. Barriers in the mind: promoting an economic case for mental health in low- and middle-income countries. *World Psychiatry: official journal of the World Psychiatric Association (WPA)*, 2008,7:79-86. PMID:18560485

33.   Becker D et al. Long-term employment trajectories among participants with severe mental illness in supported employment. *Psychiatric Services (Washington, D.C.)*, 2007,58:922-928. PMID:17602007

34.   Stapleton D et al. *Exploratory study of health care coverage and employment of people with disabilities: literature review*. Washington, United States Department of Health and Human Services, 1997 (http://aspe.hhs.gov/daltcp/Reports/eshc-clit.htm, accessed 3 July 2009).

35.   Kemp PA, Sundén A, Bakker Tauritz B, eds. *Sick societies? Trends in disability benefits in post-industrial welfare states*. Geneva, International Social Security Association, 2006.

36.   Baldwin ML, Johnson WG. Labor market discrimination against men with disabilities. *The Journal of Human Resources*, 1994,29:1-19. doi:10.2307/146053

37.   Montes A, Massiah E. *Disability data: survey and methods issues in Latin America and the Caribbean*. Washington, Inter-American Development Bank, 2002.

38.   *Transforming disability into ability: policies to promote work and income security for disabled people*. Paris, Organisation for Economic Co-Operation and Development, 2003.

39.   Maldonado Zambrano S. *Trabajo y discapacidad en el Perú: mercado laboral, políticas públicas e inclusión social (Work and disability in Peru: labour market, public policies and social inclusion)*. Lima, Fodo Editorial del Congreso del Perú, 2006.

40.   Houtenville AJ, Erickson WA, Lee CG. *Disability statistics from the American Community Survey (ACS)*. Ithaca, Cornell University Rehabilitation Research and Training Center on Disability Demographics and Statistics, 2007.

41.   Loeb ME, Eide AH. *Living conditions among people with activity limitations in Malawi: a national representative study*. Oslo, SINTEF, 2004.

42.   Eide AH, Loeb ME. *Living conditions among people with activity limitations in Zambia: a national representative study*. Oslo, SINTEF, 2006.

43. *World Health Survey*. Geneva, World Health Organization, 2002–2004 (http://www.who.int/healthinfo/survey/en/, accessed 2 February 2011).

44. Thornicroft G. *Shunned: discrimination against people with mental illness*. London, Oxford University Press, 2006.

45. Jones MK, Latreille PL, Sloane PJ. Disability, gender and the British labour market. *Oxford Economic Papers*, 2006,58:407-449. doi:10.1093/oep/gpl004

46. Verdonschot MM et al. Community participation of people with an intellectual disability: a review of empirical findings. *Journal of Intellectual Disability Research: JIDR*, 2009,53:303-318. doi:10.1111/j.1365-2788.2008.01144.x PMID:19087215

47. Mitra S, Sambamoorthi U. Government programmes to promote employment among persons with disabilities in India. *Indian Journal of Social Development*, 2006,b6:195-213.

48. Schur L. Barriers or opportunities? The causes of contingent and part-time work among people with disabilities. *Industrial Relations*, 2003,42:589-622.

49. *Microfinance and people with disabilities* [Social Finance Highlight 1]. Geneva, International Labour Organization, 2007.

50. Mitra S, Sambamoorthi U. Disability and the rural labour market in India: evidence for males in Tamil Nadu. *World Development*, 2008,36:934-952. doi:10.1016/j.worlddev.2007.04.022

51. Mitra S, Sambamoorthi U. Wage differential by disability status in an agrarian labour market in India. *Applied Economics Letters*, 2009,16:1393-1398. doi:10.1080/13504850802047011

52. *Skills development through community-based rehabilitation*. Geneva, International Labour Organization, 2008.

53. *Vocational rehabilitation and employment of people with disabilities* [Report of a European conference,Warsaw–Konstancin Jeziorna, Poland, 23–25 October 2003]. Geneva, International Labour Organization, 2004 (http://www.ilo.org/skills/what/pubs/lang — en/docName — WCMS_106627/index.htm, accessed 23 June 2009).

54. *Strategies for skills acquisition and work for people with disabilities: a report submitted to the International Labour Organization*. Geneva, International Labour Organization, 2006 (http://www.hsrc.ac.za/research/output/outputDocuments/4388_Schneider_Strategiesforskills.pdf, accessed 23 June 2009).

55. Russell C. *Education, employment and training policies and programmes for youth with disabilities in four European countries*. Geneva, International Labour Organization, 1999.

56. Burchardt T. *The education and employment of disabled young people*. York, Joseph Rowntree Foundation, 2004.

57. Eide AH, et al. *Living conditions among people with activity limitations in Zimbabwe: a national representative study*. Oslo, SINTEF, 2003.

58. *Policy recommendations*. Measuring Health and Disability in Europe, 2008 (http://www.mhadie.it/home3.aspx, accessed 24 June 2009).

59. Roberts P, Babinard J. *Transport strategy to improve accessibility in developing countries*. Washington, World Bank, 2004 (http://siteresources.worldbank.org/INTTSR/Resources/accessibility-strategy.pdf, accessed 17 January 2011).

60. Butler SE et al. Employment barriers: access to assistive technology and research needs. *Journal of Visual Impairment & Blindness*, 2002,96:664-667.

61. Shier M, Graham J, Jones M. Barriers to employment as experienced by disabled people: a qualitative analysis in Calgary and Regina, Canada. *Disability & Society*, 2009,24:63-75. doi:10.1080/09687590802535485

62. Gartrell A. 'A frog in a well': the exclusion of disabled people from work in Cambodia. *Disability & Society*, 2010,25:289-301. doi:10.1080/09687591003701207

63. Waghorn G, Lloyd C. The employment of people with mental illness. *Australian e-Journal for the Advancement of Mental Health*, 2005, 4 (http://www.auseinet.com/journal/vol4iss2suppl/waghornlloyd.pdf, accessed 3 July 2009).

64. Baldwin ML, Marcus SC. Perceived and measured stigma among workers with serious mental illness. *Psychiatric Services (Washington, D.C.)*, 2006,57:388-392. PMID:16524998

65. Thornicroft G et al. INDIGO Study GroupGlobal pattern of experienced and anticipated discrimination against people with schizophrenia: a cross-sectional survey. *Lancet*, 2009,373:408-415. doi:10.1016/S0140-6736(08)61817-6 PMID:19162314

66. Kuddo A. *Labor Laws in Eastern European and Central Asian Countries: minimum norms and practices* [SP Discussion Paper 0920]. Washington, World Bank, 2009

67. Acemoglu D, Angrist J. Consequences of employment protection? The case of the Americans with Disabilities Act. *The Journal of Political Economy*, 2001,109:915-957. doi:10.1086/322836

68. Mitra S, Stapleton D. Disability, work and return to work. In: Lewin D, ed. *Contemporary issues in industrial relations, labor and employment relations*. Ithaca, Cornell University Press, 2006:251–284.

69. Houtenville AJ, Burkhauser RV. *Did the employment of people with disabilities decline in the 1990s, and was the ADA responsible? A replication and robustness check of Acemoglu and Angrist (2001)* [Research brief]. Ithaca, Cornell University, Employment and Disability Institute, 2004 (http://digitalcommons.ilr.cornell.edu/edicollect/91, accessed 15 May 2009).

70. Bell D, Heitmueller A. The Disability Discrimination Act in the UK: helping or hindering employment among the disabled? *Journal of Health Economics*, 2009,28:465-480. doi:10.1016/j.jhealeco.2008.10.006 PMID:19091434

71. Degener T. Disability discrimination law: a global comparative approach. In: Lawson A Gooding C, eds. *Disability rights in Europe: from theory to practice*. Portland, Hart Publishing, 2005.

72. Opini BM. A review of the participation of disabled persons in the labour force: the Kenyan context *Disability & Society*, 2010,25:271-287. doi:10.1080/09687591003701181

73. Mont D. *Disability employment policy* [SP Discussion Paper 0413]. Washington, World Bank, 2004.

74. *Enforcement guidance on reasonable accommodation and undue hardship under the Americans with Disabilities Act*. Washington, Equal Employment Opportunity Commission, 2002 (http://www.eeoc.gov/policy/docs/accommodation.html, accessed 3 June 2009).

75. Stapleton DC, Burkhauser RV, eds. *The decline in employment of people with disabilities: a policy puzzle*. Kalamazoo, UpJohn Institute, 2003.

76. Jones MK. Is there employment discrimination against the disabled? *Economics Letters*, 2006,92:32-37. doi:10.1016/j.econlet.2006.01.008

77. *Council Directive 2000/78/EC of 27 November 2000, establishing a general framework for equal treatment in employment and occupation*. Brussels, European Union, 2000 (http://ec.europa.eu/employment_social/news/2001/jul/directive78ec_en.pdf, accessed 15 June 2009).

78. Pereira de Melo H. *Article 13 network of disability discrimination law experts. Country: Portugal*. Oporto, Department of Bioethics and Ethical Medics, Oporto University, 2004.

79. *Israel: 2003 IDRM [International Disability Rights Compendium] Compendium Report*. Chicago, Center for International Rehabilitation, 2003 (http://www.ideanet.org/content.cfm?id=5B5C76, accessed 22 June 2009).

80. Waldschmidt A, Lingnau K. *Report on the employment of disabled people in European countries: Germany*. Academic Network of European Disability Experts, 2007 (http://www.disability-europe.net/content/pdf/DE%20Employment%20report.pdf, accessed 15 June 2009).

81. Commission for Employment Equity. *Annual report 2007–2008*. Pretoria, Department of Labour, 2008 (http://www.info.gov.za/view/DownloadFileAction? id=90058, accessed 2 February 2009).

82. Thornton P. *Employment quotas, levies, and national rehabilitation funds for persons with disabilities: pointers for policy and practice*. Geneva, International Labour Organization, 1998 (http://digitalcommons.ilr.cornell.edu/cgi/viewcontent.cgi?article=1083&context=gladnetcollect, accessed 17 March 2008).

83. Heyer K. From special needs to equal rights: Japanese disability law. *Asian-Pacific Law and Policy Journal*, 2000, 7.

84. Waddington L, Diller M. Tensions and coherence in disability policy: the uneasy relationship between social welfare and civil rights models of disability in American, European and international employment law. In: Breslin ML, Yee S, eds. *Disability rights law and policy*. Ardsley, Transnational Publishers, 2002.

85. *Tax incentives*. Job Accommodation Network, ADA Library (online), undated (http://www.jan.wvu.edu/media/tax.html, accessed 7 December 2008).

86. *Funding assistive technology and accommodations*. Boston, National Center on Workforce and Disability, 2008 (http://www.onestops.info/article.php?article_id=22, accessed 7 December 2008).

87. Mungovan A et al. *Education to employment package: a website for graduates with disabilities and employers*. Sydney, Workplace Modification Scheme, New South Wales Department of Education and Training, University of Western Sydney, 1998 (http://pubsites.uws.edu.au/rdlo/employment/tafe/services/T_S_work_mod.htm, accessed 7 December 2008).

88. *What is supported employment*? Washington, United States Department of Labor, Office of Disability Employment Policy, 1993 (http://www.dol.gov/odep/archives/fact/supportd.htm, accessed 18 October 2007).

89. *Handbook: supported employment*. Willemstad, World Organization for Supported Employment (http://www.wase.net/handbookSE.pdf, accessed 17 March 2008).

90. Crowther RE et al. Helping people with severe mental illness to obtain work: systematic review. *BMJ (Clinical Research Ed.)*, 2001,322:204-208. doi:10.1136/bmj.322.7280.204 PMID:11159616

91. Wehman P, Revell G, Kregel J.. Supported employment: a decade of rapid growth and impact. *American Rehabilitation*, 1998,

92. Cook JA et al. Integration of psychiatric and vocational services: a multisite randomized, controlled trial of supported employment. *The American Journal of Psychiatry*, 2005,162:1948-1956. doi:10.1176/appi.ajp.162.10.1948 PMID:16199843

93. Secker J, Dass S, Grove B. Developing social firms in the UK: a contribution to identifying good practice. *Disability & Society*, 2003,18:659-674. doi:10.1080/0968759032000097870

94. Warner R, Mandiberg J. An update on affirmative businesses or social firms for people with mental illness. *Psychiatric Services (Washington, D.C.)*, 2006,57:1488-1492. PMID:17035570

95. Social Firms Europe CEFEC [web site]. (http://www.socialfirmseurope.org/, accessed 18 March 2011).

96. Durie S, Wilson L. *Six Mary's place: social return on investment report*. Edinburgh, Forth Sector, 2007 (Series Report No. 1). (http://www.socialfirms.org.uk/FileLibrary/Resources/Quality%20&%20Impact/SROI%20report%20-%20Six%20Marys%20Place.pdf, accessed 19 January 2011).

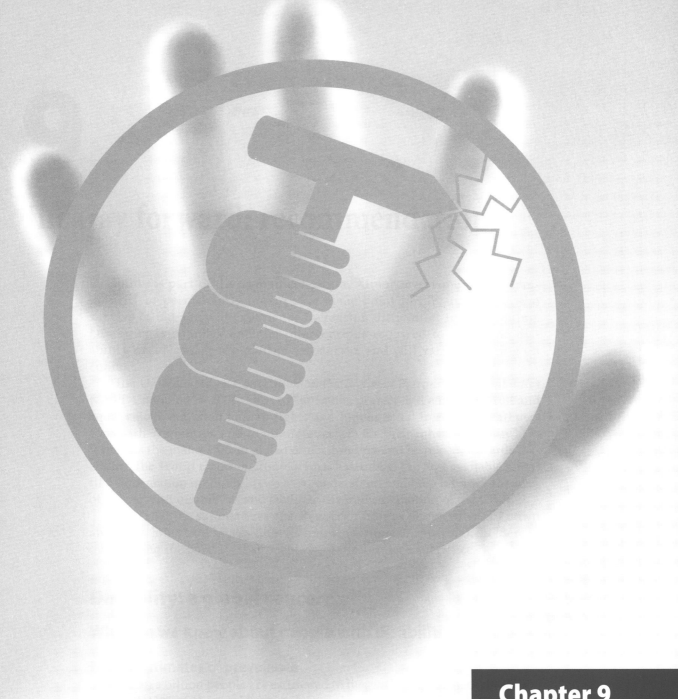

Chapter 9

The way forward: recommendations

or blindness. Only the *Global Burden of Disease* measures childhood disability (0–14 years) which is estimated to be 95 million (5.1%) children of which 13 million (0.7%) have "severe disability".

Growing numbers

The number of people with disabilities is growing. There is a higher risk of disability at older ages, and national populations are growing older at unprecedented rates. There is also a global increase in chronic health conditions, such as diabetes, cardiovascular diseases, and mental disorders, which will influence the nature and prevalence of disability. Patterns of disability in a particular country are influenced by trends in health conditions and trends in environmental and other factors – such as road traffic crashes, natural disasters, conflict, diet, and substance abuse.

Diverse experiences

The disability experience resulting from the interaction of health conditions, personal factors, and environmental factors varies greatly. While disability correlates with disadvantage, not all people with disabilities are equally disadvantaged. Women with disabilities experience gender discrimination as well as disabling barriers. School enrolment rates also differ among impairments, with children with physical impairment generally faring better than those with intellectual or sensory impairments. Those most excluded from the labour market are often those with mental health difficulties or intellectual impairments. People with more severe impairments often experience greater disadvantage.

Vulnerable populations

Disability disproportionately affects vulnerable populations. There is a higher disability prevalence in lower-income countries than in higher-income countries. People from the poorest wealth quintile, women, and older people have a higher prevalence of disability. People who have a low income, are out of work, or have low educational qualifications are at an increased risk of disability. Data from selected countries show that children from poorer households and those in ethnic minority groups are at significantly higher risk of disability than other children.

What are the disabling barriers?

The CRPD and the *International Classification of Functioning, Disability and Health* (ICF) both highlight the environmental factors that restrict participation for people with disabilities. This Report has documented widespread evidence of barriers, including the following.

- **Inadequate policies and standards.** Policy design does not always take into account the needs of people with disabilities, or existing policies and standards are not enforced. Examples include a lack of clear policy of inclusive education, a lack of enforceable access standards in physical environments, and the low priority accorded to rehabilitation.
- **Negative attitudes.** Beliefs and prejudices constitute barriers when health-care workers cannot see past the disability, teachers do not see the value in teaching children with disabilities, employers discriminate against people with disabilities, and family members have low expectations of their relatives with disabilities.
- **Lack of provision of services.** People with disabilities are particularly vulnerable to deficiencies in services such as health care, rehabilitation, or support and assistance.
- **Problems with service delivery.** Issues such as poor coordination among services, inadequate staffing, staff competencies, and training affect the quality and adequacy of services for persons with disabilities.
- **Inadequate funding.** Resources allocated to implementing policies and plans are often inadequate. Strategy papers on poverty reduction, for instance, may mention disability but without considering funding.

- **Lack of accessibility.** Built environments (including public accommodations) transport systems and information are often inaccessible. Lack of access to transport is a frequent reason for a person with a disability being discouraged from seeking work or prevented from accessing health care. Even in countries with laws on accessibility, compliance in public buildings is often very low. The communication needs of people with disabilities are often unmet. Information is frequently unavailable in accessible formats, and some people with disabilities are unable to access basic information and communication technologies such as telephones and television.
- **Lack of consultation and involvement.** Often people with disabilities are excluded from decision-making in matters directly affecting their lives.
- **Lack of data and evidence.** A lack of rigorous and comparable data on disability and evidence on programmes that work often impedes understanding and action.

How are the lives of people with disabilities affected?

These barriers contribute to the disadvantages experienced by people with disabilities, such as the following.

- **They have poor health outcomes.** Depending on the group and setting, persons with disabilities may experience greater vulnerability to preventable secondary conditions and co-morbidities, untreated mental health conditions, poor oral health, higher rates of HIV infection, higher rates of obesity, and premature mortality.
- **They have lower educational achievements.** Children with disabilities are less likely to start school than their peers without disabilities. They also have lower rates of staying in school and of being promoted, as well as lower transition rates to post-school education.

- **They are less economically active.** People with disabilities have lower employment rates than people without disabilities. Where people with disabilities are employed, they commonly earn less than their counterparts without disabilities.
- **They experience higher rates of poverty.** Households with a person with a disability have higher rates of poverty than households without disabled members. As a group and across settings, people with disabilities have worse living conditions and fewer assets. Poverty may lead to disability, through malnutrition, poor health care, and dangerous working or living conditions. Disability may lead to poverty through lost earnings, due to lack of employment or underemployment, and through the additional costs of living with disability, such as extra medical, housing, and transport costs.
- **They cannot always live independently or participate fully in community activities.** Reliance on institutional solutions, lack of community living, inaccessible transport and other public facilities, and negative attitudes leave people with disabilities dependent on others and isolated from mainstream social, cultural, and political opportunities.

Recommendations

The evidence in this Report suggests that many of the barriers people with disabilities face are avoidable and the disadvantages associated with disability can be overcome. The following nine recommendations for action are cross-cutting and guided by the more specific recommendations at the end of each chapter.

Implementing the recommendations requires involving different *sectors* – health, education, social protection, labour, transport, housing – and different *actors* – governments, civil society organizations (including disabled people's organizations), professionals, the

> **Box 9.1. An example of inclusive international cooperation**
>
> In November 2008 the Australian Government launched its strategy *"Development for all: towards a disability-inclusive Australian aid program"*. The strategy marks a significant change in the way Australia's aid is designed and delivered. *Development for All* is about improving the reach and effectiveness of development assistance by ensuring that people with disabilities are included, contribute and benefit equally from development efforts.
>
> In preparing the strategy AusAID, the Australian government's development aid agency, conducted consultations in most of the developing countries where AusAID works, involving people with disabilities, their families and caregivers, government representatives, nongovernmental organizations, and service providers. Almost 500 written submissions were received in the process.
>
> During the consultations overseas-based AusAID staff – often with little experience of relating to people with disabilities – were supported to engage with local disabled people's organizations. The direct involvement of AusAID staff was an important step in commencing the process of building institutional understanding of the importance of disability-inclusive development. Many came away better informed about disability issues and more confident about spending time with people with disabilities.
>
> Two years into implementation, there are strong signs that the strategy is working:
>
> - People with disabilities are more visible and taking a central role in decision- making, ensuring that Australia's development policies and programmes are shaped to better take account of their requirements.
> - Australia's support is bolstering partner Government's efforts, such as in Papua New Guinea, Cambodia and Timor-Leste, towards more equitable national development that benefits all citizens, including people with disability.
> - Investments in leadership by people with disabilities, together with advocacy by Australian leaders internationally, is helping to increase the priority and resources for inclusive development globally.
> - AusAID's processes, systems and information about the aid programme are more accessible to people with disabilities. Key programme areas such as scholarships have revised guidelines resulting in increased number of scholars with disabilities.
>
> The strategy takes a rights-based approach, is sensitive to the diversity of people with disabilities, gender issues, and focuses on children with disabilities.

private sector, and people with disabilities and their families.

It is essential that countries tailor their actions to their specific contexts. Where countries are limited by resource constraints, some of the priority actions, particularly those requiring technical assistance and capacity-building, can be included within the framework of international cooperation (see Box 9.1).

Recommendation 1: Enable access to all mainstream policies, systems and services

People with disabilities have ordinary needs – for health and well-being, for economic and social security, to learn and develop skills, and to live in their communities. These needs can and should be met in mainstream programmes and services. Mainstreaming not only fulfils the human rights of persons with disabilities, it is also more effective.

Mainstreaming is the process by which governments and other stakeholders ensure that persons with disabilities participate equally with others in any activity and service intended for the general public, such as education, health, employment, and social services. Barriers to participation need to be identified and removed, possibly requiring changes to laws, policies, institutions, and environments.

Mainstreaming requires a commitment at all levels, and needs to be considered across all sectors and built into new and existing legislation, standards, policies, strategies, and plans. Adopting universal design and implementing reasonable accommodations are two important strategies. Mainstreaming also requires effective planning, adequate human resources, and sufficient financial investment – accompanied by specific measures such as targeted programmes and services (see Recommendation 2) to ensure that the diverse needs of people with disabilities are adequately met.

Recommendation 2: Invest in specific programmes and services for people with disabilities

In addition to mainstream services, some people with disabilities may require access to specific measures, such as rehabilitation, support services, or training. Rehabilitation – including assistive technologies such as wheelchairs, hearing aids, and white canes – improves functioning and independence. A range of well-regulated assistance and support services in the community can meet needs for care, enabling people to live independently and to participate in the economic, social, and cultural lives of their communities. Vocational rehabilitation and training can open labour market opportunities.

While there is a need for more services, there is also a need for better, more accessible, flexible, integrated, and well-coordinated multidisciplinary services, particularly at times of transition such as between child and adult services. Existing programmes and services need to be reviewed to assess their performance and make changes to improve their coverage, effectiveness, and efficiency. The changes should be based on sound evidence, appropriate in terms of culture and other local contexts, and tested locally.

Recommendation 3: Adopt a national disability strategy and plan of action

While disability should be a part of all development strategies and action plans, it is also recommended that a national disability strategy and plan of action be adopted. A national disability strategy sets out a consolidated and comprehensive long-term vision for improving the well-being of persons with disabilities and should cover both mainstream policy and programme areas and specific services for persons with disabilities.

The development, implementation, and monitoring of a national strategy should bring together a broad range of stakeholders including relevant government ministries, nongovernmental organizations, professional groups, disabled people and their representative organizations, the general public, and the private sector.

The strategy and action plan should be informed by a situation analysis, taking into account such factors as the prevalence of disability, needs for services, social and economic status, effectiveness and gaps in current services, and environmental and social barriers. The strategy should establish priorities and have measurable outcomes. The plan of action operationalizes the strategy in short and medium terms by laying out concrete actions and timelines for implementation, defining targets, assigning responsible agencies, and planning and allocating needed resources.

Mechanisms are needed to make it clear where the responsibility lies for coordination, decision-making, regular monitoring and reporting, and control of resources.

Recommendation 4: Involve people with disabilities

People with disabilities often have unique insights about their disability and their situation. In formulating and implementing policies, laws, and services, people with disabilities should be consulted and actively involved.

Disabled people's organizations may need capacity-building and support to empower people with disabilities and advocate for their needs. When suitably developed and funded, they can also play a role in service delivery – for example, in information provision, peer support, and independent living.

At an individual level, persons with disabilities are entitled to control over their lives and therefore need to be consulted on issues that concern them directly – whether in health, education, rehabilitation, or community living. Supported decision-making may be necessary to enable some individuals to communicate their needs and choices.

Recommendation 5: Improve human resource capacity

The attitudes and knowledge of people working in, for example, education, health care, rehabilitation, social protection, labour, law enforcement, and the media are particularly important for ensuring non-discrimination and participation.

Human resource capacity can be improved through effective education, training, and recruitment. A review of the knowledge and competencies of staff in relevant areas can provide a starting point for developing appropriate measures to improve them. Relevant training on disability, which incorporates human rights principles, should be integrated into current curricula and accreditation programmes. In-service training should be provided to current practitioners providing and managing services. For example, strengthening the capacity of primary health care workers, and ensuring availability of specialist staff where required, contribute to effective and affordable health care for people with disabilities.

Many countries have too few staff working in fields such as rehabilitation and special education. Developing standards in training for different types and levels of rehabilitation personnel can assist in addressing resource gaps. There are also shortages of care workers and sign language interpreters. Measures to improve staff retention may be relevant in some settings and sectors.

Recommendation 6: Provide adequate funding and improve affordability

Existing public services for people with disabilities are often inadequately funded, affecting the availability and quality of such services. Adequate and sustainable funding of publicly provided services is needed to ensure that they reach all targeted beneficiaries and that good quality services are provided. Contracting out service provision, fostering public-private partnerships, notably with not-for profit organizations, and devolving budgets to persons with disabilities for consumer-directed care can contribute to better service provision.

During the development of the national disability strategy and related action plans, the affordability and sustainability of the proposed measures should be considered and adequately funded through relevant budgets. Programme costs and outcomes should be monitored and evaluated, so that more cost-effective solutions are developed and implemented.

Often people with disabilities and their families have excessive out-of-pocket expenses. To improve the affordability of goods and services for people with disabilities and to offset the extra costs associated with disability, particularly for poor and vulnerable persons with disabilities, consideration should be given to expanding health and social insurance coverage, ensuring that people with disabilities have equal access to public social services, ensuring that poor and vulnerable people with disabilities benefit from poverty-targeted safety net programmes, and introducing fee-waivers, reduced transport fares, and reduced import taxes and duties on assistive technologies.

Recommendation 7: Increase public awareness and understanding of disability

Mutual respect and understanding contribute to an inclusive society. Therefore it is vital to improve public understanding of disability, confront negative perceptions, and represent disability fairly. For example, education authorities should ensure that schools are inclusive and have an ethos of valuing diversity. Employers should be encouraged to accept their responsibilities towards staff with disabilities.

Collecting information on knowledge, beliefs and attitudes about disability can help identify gaps in public understanding that can be bridged through education and public information. Governments, voluntary organizations, and professional associations should consider running social marketing campaigns that change attitudes on stigmatized issues such as HIV, mental illness, and leprosy. Involving the media is vital to the success of these campaigns and to ensuring the dissemination of positive stories about persons with disabilities and their families.

Recommendation 8: Improve disability data collection

Internationally, methodologies for collecting data on people with disabilities need to be developed, tested cross-culturally, and applied consistently. Data need to be standardized and internationally comparable for benchmarking and monitoring progress on disability policies, and for the implementation of the CRPD nationally and internationally.

Nationally, disability should be included in data collection. Uniform definitions of disability, based on the ICF, can allow for internationally comparable data. Understanding the numbers of people with disabilities and their circumstances can improve country efforts to remove disabling barriers and provide appropriate services for people with disabilities. As a first step, national population census data can be collected in line with recommendations from the United Nations Washington Group on Disability and the United Nations Statistical Commission. A cost-effective and efficient approach is to include disability questions – or a disability module – in existing sample surveys such as a national household survey, national health survey, general social survey, or labour force survey. Data need to be disaggregated by population features, such as age, sex, race, and socioeconomic status, to uncover patterns, trends, and information about subgroups of persons with disabilities.

Dedicated disability surveys can also gain more comprehensive information on disability characteristics, such as prevalence, health conditions associated with disability, and use of and need for services including rehabilitation. Administrative data collection can be a useful source of information on users and on types, amounts, and cost of services, if standard disability identifiers are included.

Recommendation 9: Strengthen and support research on disability

Research is essential for increasing public understanding about disability issues, informing disability policy and programmes, and efficiently allocating resources.

This Report recommends several areas for research on disability including:

- the impact of environmental factors (policies, physical environment, attitudes) on disability and how to measure it;
- the quality of life and well-being of people with disabilities;
- barriers to mainstream and specific services, and what works in overcoming them in different contexts;
- accessibility and universal design programmes appropriate for low-income settings;
- the interactions among environmental factors, health conditions, and disability – and between disability and poverty;

Communities can:

- Challenge and improve their own beliefs and attitudes.
- Protect the rights of persons with disabilities.
- Promote the inclusion and participation of disabled people in their community.
- Ensure that community environments are accessible for people with disabilities, including schools, recreational areas and cultural facilities.
- Challenge violence against and bullying of people with disabilities.

People with disabilities and their families can:

- Support other people with disabilities through peer support, training, information, and advice.
- Promote the rights of persons with disabilities within their local communities – for example by conducting access audits, delivering disability equality training, and campaigning for human rights.
- Become involved in awareness-raising and social marketing campaigns.
- Participate in forums (international, national, local) to determine priorities for change, to influence policy, and to shape service delivery.
- Participate in research projects.

References

1. *Convention on the Rights of Persons with Disabilities*. Geneva, United Nations, 2006 (http://www2.ohchr.org/english/law/disabilities-convention.htm, accessed 10 March 2011).

Technical appendix A

Estimates of disability prevalence (%) and of years of health lost due to disability (YLD), by country

	Member State	Disability prevalence from WHS, 2002–2004[a]	Census			Disability survey or component in other surveys			YLDs per 100 persons in 2004
			Year	ICF component	Prevalence	Year	ICF component	Prevalence	
1	Afghanistan					2005	Imp, AL, PR	2.7 (1)	15.3
2	Albania					2008	Imp	3.4 (2)	7.8
3	Algeria					1992		1.2 (3)	8.0
4	Andorra								6.8
5	Angola								14.4
6	Antigua and Barbuda								8.8
7	Argentina		2001	Imp, AL	7.1 (4)				8.7
8	Armenia								7.9
9	Australia		2006		4.4 (5)	2003		20.0 (6)	6.8
10	Austria					2002	Imp, AL, PR	12.8 (7)	6.7
11	Azerbaijan								8.2
12	Bahamas		2000	Imp	4.3 (8)	2001	Imp	5.7 (9)	9.0
13	Bahrain		1991	Imp	0.8 (10)				7.6
14	Bangladesh	31.9				2005	Imp	2.5 (11)	10.1
15	Barbados		2000	Imp	4.6 (12)				8.5
16	Belarus								8.4
17	Belgium					2002	Imp, AL, PR	18.4 (7)	6.9
18	Belize		2000	Imp, AL, PR	5.9 (13)				10.0
19	Benin		2002	Imp	2.5 (14)	1991		1.3 (10)	11.0
21	Bhutan		2005	Imp	3.4 (15)	2000	Imp	3.5 (16)	9.5
22	Bolivia (Plurinational State of)		2001	Imp	3.1 (17)	2001	Imp	3.8 (18)	10.8
23	Bosnia and Herzegovina	14.6							7.6
24	Botswana		2001	Imp	3.5 (19)				13.8
25	Brazil	18.9	2000	Imp	14.9 (20)	1981	Imp	1.8 (10)	10.1
26	Brunei Darussalam								7.4
27	Bulgaria								7.9
28	Burkina Faso	13.9							12.1
29	Burundi								13.5

continues ...

... continued

	Member State	Disability prevalence from WHS, 2002–2004[a]	Census			Disability survey or component in other surveys			YLDs per 100 persons in 2004
			Year	ICF component	Prevalence	Year	ICF component	Prevalence	
30	Cambodia		2008		1.4 (21)	1999	Imp	2.4 (11)	10.8
31	Cameroon								11.7
32	Canada		2001	Imp, AL, PR	18.5 (22)	2006	Imp, AL, PR	14.3 (23)	6.9
33	Cape Verde		1990	Imp	2.6 (10)				8.1
34	Central African Republic		1988		1.5 (10)				13.1
35	Chad	20.9							13.6
36	Chile		2002	Imp	2.2 (24)	2004	Imp, AL, PR	12.9 (25)	8.1
37	China					2006	Imp	6.4 (26)	7.7
38	Colombia		2005	Imp, AL, PR	6.4 (27)	1991	Imp	5.6 (10)	10.2
39	Comoros		1980		1.7 (10)				10.0
40	Congo		1974		1.1 (10)				11.0
41	Cook Islands								7.7
42	Costa Rica		2000	Imp	5.4 (28)	1998	Imp	7.8 (28)	7.9
43	Côte d'Ivoire								13.8
44	Croatia	13.9	2001	Imp	9.7 (29)	2009	Imp, AL, PR	11.3 (30)	7.4
45	Cuba		2003	Imp	4.2 (31)	2000	Imp	7.0 (31)	8.2
46	Cyprus		1992	AL	6.4 (32)	2002	Imp, AL, PR	12.2 (7)	7.4
47	Czech Republic	11.7				2007	Imp, AL, PR	9.9 (33)	7.0
48	Democratic People's Republic of Korea								9.5
49	Democratic Republic of the Congo								13.6
50	Denmark					2002	Imp, AL, PR	19.9 (7)	7.1
51	Djibouti								10.5
52	Dominica		2002	Imp	6.1 (34)				8.8
53	Dominican Republic	11.1	2002	Imp	4.2 (35)	2007	Imp	2.0 (36)	9.8
54	Ecuador	13.6	2001	Imp	4.6 (37)	2005	Imp, AL, PR	12.1 (37)	9.2
55	Egypt		2006		1.2 (38)	1996	Imp	4.4 (38)	8.6
56	El Salvador		1992	Imp	1.8 (39)	2003	Imp, AL	1.5 (39)	9.8
57	Equatorial Guinea								12.3
58	Eritrea								9.5
59	Estonia	11.0	2000	Imp	7.5 (40)	2008	Imp, AL, PR	9.9 (40)	7.9
60	Ethiopia	17.6	1984		3.8 (10)				11.3
61	Fiji		1996	Imp, AL	13.9 (11)				8.6
62	Finland	5.5				2002	Imp, AL, PR	32.2 (7)	7.2
63	France	6.5				2002	Imp, AL, PR	24.6 (7)	6.8
64	Gabon								11.0
65	Gambia								11.0
66	Georgia	15.6							7.6
67	Germany		2007	Imp	8.4 (41)	2002	Imp, AL, PR	11.2 (7)	6.7

continues ...

... continued

	Member State	Disability prevalence from WHS, 2002–2004[a]	Census			Disability survey or component in other surveys			YLDs per 100 persons in 2004
			Year	ICF component	Prevalence	Year	ICF component	Prevalence	
68	Ghana	12.8							11.1
69	Greece					2002	Imp, AL, PR	10.3 (*7*)	6.3
70	Grenada								8.9
71	Guatemala		2002	Imp	6.2 (*42*)	2005	Imp, AL, PR	3.7 (*42*)	10.0
72	Guinea								11.7
73	Guinea-Bissau								12.7
74	Guyana		2002	Imp, AL, PR	2.2 (*43*)				11.5
75	Haiti		2003	Imp	1.5 (*44*)				11.7
76	Honduras		2000	Imp	1.8 (*45*)	2002	Imp, AL, PR	2.6 (*46*)	9.5
77	Hungary	10.5	2001	Imp	3.1 (*47*)	2002	Imp, AL, PR	11.4 (*7*)	7.9
78	Iceland					2008		7.4 (*48*)	6.0
79	India	24.9	2001	Imp	2.1 (*49*)	2002	Imp	1.7 (*11*)	10.5
80	Indonesia					2007	Imp, AL, PR	21.3 (*50*)	10.4
81	Iran (Islamic Republic of)		2006	Imp	1.5 (*51*)				9.3
82	Iraq		1977	Imp	0.9 (*10*)				19.4
83	Ireland	4.3	2006	Imp, AL, PR	9.3 (*52*)	2006	Imp, AL, PR	18.5 (*53*)	6.7
84	Israel	15.8							6.2
85	Italy					2002	Imp, AL, PR	6.6 (*7*)	6.1
86	Jamaica		2001	Imp	6.2 (*54*)				8.7
87	Japan					2005		5.0 (*55*)	5.5
88	Jordan		1994	Imp	1.2 (*10*)	2001		12.6 (*56*)	7.9
89	Kazakhstan	14.2	2006		3.0 (*11*)				10.1
90	Kenya	15.2	1989	Imp	0.7 (*10*)				10.8
91	Kiribati					2004	Imp	3.8 (*11*)	9.6
92	Kuwait								6.9
93	Kyrgyzstan					2008	Imp, AL, PR	20.2 (*57*)	9.6
94	Lao People's Democratic Republic	8.0	2004		8.0 (*11*)				10.5
95	Latvia	18.0				2009		5.2 (*16*)	8.0
96	Lebanon					2002		1.5 (*58*)	9.1
97	Lesotho								11.4
98	Liberia		1971		0.8 (*10*)	1997	Imp	16.4 (*59*)	13.9
99	Libyan Arab Jamahiriya		1984	Imp	1.5 (*10*)	1995		1.7 (*10*)	7.8
100	Lithuania		2001	Imp	7.5 (*60*)	2002	Imp, AL, PR	8.4 (*7*)	8.0
101	Luxembourg	10.2				2002	Imp, AL, PR	11.7 (*7*)	6.8
102	Madagascar					2003	Imp, AL	7.5 (*61*)	10.7
103	Malawi	14.0	1983		2.9 (*10*)	2004	Imp, AL, PR	10.6 (*62*)	13.1
104	Malaysia	4.5				2000		0.4 (*63*)	8.0
105	Maldives		2003	Imp	3.4 (*11*)				10.2
106	Mali	9.8	1987		2.7 (*10*)				13.0

continues ...

... continued

Member State	Disability prevalence from WHS, 2002–2004[a]	Census			Disability survey or component in other surveys			YLDs per 100 persons in 2004
		Year	ICF component	Prevalence	Year	ICF component	Prevalence	
107 Malta		2005	Imp, AL. PR	5.9 (*64*)	2002	Imp, AL, PR	8.5 (*7*)	6.3
108 Marshall Islands		1999	Imp	1.6 (*65*)				8.2
109 Mauritania	24.9	1988		1.5 (*10*)				11.0
110 Mauritius	13.1	2000	Imp	3.5 (*66*)				9.1
111 Mexico	7.5	2000	Imp	1.8 (*67*)	2002	AL. PR	8.8 (*68*)	8.2
112 Micronesia (Federated States of)								7.0
113 Monaco								6.5
114 Mongolia					2005		3.5 (*11*)	9.0
115 Montenegro								7.4 (*69*)
116 Morocco	32.0	1982		1.1 (*10*)	2004		5.12 (*70*)	8.7
117 Mozambique		1997	Imp	1.9 (*71*)	2009	Imp, AL, PR	6.0 (*72*)	12.5
118 Myanmar	6.4	1985	Imp	2.0 (*73*)	2007	Imp	2.0 (*16*)	9.8
119 Namibia	21.4	2001	Imp	5.0 (*74*)	2002	Imp, AL, PR	1.6 (*75*)	10.2
120 Nauru								9.5
121 Nepal	21.7	2001	Imp	0.5 (*76*)	2001	Imp	1.6 (*11*)	11.1
122 Netherlands					2002	Imp, AL, PR	25.6 (*7*)	6.4
123 New Zealand					2001	Imp, AL, PR	20.0 (*77*)	6.9
124 Nicaragua					2003	Imp, AL, PR	10.3 (*78*)	8.5
125 Niger		1988		1.3 (*10*)				13.7
126 Nigeria		1991		0.5 (*10*)				13.2
127 Niue								8.4
128 Norway	4.3				2002	Imp, AL, PR	16.4 (*7*)	6.8
129 Oman		2005		0.5 (*79*)				7.2
130 Pakistan	13.4	1998	Imp	2.5 (*80*)				9.6
131 Palau								7.8
132 Panama		2000	Imp	1.8 (*81*)	2005	Imp, AL, PR	11.3 (*81*)	8.4
133 Papua New Guinea								9.4
134 Paraguay	10.4	2002	Imp	1.1 (*82*)	2002	Imp, AL	3.0 (*82*)	9.4
135 Peru		2007	Imp, AL, PR	10.9 (*83*)	2006	Imp, AL, PR	8.7 (*84*)	9.4
136 Philippines	28.8	2000	Imp	1.2 (*85*)				9.2
137 Poland		2002	AL	14.3 (*86*)				7.3
138 Portugal	11.2	2001	Imp	6.2 (*87*)	2002	Imp, AL, PR	19.9 (*7*)	7.0
139 Qatar		1986		0.2 (*10*)				7.1
140 Republic of Korea		2005	Imp	4.6 (*11*)				7.6
141 Republic of Moldova								8.6
142 Romania					2009	Imp, AL, PR	19.0 (*88*)	7.9
143 Russian Federation	16.4							10.0
144 Rwanda								13.3
145 Saint Kitts and Nevis								9.0

continues ...

... continued

	Member State	Disability prevalence from WHS, 2002–2004[a]	Census			Disability survey or component in other surveys			YLDs per 100 persons in 2004
			Year	ICF component	Prevalence	Year	ICF component	Prevalence	
146	Saint Lucia		2001	Imp	5.1 (*89*)				8.7
147	Saint Vincent and the Grenadines		2001	imp	4.6 (*89*)				9.0
148	Samoa					2002		3.0 (*90*)	7.0
149	San Marino								6.2
150	Sao Tome and Principe		1991		4.0 (*10*)				10.0
151	Saudi Arabia					1996	Imp	4.5 (*91*)	8.1
152	Senegal	15.5	1988		1.1 (*10*)				11.3
153	Serbia					2008	Imp, AL, PR	7.4 (*92*)	7.4 (*93*)
154	Seychelles					2007	Imp	1.3 (*16*)	8.8
155	Sierra Leone		2004		2.4 (*94*)				14.7
156	Singapore					2003	Imp	3.0 (*11*)	6.6
157	Slovakia	12.1				2002	Imp, AL, PR	8.2 (*7*)	7.7
158	Slovenia					2002	Imp, AL, PR	19.5 (*7*)	7.1
159	Solomon Islands					2004	Imp	3.5 (*11*)	7.9
160	Somalia								14.3
161	South Africa	24.2	2001	Imp, PR	5.0 (*95*)	1998	Imp, AL, PR	5.9 (*96*)	12.2
162	Spain	9.5				2008	Imp, AL	8.5 (*97*)	6.2
163	Sri Lanka	12.9	2001	Imp	1.6 (*98*)	1986	Imp	2.0 (*10*)	11.5
164	Sudan		1993		1.6 (*10*)	1992		1.1 (*10*)	12.2
165	Suriname		1980	Imp	2.8 (*99*)				10.1
166	Swaziland	35.9		1986	2.2 (*10*)				13.0
167	Sweden	19.3				2002	Imp, AL, PR	19.9 (*7*)	6.5
168	Switzerland					2007	Imp, AL, PR	14.0 (*100*)	6.2
169	Syrian Arab Republic		1981		1.0 (*10*)	1993		0.8 (*10*)	7.7
170	Tajikistan					2007		1.9 (*101*)	8.7
171	Thailand					2007	Imp, AL, PR	2.9 (*102*)	9.4
172	The former Yugoslav Republic of Macedonia								7.3
173	Timor Leste					2002		1.5 (*11*)	11.0
174	Togo		1970		0.6 (*10*)				11.4
175	Tonga					2006		2.8 (*103*)	6.9
176	Trinidad and Tobago		2000	Imp, AL	4.2 (*104*)				9.2
177	Tunisia	16.3	1994		1.2 (*10*)	1989		0.9 (*10*)	7.5
178	Turkey	20.6				2002	Imp, AL	12.3 (*105*)	7.5
179	Turkmenistan								9.1
180	Tuvalu								8.0
181	Uganda		2002	Imp	3.5 (*106*)	2006	Imp	7.2 (*107*)	12.7
182	Ukraine	14.8							8.8
183	United Arab Emirates	10.8							7.3

continues ...

... continued

	Member State	Disability prevalence from WHS, 2002–2004[a]	Census			Disability survey or component in other surveys			YLDs per 100 persons in 2004
			Year	ICF component	Prevalence	Year	ICF component	Prevalence	
184	United Kingdom of Great Britain and Northern Ireland		2001	Imp, AL, PR	17.6 (*108*)	2002	Imp, AL, PR	27.2 (*7*)	7.1
185	United Republic of Tanzania					2008	Imp, AL, PR	7.8 (*109*)	12.7
186	United States of America		2000	Imp, AL, PR	19.3 (*110*)	2007	Imp, AL, PR	14.9 (*111*)	7.9
187	Uruguay	4.6				2004	Imp, AL, PR	7.6 (*112*)	9.0
188	Uzbekistan								8.0
189	Vanuatu					1999		1.4 (*113*)	7.6
190	Venezuela (Bolivarian Republic of)		2001	Imp	4.2 (*114*)				9.1
191	Viet Nam	5.8				2005		6.4 (*11*)	7.8
192	Yemen		2004	Imp	1.9 (*115*)	1998		1.7 (*56*)	12.9
193	Zambia	14.8	2000	Imp	2.7 (*10*)	2006	Imp, AL, PR	11.0 (*116*)	14.2
194	Zimbabwe	16.9				2003	Imp, AL, PR	18.0 (*117*)	12.3

(a) WHS results are weighted and age standardized

Abbreviations for ICF components: AL=activity limitations; Imp=impairments; PR=participation restrictions.

References

1. Islamic State of Afghanistan, and Handicap International. *National Disability Survey in Afghanistan. Towards well-being for Afghans with disabilities: the health challenge.* Lyon, Handicap International, 2005 (http://www.handicap-international.fr/uploads/media/HI_HEALTH_REPORTFINAL2_01.pdf, accessed 27 January 2010).

2. *Disability in Albania: annual report 2007–2008.* Tirana, Ministry of Labour, Social Affairs and Equal Opportunities Department and National Observatory of Persons with Disabilities, 2008.

3. *Human functioning and disability: Algeria, 1992 survey.* New York, Statistics Division, United Nations (http://unstats.un.org/unsd/demographic/sconcerns/disability/disab2.asp, accessed 27 January 2010).

4. *National survey of persons with disabilities (2002–2003).* Buenos Aires, National Institute of Statistics and Censuses, 2003 (http://www.indec.mecon.ar/, accessed 27 January 2010).

5. *People with a need for assistance: a snapshot, 2006.* Canberra, Australian Bureau of Statistics, 2008 (http:www.abs.gov.au/AUSSTATS/abs@.nsf/Lookup/4445.0Main+Features12006?OpenDocument, accessed 27 January 2010).

6. *Disability, ageing and carers: summary of findings, 2003.* Canberra, Australian Bureau of Statistics, 2004 (http://tinyurl.com/ykbapow, accessed 25 March 2010).

7. *Living conditions in Europe: data 2002–2005.* Luxembourg, EUROSTAT, 2007 (http://tinyurl.com/yab3l94, accessed 25 March 2010). [Note: Prevalence data are valid for people aged 16–64 years.]

8. *The 2000 census of population and housing report.* Nassau, Department of Statistics (http://statistics.bahamas.gov.bs/download/022740800.pdf, accessed 6 March 2010).

9. *Bahamas living conditions survey 2001.* Nassau, Department of Statistics, 2004. (http://statistics.bahamas.gov.bs/archives.php?cmd=view&id=3, accessed 2 February 2010).

10. *Bahrain: 1991 census.* New York, United Nations Disability Statistics Database (http://unstats.un.org/unsd/demographic/sconcerns/disability/disab2.asp, accessed 2 February 2010).

11. *Disability at a glance: a profile of 28 countries and areas in Asia and the Pacific.* Bangkok, United Nations Economic and Social Commission for Asia and the Pacific, 2006 (http://unescap.org/esid/psis/disability/publications/glance/disability%20at%20a%20glance.pdf, accessed 2 February 2010).

12. Trevor D. *Disability statistics in Barbados* [Datos de discapacidad en el Caribe]. Kingston, Inter-American Development Bank, 2005 (http://tinyurl.com/ylgft9x, accessed 2 February 2010).

13. Statistical Institute of Belize [web site]. (http://www.statisticsbelize.org.bz/, accessed 2 February 2010).

14. Institut National de la Statistique et de l'Analyse Economique [web site]. (http://www.insae-bj.org, accessed 2 February 2010).

15. *Disability at a glance: a profile of 28 countries and areas in Asia and the Pacific.* Bangkok, United Nations Economic and Social Commission for Asia and the Pacific, 2006 (http://unescap.org/esid/psis/disability/publications/glance/disability%20at%20a%20glance.pdf, accessed 2 February 2010).

16. From official statistics provided to the WHO regional office.

17. Chumacero Viscarra M. *Statistics on persons with disability in Bolivia* [Datos de discapacidad en la región Andina]. Lima, Inter-American Development Bank, 2005 (http://tinyurl.com/ylgft9x, accessed 2 February 2010).

18. National Statistics Office [web site]. (http://www.ine.gov.bo/default.aspx, accessed 2 February 2010).

19. *2001 Population census atlas: Botswana.* Gaborone, Botswana Central Statistics Office, 2005 (http://www.cso.gov.bw/images/stories/Census_Publication/pop%20atlas.pdf, accessed 6 March 2010).

20. Instituto Brasileiro de Geografia e Estatística [web site]. (http://www.ibge.gov.br/english/estatistica/populacao/censo2000/default_populacao.shtm, accessed 2 February 2010).

21. *General population census of Cambodia 2008.* Phnom Penh, National Institute of Statistics, 2008.

22. *Census of Canada.* Ottawa, Statistics Canada, 2001 (http://www12.statcan.ca/english/census01/home/index.cfm, accessed 6 March 2010).

23. *Prevalence of disability in Canada 2006.* Ottawa, Statistics Canada (http://www.statcan.gc.ca/pub/89-628-x/2007002/4125019-eng.htm, accessed 2 February 2010).

24. Zepeda M. *First national study on disability: summary of results* [Estadísticas de discapacidad en el Cono Sur]. Buenos Aires, Inter-American Development Bank, 2005 (http://tinyurl.com/ylgft9x, accessed 2 February 2010).

25. *First national study on disability.* Santiago, Government of Chile, 2004 (http://www.ine.cl/canales/chile_estadistico/encuestas_discapacidad/pdf/estudionacionaldeladiscapacidad(ingles).pdf, accessed 2 February 2010).

26. National Bureau of Statistics of China [web site]. (http://www.stats.gov.cn, accessed 2 February 2010).

27. González CI. *First meeting on disability statistics in the Andean region* [Datos de discapacidad en la región Andina]. Lima, Inter-American Development Bank, 2005 (http://tinyurl.com/ylgft9x, accessed 2 February 2010).

28. González ME. *Disability statistics: experiences since the implementation of the household survey and population census* [Estadística sobre personas con discapacidad en Centroamérica]. Managua, Inter-American Development Bank, 2004 (http://tinyurl.com/ylgft9x, accessed 2 February 2010).

29. Republic of Croatia, Central Bureau of Statistics [web site]. (http://www.dzs.hr, accessed 3 February 2010).

30. Benjak T, Petreski N. *Izvješće o osobama s invaliditetom u Republici Hrvatskoj.* Zagreb, Croatian National Institute of Public Health, 2009 (http://www.hzjz.hr/epidemiologija/kron_mas/invalidi08.pdf, accessed 3 February 2010).

31. Oficina Nacional de Estadísticas [web site]. (http://www.one.cu, accessed 3 February 2010).

32. *Census 1992.* Nicosia, Statistical Service of the Republic of Cyprus (http://www.mof.gov.cy/mof/cystat/statistics.nsf/index_gr/index_gr?OpenDocument, accessed 3 February 2010).

33. Czech Statistical Office [web site]. (http://www.czso.cz/csu/2008edicniplan.nsf/p/3309-08, accessed 3 February 2010).

34. Government of the Commonwealth of Dominica [web site]. (http://www.dominica.gov.dm/cms/index.php?q=node/28, accessed 3 February 2010).

35. *La discapacidad en República Dominicana: un perfil a partir de datos censales.* Santo Domingo, National Disability Council and Pan American Health Organization, 2006.

36. *Encuesta de demografía y salud: República Dominicana.* Calverton, Centro de Estudios Sociales y Demográficos and ORC Macro, 2007.

37. Parrales EMM. *Disability statistics in the 2001 census* [Datos de discapacidad en la región Andina]. Lima, Inter-American Development Bank, 2005 (http://tinyurl.com/ylgft9x, accessed 3 February 2010).

38. *Population and housing census 2006: population distribution by physical status.* Cairo, Central Agency for Mobilization and Statistics, 2006 (http://www.msrintranet.capmas.gov.eg/ows-img2/pdf/tab10_e.pdf, accessed 3 February 2010).

39. Corleto MA. *Characterization of disability in El Salvador following the EHPM 2003* [Estadística sobre personas con discapacidad en Centroamérica]. Managua, Inter-American Development Bank, 2005 (http://tinyurl.com/ylgft9x, accessed 3 February 2010).

40. *Limitations of everyday activities of persons aged 16 and older due to health problems by sex and age group.* Tallinn, Population and Social Statistics Department, 2008 (http://pub.stat.ee/px-web.2001/Dialog/varval.asp?ma=PH81&ti=LIMITATIONS+OF+EVERYDAY+ACTIVITIES+OF+PERSONS+AGED+16+AND+OLDER+DUE+TO+HEALTH+PROBLEMS+BY+SEX+AND+AGE+GROUP&path=./I_Databas/Social_life/05Health/05Health_status/&lang=1, accessed 3 February 2010).

41. Statistisches Bundesamt Deutschland [web site]. (http://www.destatis.de/jetspeed/portal/cms/Sites/destatis/Internet/DE/Presse/pm/2008/07/PD08__258__227.psml, accessed 3 February 2010). [Note: Prevalence rate refers only to persons with severe disability (more than 50% of "degree of disability").]

42. Lee Leiva JRS. *Planning the first national survey on disability* [Armonización regional de la definición de discapacidad]. Buenos Aires, Inter-American Development Bank, 2005 (http://tinyurl.com/ylgft9x, accessed 3 February 2010).

43. Luke DA. *Disability data: census and other sources* [Datos de discapacidad en el Caribe]. Kingston, Inter-American Development Bank, 2005 (http://tinyurl.com/ylgft9x, accessed 3 February 2010).

44. L'Institut Haïtien de Statistique et d'Informatique [web site]. (http://www.mefhaiti.gouv.ht/ihsi.htm, accessed 3 February 2010).

45. García M, Rodriguez RD. *Harmonization of the definition of disability* [Armonización regional de la definición de discapacidad]. Buenos Aires, Argentina Inter-American Development Bank, 2005 (http://tinyurl.com/ylgft9x, accessed 3 February 2010).

46. García M. Data on disability in Honduras [Datos sobre discapacidad en Honduras]. Tegucigalpa, Instituto Nacional de Estadística and Inter-American Development Bank, 2002 (http://www.iadb.org/sds/SOC/publication/gen_6191_4149_s.htm, accessed 4 April 2010).

47. Hungarian Central Statistical Office [web site]. (http://portal.ksh.hu, accessed 3 February 2010).

48. *Social insurance administration, invalidity and rehabilitation pensioners and recipients of invalidity allowances 1986–2008*. Reykjavik, Tryggingastofnun, 2009 (http://www.tr.is/media/frettir/stadtolur//2008_Tafla1_22_net.xls, accessed 3 February 2010). [Note: Prevalence rate refers only to persons with severe disability (more than 50% of "degree of disability").].

49. *Census of India*. New Delhi, Office of the Registrar General (http://www.censusindia.net, accessed 3 February 2010).

50. *Report of baseline health research*. Jakarta, National Institute of Health Research and Development, Ministry of Health, 2008.

51. *General results of Iran census 2006: population and housing*. Tehran, National Statistics Office, Statistical Centre of Iran, 2006.

52. *Census 2006: principal socio-economic results*. Dublin, Central Statistics Office, 2006 (http://www.cso.ie/census/census2006results/PSER/PSER_Tables%2031-38.pdf, accessed 3 February 2010).

53. *National disability survey*. Dublin, Central Statistics Office, 2008 (http://www.cso.ie/releasespublications/documents/other_releases/nationaldisability/National%20Disability%20Survey%202006%20First%20Results%20full%20report.pdf, accessed 3 February 2010).

54. Bartley M. *Measurement of disability data: Jamaica's experience with censuses and surveys* [Estadísticas de discapacidad en el Cono Sur]. Buenos Aires, Inter-American Development Bank, 2005 (http://tinyurl.com/ylgft9x, accessed 3 February 2010).

55. *Annual report on government measures for persosn with disabilities*. Tokyo, Cabinet Office, 2005 (http://www8.cao.go.jp/shougai/english/annualreport/2005/h17_report.pdf, accessed 3 February 2010).

56. *A note on disability issues in the Middle East and North Africa*. Washington, World Bank, 2005 (http://siteresources.worldbank.org/DISABILITY/Resources/Regions/MENA/MENADisabilities.doc, accessed 3 February 2010).

57. Disability data from the annual report of the Ministry of Health and the Republican Medical Information Centre: *Health of the population and functioning of health facilities in 2008*. Bishkek, Ministry of Health, 2009. Population data from: *Main social and demographic characteristics of population and number of housing units*. Bishkek, National Statistical Committee of the Kyrgyz Republic, 2009.

58. *National human development report: Lebanon 2001–2002*. Beirut, United Nations Development Programme, 2002.

59. *National needs assessment survey of the injured and disabled*. Monrovia, Centers for the Rehabilitation of the Injured and Disabled, 1997.

60. Statistikos Departmentas [web site]. (http://db1.stat.gov.lt/statbank/default.asp?w=1680, accessed 3 February 2010).

61. Rapport d'enquête: coordination des soins aux personnes handicapées. Antananarivo, Ministère de la Santé, 2003.

62. Loeb ME, Eide AE. *Living conditions among people with activity limitations in Malawi: a national representative study*. Trondheim, SINTEF, 2004 (http://www.safod.org/Images/LCMalawi.pdf, accessed 3 February 2010).

63. *Country profile: Malaysia*. Bangkok, Asia-Pacific Development Center on Disability, 2006 (http://www.apcdfoundation.org/countryprofile/malaysia/index.html, accessed 25 March 2010). [Note: "Prevalence data" refers to registered persons with disabilities.]

64. National Statistics Office of Malta [web site]. (http://www.nso.gov.mt, accessed 3 February 2010).

65. *Census 1999*. Majuro, Republic of the Marshall Islands Census, 1999 (http://www.pacificweb.org/DOCS/rmi/pdf/99census.pdf, accessed 6 March 2010).

66. Central Statistics Office. Republic of Mauritius [web site]. (http://www.gov.mu/portal/goc/cso/census_1.htm, accessed 3 February 2010).

67. Lerma RV. *Generating disability data in Mexico* [Estadística sobre personas con discapacidad en Centroamérica]. Managua, Inter-American Development Bank, 2004 (http://tinyurl.com/ylgft9x, accessed 3 February 2010).

68. *Bases de datos en formato de cubo dinámico*. Mexico City, Sistema Nacional de Información en Salud, 2008 (http://dgis.salud.gob.mx/cubos.html, accessed 3 February 2010).

69. The YLD estimate for 2004 is reported for Serbia and Montenegro.

70. *Enquête nationale sur le handicap*. Rabat, Secrétariat d'Etat chargé de la Famille, de l'Enfance et des Personnes Handicapées, 2006 (http://www.alciweb.org/websefsas/index.htm, accessed 10 March 2010).

71. *Disability*. Maputo, Instituto Nacional de Estatística (http://www.ine.gov.mz/Ingles/censos_dir/recenseamento_geral/ deficiencia, accessed 3 February 2010).

72. Eide HE, Kamaleri Y. *Health research, living conditions among people with disabilities in Mozambique: a national representative study*. Oslo, SINTEF, 2009 (http://www.sintef.no/upload/Helse/Levekår%20og%20tjenester/LC%20Report%20 Mozambique%20-%202nd%20revision.pdf, accessed 4 April 2010).

73. Department of Statistics. Malaysia [web site]. (http://www.statistics.gov.my, accessed 3 February 2010).

74. *Namibia 2001: population and housing census*. Windhoek, National Planning Commission (http://www.npc.gov.na/census/ index.htm, accessed 3 February 2010).

75. Eide AH, van Rooy G, Loeb ME. *Living conditions among people with activity limitations in Namibia: a representative, national study*. Oslo, SINTEF, 2003 (http://www.safod.org/Images/LCNamibia.pdf, accessed 3 February 2010).

76. *Table 22: Population by type of disability, age groups and sex for regions*. Kathmandu, National Planning Commission Secretariat, Central Bureau of Statistics (http://www.cbs.gov.np/Population/National%20Report%202001/tab22.htm, accessed 3 February 2010).

77. *Disability counts 2001*. Wellington, Statistics New Zealand, 2002 (http://www2.stats.govt.nz/domino/external/pasfull/ pasfull.nsf/0/4c2567ef00247c6acc256e6e006bcf1f/$FILE/DCounts01.pdf, accessed 3 February 2010).

78. Paguaga ND. *Statistics on persons with disabilities* [Estadística sobre personas con discapacidad en Centroamérica]. Managua, Inter-American Development Bank, 2004 (http://tinyurl.com/ylgft9x, accessed 3 February 2010).

79. *Number of recipients of social welfare by case (various years)*. Muscat, National Statistics, 2006 (http://www.moneoman.gov. om/stat_book/2006/fscommand/SYB_2006_CD/social/social_4-20.htm, accessed 3 February 2010).

80. *Population census organization*. Islamabad, Statistics Division, 2004 (http://www.statpak.gov.pk/depts/fbs/publications/ compendium_gender2004/gender_final.pdf, accessed 10 March 2010).

81. Quesada LE. *Statistics on persons with disabilities* [Estadística sobre personas con discapacidad en Centroamérica]. Managua, Inter-American Development Bank, 2004 (http://tinyurl.com/ylgft9x, accessed 3 February 2010).

82. Barrios O. *Regional harmonization of the definition of disability* [Armonización regional de la definición de discapacidad]. Buenos Aires, Inter-American Development Bank, 2005 (http://tinyurl.com/ylgft9x, accessed 3 February 2010).

83. *Census 2007*. Lima, National Statistics Office, 2008 (http://www.inei.gob.pe/, accessed 25 March 2010). [Note: data correspond to percentage of surveyed homes with a person with disability.]

84. Araujo GR. *Various statistics on disability in Peru* [Datos de discapacidad en la región Andina]. Lima, Inter-American Development Bank, 2005 (http://tinyurl.com/ylgft9x, accessed 3 February 2010).

85. *A special release based on the results of Census 2000*. Manila, National Statistics Office, 2005 (http://www.census.gov.ph/data/ sectordata/sr05150tx.html, accessed 10 March 2010).

86. Central Statistical Office [web site]. (http://www.stat.gov.pl, accessed 4 February 2010).

87. Instituto Nacional de Estatística [web site] (http://www.ine.pt, accessed 4 February 2010).

88. *Statistics annual book*. Bucharest, Ministry of Health, 2008.

89. *The Caribbean* (Studies and Perspectives Series, No. 7). Port of Spain, United Nations Economic Commission for Latin America and the Caribbean, Statistics and Social Development Unit, 2008.

90. *Country profile: Samoa*. Bangkok, Asia-Pacific Development Center on Disability, 2006 (http://www.apcdfoundation.org/ countryprofile/samoa/index.html, accessed 25 March 2010). [Note: "Prevalence data" refers to people aged 15 years and older.]

91. *Country profile on disability: Kingdom of Saudi Arabia*. Washington, World Bank and JICA Planning and Evaluation Department, 2002 (http://siteresources.worldbank.org/DISABILITY/Resources/Regions/MENA/JICA_Saudi_Arabia.pdf, accessed 4 February 2010).

92. From official statistics provided by the Ministry of Health to the WHO regional office. Note: data only valid for age group 16–64 years and only in relation to disabilities recorded in the occupational statistics.

93. The YLD estimate for 2004 is reported for Serbia and Montenegro.

94. *2004 population and housing census: mortality and disability*. Freetown, Statistics Sierra Leone and UNFPA, 2006 (http://www. sierra-leone.org/Census/Mortality and Disability.pdf, accessed 4 February 2010).

95. *Prevalence of disability in South Africa*, Census 2001. Pretoria, Statistics South Africa, 2005 (http://www.statssa.gov.za/ PublicationsHTML/Report-03-02-44/html/Report-03-02-44.html, accessed 4 February 2010).

96. Department of Health Facts and Statistics [web site]. (http://www.doh.gov.za/facts/index.html, accessed 4 February 2010).

97. Instituto Nacional de Estadística, [web site] (http://www.ine.es/en/inebmenu/mnu_salud_en.htm, accessed 4 February 2010).
98. *Census of population and housing 2001: disabled persons by type and disability, age and sex.* Colombo, National Statistics Office, 2001 (http://www.statistics.gov.lk/PopHouSat/PDF/Disability/p11d2%20Disabled%20persons%20by%20Age%20and%20Sex.pdf, accessed 4 February 2010).
99. Hunte A. *Disability studies in Suriname* [Datos de discapacidad en el Caribe]. Kingston, Inter-American Development Bank, 2005 (http://tinyurl.com/ylgft9x, accessed 4 February 2010).
100. National Statistics Office of Switzerland [web site]. (http://www.bfs.admin.ch/bfs/portal/fr/index/themen/20/06.html, accessed 4 February 2010).
101. From official statistics provided to the WHO regional office. Note: data refer to working-age population.
102. National Statistics Office of Thailand [web site]. (http://portal.nso.go.th/otherWS-world-context-root/index.jsp, accessed 4 February 2010).
103. *National disability identification survey.* Nuku'alofa, Tonga Department of Statistics, 2006 (http://www.spc.int/prism/Country/to/Stats/pdfs/Disability/NDIS06.pdf, accessed 4 February 2010).
104. Schmid K, Vézina S, Ebbeson L. *Disability in the Caribbean. A study of four countries: a socio-demographic analysis of the disabled.* UNECLAC Statistics and Social Development Unit, 2008 (http://www.eclac.org/publicaciones/xml/2/33522/L.134.pdf, accessed 4 February 2010).
105. *Turkey disability survey.* Ankara, Turkish Statistical Institute, 2002 (http://www.turkstat.gov.tr/VeriBilgi.do?tb_id=5&ust_id=1, accessed 4 February 2010).
106. *Census 2002.* Kampala, Uganda Bureau of Statistics (http://www.ubos.org/index.php?st=pagerelations2&id=16&p=related%20pages%202:2002Census%20Results, accessed 10 March 2010).
107. *Uganda national household survey 2005–2006: report on the socio-economic module.* Kampala, Uganda Bureau of Statistics, 2006 (http://www.ubos.org/onlinefiles/uploads/ubos/pdf%20documents/UNHSReport20052006.pdf, accessed 4 April 2010).
108. United Kingdom National Statistics [web site]. (http://www.statistics.gov.uk, accessed 4 February 2010).
109. *Tanzania disability survey 2008.* Dar es Salaam, National Bureau of Statistics, 2008. (http://www.nbs.go.tz/index.php?option=com_phocadownload&view=category&id=71:dissability&Itemid=106#, accessed 10 March 2010).
110. *Census 2000.* Washington, United States Census Bureau (http://www.census.gov/main/www/cen2000.html, accessed 6 March 2010).
111. *American community survey 2007.* Washington, United States Census Bureau (http://www.census.gov/acs/, accessed 4 February 2010). [Note: Prevalence data are valid for people aged 5 years and older.]
112. Damonte AM. *Regional harmonization of the definition of disability* [Armonización regional de la definición de discapacidad]. Buenos Aires, Inter-American Development Bank, 2005 (http://tinyurl.com/ylgft9x, accessed 4 February 2010).
113. *Vanuatu: disability country profile.* Suva, Pacific Islands Forum Secretariat, 2009 (http://www.forumsec.org/pages.cfm/strategic-partnerships-coordination/disability/, accessed 2 June 2009).
114. León A. *Venezuela: characterization of people with disability, Census 2001* [Datos de discapacidad en la región Andina]. Lima, Inter-American Development Bank, 2005 (http://tinyurl.com/ylgft9x, accessed 4 February 2010).
115. Central Statistical Organization [web site]. (http://www.cso-yemen.org/publication/census/second_report_demography_attached.pdf, accessed 4 February 2010).
116. Eide AH, Loeb ME, eds. *Living conditions among people with activity limitations in Zambia: a national representative study.* Oslo, SINTEF, 2006 (http://www.sintef.no/upload/Helse/Levekår%20og%20tjenester/ZambiaLCweb.pdf, accessed 7 December 2009).
117. Eide AH et al. *Living conditions among people with activity limitations in Zimbabwe: a representative regional survey.* Oslo, SINTEF, 2003 (http://www.safod.org/Images/LCZimbabwe.pdf, accessed 4 February 2010).

Technical appendix B

Overview of global and regional initiatives on disability statistics

There are numerous databases (including web sites) and studies of various international and national organizations that have compiled disability statistics (*1–9*).

To illustrate some of the current initiatives to improve disability statistics, the work of five organizations is described here. They are:

- The United Nations Washington Group on Disability Statistics.
- The United Nations Economic and Social Commission for Asia and the Pacific (UNESCAP).
- The WHO Regional Office for the Americas/Pan American Health Organization (PAHO).
- The European Statistical System (ESS).
- The United Nations Economic Commission for Europe (UNECE).

The United Nations Washington Group on Disability Statistics

The Washington Group was set up by the United Nations Statistical Commission in 2001 as an international, consultative group of experts to facilitate the measurement of disability and the comparison of data on disability across countries (*10*). At present, 77 National Statistical Offices are represented in the Washington Group, as well as seven international organizations, six organizations that represents people with disabilities, the United Nations Statistics Division, and three other United Nations-affiliated bodies.

As described in Chapter 2, the Washington Group created a short set of six questions for use in censuses and surveys, following the Fundamental Principles of Official Statistics and consistent with the *International Classification of Functioning, Disability and Health* (ICF) (*11*). These questions, when used in combination with other census data, assess the degree of participation of people with disabilities in education, employment, and social life – and can be used to inform policy on equalization of opportunities. The United Nations *Principles and Recommendations for Population and Housing Censuses* incorporates the approach taken by the Washington Group (*12*).

The recommended Washington Group short set of questions thus aims to identify the majority of the population with difficulties in functioning in six core domains of functioning (seeing, hearing, mobility, cognition, self-care, communication); difficulties that have the potential to limit independent living or social integration if appropriate accommodation is not made. The Washington Group short set of census questions underwent a series of cognitive and field tests in 15 countries before being finalized (13).

A second priority was to recommend one or more extended sets of survey items to measure the different aspects of disability, or principles for their design, that could be used as components of population surveys or as supplements to special surveys. The extended set of questions has undergone cognitive testing in 10 countries, with further field-testing taking place in five countries in Asia and the Pacific – in collaboration with the UNESCAP Statistical Division – and one in Europe.

The Washington Group is also involved in building capacity in developing countries to collect data on disability, for example by training government statisticians on disability measurement methodology. In addition, it has produced a series of papers that:

- describe its work for disabled peoples' organizations (14);
- can assist national statistical offices (15);
- show how disability is interpreted using the short set of six questions (16);
- give examples of how the short set of questions can be used to monitor the United Nations *Convention on the Rights of Persons with Disabilities* (CRPD) (17).

United Nations Economic and Social Commission for Asia and the Pacific

The UNESCAP has been working to improve disability measurement and statistics in line with the Biwako "Millennium Framework for Action towards an Inclusive, Barrier-Free and Rights-Based Society". They have implemented a joint ESCAP/WHO disability project (2004–06) – based on the ICF – to improve the availability, quality, comparability, and policy relevance of disability statistics in the region.

An ongoing project entitled – *Improvement of Disability Measurement and Statistics in Support of the Biwako Millennium Framework and Regional Census Programme* – funded by the United Nations Development Account builds on the momentum generated by the earlier project. The project – implemented by the UNESCAP's Statistics Division in close collaboration with internal and external partners including the United Nations Statistics Division, the Washington Group, World Health Organization (WHO), and selected national statistical offices in the region (18) – is designed to be linked to other global initiatives involving disability data collection through population censuses and surveys such as the Washington Group. The project combines several components including:

- country pilot tests of standard question sets;
- targeted training of statistical experts and health professionals;
- country advisory services;
- development of knowledge management tools and the establishment of a regional network of national disability statistics experts working within governments, to facilitate cross-country cooperation.

The Pan American Health Organization

In Latin America and the Caribbean, PAHO has established a strategic initiative to improve and standardize disability data through the application of the ICF. The initiative takes the form of a network of governmental and non-governmental organizations involved in the collection and use of disability data. It serves two broad purposes. At country level, the focus is on building capacity and providing technical assistance for disability information systems. At the regional level, the initiative promotes the sharing of knowledge and best practice and the development of standard measurement and operational guidelines (*19*).

The European Statistical System

Over the past decade, ESS has undertaken a project in the European Union to achieve comparable statistics on health and disability through surveys (*20*). As a result, a consistent framework of household and individual surveys measuring health and disability is now being implemented within the European Union. Common questions on disability have been integrated into the various European-wide surveys. Several general questions, for instance, have been included on activity restrictions in the European Union–Statistics on Income and Living Conditions (EU–SILC) surveys which replaced the European Community Household Panel. The EU–SILC includes a "disability" question on "longstanding limitations in activities due to a health problem" (known as the Global Activity Limitation Indicator – GALI – question) that is used in the calculation of the Healthy Life Years structural indicator. Special surveys, such as the European Health Interview Survey (EHIS), and the European Survey on Health and Social Integration (ESHSI) – have also been developed. The EHIS in its first round (2008–10) included questions on domains of functioning including seeing, hearing, walking, self-care, and domestic life. The ESHSI addresses additional domains of functioning as well as environmental factors including mobility, transport, accessibility to buildings, education and training, employment, internet use, social contact and support, leisure pursuits, economic life, attitudes, and behaviour.

Variables and questions for these different surveys all are linked to the ICF structure.

Each of these surveys also contains the European Union's core set of social variables, which allows for a breakdown by socioeconomic factors. Importance has been attached to translating the common questions into the various languages of the European Union, to testing the questions and to using a common implementation schedule and methodology. Results from a special survey, the European Health Interview Survey, will gradually become available in the coming years. The ESHSI is planned for implementation in 2012.

United Nations Economic Commission for Europe – Budapest Initiative on Measuring Health Status

In 2004, under the aegis of UNECE, a Joint Steering Group and Task Force on Measuring Health Status was set up with the UNECE, the Statistical Office of the European Union (EUROSTAT) and WHO. The Task Force has been known as the Budapest Initiative since its first meeting in Budapest in 2005 (*21*).

The main purpose of the Budapest Initiative was to develop a new common instrument, based on the ICF, to measure health state suitable for inclusion in interview surveys. The objectives were to obtain basic information on population health which can also be used to describe trends in health over time within a country, across subgroups of the population and across countries within the framework of official national statistical systems. Health state measures functional ability in terms of capacity – and not other aspects of health such as determinants and risk factors, disease states, use of health care, and environmental barriers and facilitators (*21, 22*). This information is useful for both the profiling of health of different populations, and also for subsequent development of summary indices of population health such as those used by the *Global Burden of Disease*. The Budapest Initiative questions cover vision, hearing, walking and mobility, cognition, affect (anxiety and depression), and pain – and use different response categories relevant to the particular domain (*23*).

The Budapest initiative also works to coordinate with existing groups and build on existing work carried out by the ESS, the *World*

Health Survey, the joint United States of America and Canada survey and the Washington Group. For example, the Washington Group and the Budapest Initiative – with support from UNESCAP – are carrying out cognitive and field testing of an extended question set developed by the Washington Group/Budapest Initiative collaboration.

References

1. *United Nations disability statistics database (DISTAT)*. New York, United Nations, 2006 (http://unstats.un.org/unsd/demographic/sconcerns/disability/disab2.asp, accessed 9 December 2009).
2. *United Nations demographic yearbook, special issue: population ageing and the situation of elderly persons*. New York, United Nations, 1993.
3. *Human development report 1997*. New York, United Nations Development Programme and Oxford University Press, 1997.
4. Filmer D. *Disability, poverty and schooling in developing countries: results from 11 household surveys*. Washington, World Bank, 2005, (http://siteresources.worldbank.org/SOCIALPROTECTION/Resources/SP-Discussion-papers/Disability-DP/0539.pdf, accessed 9 December 2009).
5. *Statistics on the employment situation of people with disabilities: a compendium of national methodologies*. Geneva, International Labour Organization, 2003.
6. *Disability at a glance: a profile of 28 countries and areas in Asia and the Pacific*. Bangkok, United Nations Economic and Social Commission for Asia and the Pacific, 2004.
7. *Data on disability*. Washington, Inter-American Development Bank, 2005 (http://www.iadb.org/sds/soc/site_6215_e.htm#Prevalence, accessed 9 December 2009).
8. *Disability and social participation in Europe*. Brussels, EUROSTAT, 2001.
9. Lafortune G, Balestat G. *Trends in severe disability among the elderly people: assessing the evidence in 12 OECD countries and the future implications*. Paris, Organisation for Economic Co-operation and Development, 2007 (OECD Health Working Papers No. 26) (http://www.oecd.org/dataoecd/13/8/38343783.pdf, accessed 9 December 2009).
10. *Washington Group on Disability Statistics*. Atlanta, Centers for Disease Control and Prevention, 2009 (http://www.cdc.gov/nchs/washington_group.htm, accessed 9 December 2009).
11. *Statistical Commission Report on the Special Session, New York, 11–15 April 1994*. New York, United Nations Economic and Social Council, 1994 (Supplement No. 9, Series No. E/CN.3/1994/18).
12. *Principles and recommendations for population and housing censuses: revision 2*. New York, United Nations, 2008 (Statistical Papers Series M, No. 67/Rev.2) (http://unstats.un.org/unsd/demographic/sources/census/docs/P&R_Rev2.pdf).
13. Washington Group on Disability Statistics. In: *Statistical Commission forty-first session, 23–26 February 2010*. New York, United Nations Economic and Social Council, 2010 (E/CN.3/2010/20) (http://unstats.un.org/unsd/statcom/doc10/2010-20-WashingtonGroup-E.pdf, accessed 29 December 2010).
14. *Disability information from censuses*. Hyattsville, Washington Group on Disability Statistics, 2008 (http://www.cdc.gov/nchs/data/washington_group/meeting8/DPO_report.pdf, accessed 9 December 2009).
15. *Development of an internationally comparable disability measure for censuses*. Hyattsville, Washington Group on Disability Statistics, 2008 (http://www.cdc.gov/nchs/data/washington_group/meeting8/NSO_report.pdf, accessed 9 December 2009).
16. *Understanding and interpreting disability as measured using the WG short set of questions*. Hyattsville, Washington Group on Disability Statistics, 2009 (http://www.cdc.gov/nchs/data/washington_group/meeting8/interpreting_disability.pdf, accessed 9 December 2009).
17. *Monitoring the United Nations (UN) Convention on the Rights of Persons with Disabilities*. Hyattsville, Washington Group on Disability Statistics, 2008 (http://www.cdc.gov/nchs/data/washington_group/meeting8/UN_convention.htm, accessed 9 December 2009).
18. *Improvement of disability measurement and statistics in support of Biwako Millennium Framework and Regional Census Programme*. Bangkok, United Nations Economic and Social Commission for Asia and the Pacific, 2010 (http://www.unescap.org/stat/disability/index.asp#recent_activities, accessed 29 December 2010).
19. Vásquez A, Zepeda M. *An overview on the state of art of prevalence studies on disability in the Americas using the International Classification of Functioning, Disability and Health (ICF): conceptual orientations and operational guidelines with regard to the application of the ICF in population studies and projects of intervention*. Santiago, Programa Regional de Rehabilitación, Pan American Health Organization, 2008.

20. EUROSTAT. *Your key to European statistics*. Luxembourg, European Commission, n.d. (http://epp.eurostat.ec.europa.eu, accessed 9 December 2009).

21. Health state survey module: Budapest Initiative: mark 1. In: *Fifty-fifth plenary session, Conference of European Statisticians, Geneva, 11–13 June 2007*. Geneva, United Nations Economic Commission for Europe, 2007 (ECE/CES/2007/6) (http://www.unece.org/stats/documents/ece/ces/2007/6.e.pdf, accessed 29 December 2010).

22. Health as a multi-dimensional construct and cross-population comparability. In: *Conference of European Statisticians, Joint UNCE/WHO/Eurostat meeting on the measurement of health status, Budapest, Hungary, 14–16 November 2005*. United Nations Economic Commission for Europe, 2005 (Working Paper No. 1) (http://www.unece.org/stats/documents/ece/ces/ge.13/2005/wp.1.e.pdf, accessed 29 December 2010).

23. Revised terms of reference of UNECE/WHO/EUROSTAT steering group and task force on measuring health status. In: *Conference of European Statisticians, First Meeting of the 2009/2010 Bureau, Washington, D.C., 15–16 October 2009*. Geneva, United Nations Economic Commission for Europe, 2009 (ECE/CES/BUR/2009/Oct/11) (http://www.unece.org/stats/documents/ece/ces/bur/2009/mtg1/11.e.pdf, accessed 29 December 2010).

Technical appendix C

Design and implementation of the World Health Survey

The *World Health Survey* was implemented in 70 countries. The sample sizes ranged from 700 in Luxembourg to 38 746 in Mexico. The respondents were men and women older than 18 years living in private households. All samples were drawn from a current national frame using a multistage cluster design so as to allow each household and individual respondent to be assigned a known nonzero probability of selection, with the following exceptions: in China and India, the surveys were carried out in selected provinces and states; in the Comoros, the Republic of the Congo, and Côte d'Ivoire, the surveys were restricted to regions where over 80% of the population resided; in Mexico, the sample was intended to provide subnational estimates at the state level. The face-to-face interviews were carried out by trained interviewers. The individual response rates (calculated as the ratio of completed interviews among selected respondents in the sample, and excluding ineligible respondents from the denominator) ranged from 63% in Israel to 99% in the Philippines.

The health module in the *World Health Survey* was closely synchronized with the revision of the *International Classification of Functioning, Disability and Health* (ICF). The aim was not to capture individual impairments, but to provide a cross-sectional snapshot of functioning among the respondents in the different country surveys that could be aggregated to the population level. Respondents were not asked about health conditions or about the duration of their limitation in functioning.

To develop a *World Health Survey* module for health state description, an item pool was constructed and the psychometric properties of each question documented (1). Qualitative research identified the core constructs in different countries. The questionnaire was tested extensively before the start of the main study. The pilot testing was carried out initially in three countries in United Republic of Tanzania, the Philippines and Colombia and subsequently used in World Health Organization's (WHO) MultiCountry Survey Study in 71 surveys in 61 countries. Of these surveys, 14 were carried out using an extensive face-to-face interview of respondents covering

21 domains of health with sample size of more than 88 000 respondents (1). The *World Health Survey* survey instrument was then developed in several languages and further refined using cognitive interviews and cultural applicability tests. Rigorous translation protocols devised by panels of bilingual experts, focused back-translations, and in-depth linguistic analyses were used to ensure culturally relevant questions. Between February and April 2002, revised modules for health state description were further tested in China, Myanmar, Pakistan, Sri Lanka, Turkey, and the United Arab Emirates.

Short and long versions of the survey instrument were then developed. The survey instrument asked about difficulties over the last 30 days in functioning in eight life domains: mobility, self care, pain and discomfort, cognition, interpersonal activities, vision, sleep and energy, and affect. For each domain, two questions of varying difficulty were asked in the long version of the surveys, while a single question was asked in the short version. The questions in the *World Health Survey* in the different domains were very similar or identical to questions that had been asked in national and international surveys on health and disability. They spanned the levels of functioning within a given domain and focused as far as possible on the intrinsic capacities of individuals in that domain. In the case of mobility, for example, respondents were asked about difficulties with moving around and difficulties with vigorous activities. In the case of vision, they were asked about difficulties with near and distant vision. The response scale for each item was identical on a 5 point scale ranging from no difficulty (a score of 1) to extreme difficulty or cannot do (a score of 5). The prevalence of difficulties in functioning was estimated across sex, age, place of residence and wealth quintiles.

Analysis of the World Health Survey, including derivation of threshold for disability

Data from 69 countries were used in the analyses for this Report. Data from Australia were excluded as the survey was carried out partly as a drop-and-collect survey and partly as a telephone interview and it was not possible to combine these estimates due to unknown biases. Data were weighted for 59 of the 69 surveys based on complete sampling information. Individual country estimates are presented in Appendix A excluding those countries that were unweighted: Austria, Belgium, Denmark, Germany, Greece, Italy, Netherlands, and the United Kingdom of Great Britain and Northern Ireland (all short version surveys) and Guatemala and Slovenia (both long version surveys) or where the surveys were not nationally representative: China, the Comoros, the Republic of the Congo, and Côte d'Ivoire. The survey in India was carried out in six states, these estimates were weighted to provide national estimates and the results have been included in Appendix A. Pooled prevalence estimates were calculated from weighted and age-standardized data from 59 of the 69 countries

While the sample sizes in each country in the survey vary, for the purposes of the pooled estimates the post-stratified weights were used with no specific adjustment to the individual survey sample size. The United Nations population database was used for post-stratification correction of the sample weights and for the sex standardization. For age standardization, the WHO world standard population was used (2).

Detailed information on the quality metrics of each survey in terms of representativeness, response rates, item non-response and person non-response are available from the *World*

Table C.1. Proportion of respondents reporting different levels of difficulty on 16 World Health Survey domains of functioning

	None	Mild	Moderate	Severe	Extreme
Mobility					
Moving around	64.8	16.5	11.4	5.9	1.3
Vigorous activity	50.7	16.0	13.3	10.3	9.7
Self-care					
Self-care	79.8	10.7	5.9	2.6	1.0
Appearance, grooming	80.4	10.7	6.0	2.2	0.9
Pain					
Bodily aches and pains	45.2	26.3	16.8	9.5	2.2
Bodily discomfort	49.2	24.9	16.1	8.0	1.8
Cognition					
Concentrating, remembering	61.5	20.0	11.8	5.5	1.3
Learning	65.6	17.3	9.8	4.7	2.5
Interpersonal relationships					
Participation in community	76.8	13.1	6.6	2.4	1.2
Dealing with conflicts	74.4	14.4	6.7	3.0	1.5
Vision					
Distance vision	75.4	11.6	7.1	4.3	1.6
Near vision	76.3	11.9	7.0	3.8	1.0
Sleep and energy					
Falling asleep	60.9	18.9	10.0	6.6	1.6
Feeling rested	57.2	22.1	13.1	6.2	1.4
Affect					
Feeling depressed	56.1	22.5	12.9	6.6	2.0
Worry, anxiety	51.2	22.9	14.0	8.3	3.6

Health Survey web site: http://www.who.int/healthinfo/survey/whsresults/en/index.html

Respondents reporting different levels of difficulty

Data on 16 items are available from 53 countries, with the remaining 16 countries providing data on eight items. Table C.1 shows the proportion of respondents who responded in each category.

A much larger proportion of respondents reported severe (10.3%) or extreme (9.7%) difficulties with vigorous activities than in the areas of self-care and interpersonal relationships. Once vigorous activities are excluded, 8.4% of respondents reported having extreme difficulties or being unable to function in at least one area of functioning. Furthermore, 3.3% of respondents reported extreme difficulties in functioning in two or more areas and 1.7% reported extreme difficulties in functioning in three or more areas. Difficulties with self-care and interpersonal relationships, which includes participation in community and dealing with conflicts, were the least common, while difficulties with mobility and pain were among the most commonly reported. Across all domains, difficulties in functioning were more common in older age groups and among women.

Fig. C.1. Cumulative Distribution of IRT disability scores

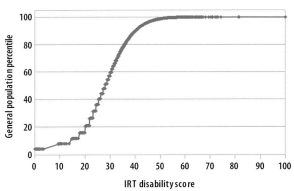

These proportions are not to be construed as the prevalence of disability in the population. Difficulties in functioning are not equivalent to specific impairments. A person with a particular health condition would be likely to experience a constellation of limitations. For the purpose of this Report and in keeping with the ICF, disability is conceptualised as a decrement in functioning above a chosen threshold. It is measured by a vector of a constellation of items that span a set of domains that measure this construct in the most parsimonious manner.

Calculating the composite score

A composite score for each individual was calculated across all the 16 items to estimate where each individual in the survey would be placed on a latent dimension of functioning. An Item Response Theory (IRT) approach using a Rasch model was used to construct this score (see Fig. C.1 for the cumulative distribution of the IRT scores). Rasch models help to transform raw data from the categorical ordered self-report scale of difficulty to an equal-interval scale. Equality of intervals is achieved through log transformations of raw data odds, and abstraction is accomplished through probabilistic equations. This transformation for the partial credit model allows not only for a hierarchical order of difficulty of the items but for different thresholds of item categories as well.

The original 16-item health module was analysed with the Rasch Rating Scale model using the WINSTEPS computer program. Surveys that used only 8 items and those that used the full 16 items were analysed together in this model to yield a common scale across all surveys. A calibration was obtained for each item. To determine how well each item contributed to the common global functioning measurement, chi squared (χ^2) goodness-of-fit statistics, known as Infit Mean Squares (MNSQ), were also calculated. The Infit MNSQ ranged from 0.77 to 1.38 (SD = 0.27). Only the domain of vision slightly exceeded the recommended item misfit threshold of 1.3, but this domain was retained in the analysis. The Dimensionality Map – a principal components factor plot on the residuals – showed no existence of a secondary factor. To test Differential Item Functioning (DIF) by country, the logistic-regression approach described by Zumbo was used (3). The pseudo-R2 change of 0.02 showed a tolerable DIF effect. Finally, to take into account each particular item calibration for the 16 health items, raw scores were transformed through Rasch modelling into a new scale of scores, with 0 = no difficulty and 100 = complete difficulty.

Determining the threshold for the prevalence of disability

Since the score range derived from the IRT model was continuous, to divide the population into "disabled" and "not disabled" groups it was necessary to decide on a threshold value.

The average of scores from respondents who reported extreme difficulties or total inability in any of the eight domains of functioning was calculated for all countries. People reporting extreme difficulties in functioning in these domains are considered disabled in most data collection strategies for estimating disability prevalence. The average scores of respondents who reported having been diagnosed with a chronic disease – such as arthritis, angina,

Table C.2. Showing different thresholds (40 and 50) and related disability prevalence rates from multidomain functioning levels in 59 countries by country level, sex, age, place of residence and wealth

Population subgroup	Threshold of 40			Threshold of 50		
	Higher income countries (standard error)	Lower income countries (standard error)	All countries (standard error)	Higher income countries (standard error)	Lower income countries (standard error)	All countries (standard error)
Sex						
Male	9.1 (0.32)	13.8 (0.22)	12.0 (0.18)	1.0 (0.09)	1.7 (0.07)	1.4 (0.06)
Female	14.4 (0.32)	22.1 (0.24)	19.2 (0.19)	1.8 (0.10)	3.3 (0.10)	2.7 (0.07)
Age group						
18–49	6.4 (0.27)	10.4 (0.20)	8.9 (0.16)	0.5 (0.06)	0.8 (0.04)	0.7 (0.03)
50–59	15.9 (0.63)	23.4 (0.48)	20.6 (0.38)	1.7 (0.23)	2.7 (0.19)	2.4 (0.14)
60 and over	29.5 (0.66)	43.4 (0.47)	38.1 (0.38)	4.4 (0.25)	9.1 (0.27)	7.4 (0.19)
Place of residence						
Urban	11.3 (0.29)	16.5 (0.25)	14.6 (0.19)	1.2 (0.08)	2.2 (0.09)	2.0 (0.07)
Rural	12.3 (0.34)	18.6 (0.24)	16.4 (0.19)	1.7 (0.13)	2.6 (0.08)	2.3 (0.07)
Wealth quintile						
Q1(poorest)	17.6 (0.58)	22.4 (0.36)	20.7 (0.31)	2.4 (0.22)	3.6 (0.13)	3.2 (0.11)
Q2	13.2 (0.46)	19.7 (0.31)	17.4 (0.25)	1.8 (0.19)	2.5 (0.11)	2.3 (0.10)
Q3	11.6 (0.44)	18.3 (0.30)	15.9 (0.25)	1.1 (0.14)	2.1 (0.11)	1.8 (0.09)
Q4	8.8 (0.36)	16.2 (0.27)	13.6 (0.22)	0.8 (0.08)	2.3 (0.11)	1.7 (0.08)
Q5(richest)	6.5 (0.35)	13.3 (0.25)	11.0 (0.20)	0.5 (0.07)	1.6 (0.09)	1.2 (0.07)
Total	11.8 (0.24)	18.0 (0.19)	15.6 (0.15)	2.0 (0.13)	2.3 (0.09)	2.2 (0.07)

Source (4).

asthma, diabetes, and depression – were also computed. The respondents diagnosed with these conditions included those with and without current treatment. Respondents in the *World Health Survey* who reported being on current treatment had a higher score than those not on current treatment. Given that these chronic diseases are associated with disability, it is justifiable to use them as indicator conditions to set a meaningful threshold for significant disability. The average score for all these groups – those reporting extreme difficulties and those reporting chronic diseases – was around 40, with a range from 0 (no functioning difficulty) to 100 (complete difficulty).

Therefore 40 was chosen as the threshold point between "disabled" and "not disabled" for all survey respondents. It should be noted that the *Global Burden of Disease* class of moderate disability, used to generate the estimates of disability from the *Global Burden of Disease* data as reported in Chapter 2, includes conditions such as arthritis and angina that were also used in the analysis of the *World Health Survey* data to set this threshold.

To assess the sensitivity of these results, the item on vigorous activities was dropped from the estimation of the score and the same steps followed for setting a threshold and deriving the proportion of those "disabled". These

Table C.3. IRT score based on different thresholds of item categories

	N	%	mean IRT	SE
None	46 069	18.59	2.49	0.03
Severe	48 678	19.53	37.45	0.04
Extreme1+	25 344	8.98	40.75	0.07
Extreme2+	11 970	3.6	45.53	0.08
Extreme3+	6 361	1.88	49.54	0.08

a. Severe difficulty in at least one item.
b. Extreme difficulty in at least one item.
c. Extreme difficulty in at least two items.
d. Extreme difficulty in three or more items.

analyses show that the disability prevalence rates dropped from 17.5% to 15.6%. Therefore, based on this sensitivity test, it was decided to drop the item for vigorous activities from the estimates.

The estimates of disability prevalence using the difficulties in functioning framework and the method described above are presented in Table C.2. The threshold of 40 produces an estimate of 15.6% of the population experiencing disability. Raising this threshold to a score of 50 (the mean score for those who report extreme difficulties in three or more items of functioning, see Table C.3) produces an estimate of 2.2% of people with very significant disability (see Table C.2).

Measuring wealth in the World Health Survey

Wealth – an indicator of the long-running economic status of households – was derived using a dichotomous hierarchical ordered probit (DIHOPIT) model.

The premise is that wealthier households are more likely to own a given set of assets, thus providing an indicator of economic status. Asset-based approaches avoid some of the reporting biases that arise from self-reported income. The method has been used in previous cross-national studies of economic status and health in developing countries (5, 6).

The effects of asset ownership and household characteristics on household wealth were simultaneously estimated using a random-effects probit model (DIHOPIT), with the hierarchical error term at the household level. The output of the model is a set of covariate coefficients and asset cut points. The covariate coefficients represent the underlying relationship between each sociodemographic predictor and the "latent wealth variable". The asset cut points represent the threshold on the wealth scale above which a household is more likely to own a particular asset. This "asset ladder" was then applied to every household in each survey to produce adjusted estimates of household wealth.

Comparison with the Global Burden of Disease

To compare the disability prevalence rates obtained from the *World Health Survey* with the estimates of "years lived with disability" (YLD) from the *Global Burden of Disease* study, a correlation coefficient was calculated. This produced a Spearman rank order correlation of 0.46 and a Pearson product moment correlation of 0.35, indicating a moderate correlation between the two approaches. While the two approaches estimate disability with different methods, the moderate degree of correlation between them suggests that these approaches, at triangulation with better primary data, could provide fairly reliable estimates of disability prevalence. It should also be noted that alternative approaches to defining and quantifying disability would produce different estimates of prevalence.

Limitations of the World Health Survey

Like all approaches to prevalence estimation, the *World Health Survey* methodology has its limitations and uncertainties. For example, there remain substantially greater variations across countries in reported disability than may be plausible. There could have been systematic reporting biases in levels of functioning and in other aspects of self-reported health. Like other household interview surveys and censuses, the *World Health Survey* is based entirely on self-report. It is quite likely that this leads to variations, because people understand questions differently and pick categories on the scale based on their experiences, expectations and culture. Despite attempts to ensure adequate conceptual translations and uniform understanding of questions and responses, these problems may not have been entirely eliminated. While IRT is supposedly population-invariant, it may not be able to adjust for these systematic reporting variations. This produces some problems in comparing results across populations. To address this issue of comparability – how different respondents used response categories – the surveys included anchoring vignettes that were intended to calibrate the respondents' description of their own functioning. Statistical methods have been developed for correcting biases (or variations) in self-reported functioning using such calibration data (7). However, while these methods have demonstrated the existence of "biases" in self-reported functioning, they have so far not been found to adequately correct for these biases.

Ideally, self-reported disability data from surveys (where responses may often reflect a concern with activity limitations or participation restrictions) should be compared and combined with independent expert assessment of functioning that measure decrements in functioning in multiple domains to validate the self-reports and correct for reporting biases.

A decision has been made in this analysis to set a threshold for disability on a continuous functioning status score that is contestable. The scores could have been affected by reporting biases; the choice of threshold; and diagnosis of chronic diseases that were based on algorithms using questions based on symptoms and were not corroborated with other tests for these chronic diseases. It is possible that both false-positives and false-negatives are included in this sample.

There are several other limitations of the *World Health Survey* data including: not all surveys were nationally representative; not all survey data were weighted; the inclusion of only two high-income countries using the long version of the survey; the choice of parsimonious domains of health could have possibly excluded respondents with functioning problems in other areas such as hearing, breathing, and so on; there were no independent validations of self-reported data through examinations or health records; and both institutionalised populations and children were excluded from the survey. Future data collection efforts on disability prevalence and determinants should attempt to address these shortcomings.

Discussion of approach

Several conceptual points will remain controversial in this approach. First, the decision on where to place the threshold is made during the analysis of the data rather than being set a priori – before or during the data collection – as would be the case, for example, if one were to use a set of impairment categories where only those individuals above a certain level of impairment were captured during data collection.

It is always necessary to set a threshold and there is no "gold standard" for where this line should be drawn. What is important is not so much where the line is drawn, as the reasons justifying that decision. This is because decisions about thresholds should be based on a range of considerations. A policy-maker, for example, needs to know the implications of each level of severity that could be chosen as a threshold in terms of pensions, health insurance and other disability-related programmes. Decisions about resource allocation cannot be avoided. The benefit of a transparent process of setting thresholds is that these decisions can be publicly debated, rather than hidden in some categorical listing of "severe disabilities".

Second, these *World Health Survey* prevalence estimates are based on averaging, and will result in a distribution around the threshold. While individuals included in this estimate of "disability" from the *World Health Survey* include individuals with severe and/or extreme difficulties in functioning in any one given domain (e.g. those likely to be captured in surveys of disability that focus predominantly on impairments), the estimate also includes some people who may have mild levels of difficulty in functioning in multiple domains who may not be considered disabled by traditional definitions. Equally, some respondents who reported severe or extreme difficulties in functioning in one domain, but who

had an overall score below the 40% threshold are excluded. For example, of the 1.4% of respondents who reported severe or extreme difficulties with moving around, 18% were below the threshold. A detailed analysis of these reporting patterns suggests that these errors of exclusion do not have a significant impact on the pooled estimates presented in the Report.

Third, the *World Health Survey* asked about decrements in functioning in the past month, thereby including those with relatively acute problems, which may be short-lived. Other approaches to disability measurement only consider chronic problems that have lasted six months or longer.

Finally, it would be desirable to incorporate measures of the attitudinal and built environment within such surveys, so as to explore the interaction between the features of the individual and the features of the environment which contribute to producing disability, and to disentangle the complexity of the experience of disability. The feasibility of such even more complex exercises need to be examined in resource constrained contexts.

References

1. Üstün TB et al. The World Health Survey. In: Murray CJL, Evans DB, eds. *Health systems performance assessment: debates, methods and empiricism*. Geneva, World Health Organization, 2003:797–808.
2. Ahmad OB et al. *Age Standardization of Rates: a new WHO standard*. Geneva, World Health Organization, 2001.
3. Zumbo BD. *A handbook on the theory and methods of Differential Item Functioning (DIF): logistic regression modeling as a unitary framework for binary and Likert-type (ordinal) item scores*. Ottawa, Directorate of Human Resources Research and Evaluation, Department of National Defence, 1999.
4. *World Health Survey*. Geneva, World Health Organization, 2002–2004.
5. Ferguson B et al. Estimating permanent income using asset and indicator variables. In: Murray CJL, Evans DB, eds. *Health systems performance assessment: debate, new methods, and new empiricism*. Geneva, World Health Organization, 2003.
6. Gakidou E et al. Improving child survival through environmental and nutritional interventions: the importance of targeting interventions toward the poor. *JAMA: Journal of the American Medical Association*, 2007,298:1876-1887. doi:10.1001/jama.298.16.1876 PMID:17954539
7. Tandon A et al. Statistical models for enhancing cross-population comparability. In: Murray CJL, Evans DB, eds. *Health systems performance assessment: debates, methods and empiricism*. Geneva, World Health Organization, 2003:727–746.

Technical appendix D

Global Burden of Disease methodology

The *Global Burden of Disease* study introduced a new metric – the "disability adjusted life year" (DALY) – to simultaneously quantify the burden of disease from premature mortality and from disability (*1*).

The DALY is a metric for lost years of healthy life from mortality and disability. For a particular disease or injury, DALYs are calculated as the sum of the years of life lost due to premature mortality (YLL) in a population, and the years of full health lost due to disability (YLD) from incident cases of the disease or injury. The years lived in states of less than full health are converted to the equivalent number of lost years of full health using health-state valuations, or "disability weights". The disability weights provide a single average numerical score between 0 (for full health) and 1 (for health states equivalent to death).

YLD have been calculated for disabling sequelae of a comprehensive set of diseases and injuries. The country-level rates of YLD given in Appendix A are estimated by imputation from regional-level estimates, making use of available country-specific estimates for around 20 causes and country-specific analyses of cause-specific mortality. They are computed by summing YLD across all diseases and injuries, for all ages and both sexes, without further adjustments for co-morbidity, and dividing the result by the total population.

The original *Global Burden of Disease* study established disability severity weights for 22 sample "indicator conditions", using an explicit "trade-off" protocol in a formal exercise involving health workers from all regions of the world. Subsequent valuation exercises carried out in various settings have closely matched the results of the original *Global Burden of Disease* exercise (*2*). The weights obtained were then grouped into seven classes, with Class I having a weight between 0.00 and 0.02 and Class VII a weight between 0.7 and 1.0 (*1*). To generate disability weights for the remainder of the approximately 500 disabling sequelae in the study, participants in the study were asked to estimate distributions across the seven classes for each sequela.

The *Global Burden of Disease* 2004 update estimated age and sex-specific prevalence for 632 disease and injury sequelae pairings for 17 subregions of the world in 2004 (*3*). These were used, together with the estimated distributions of cases across the seven disability classes, to estimate the prevalence of disability by severity class. Results are presented here for the prevalence of "severe" disability, defined as severity Classes VI and VII – the equivalent of having blindness, Down syndrome, quadriplegia, severe depression, or active psychosis. They are also presented for "moderate and severe" disability, defined as severity Classes III and higher – the equivalent of having angina, arthritis, low vision, or alcohol dependence.

The *Global Burden of Disease* prevalence estimates cannot simply be added, because they were calculated without regard for multiple pathologies or co-morbidities. In other words, it is possible for a given individual to fall within more than one disability level if they have more than one health condition. In adding the prevalence of disabilities across sequelae, an adjustment for co-morbidity has been made that takes into account the increased probability of having certain pairs of conditions (*4*). Estimates of disability from the *Global Burden of Disease* study were limited to conditions that last six months or more. The estimates therefore excluded conditions such as fractures from which most people tend to recover without residual problems in functioning.

The *Global Burden of Disease* prevalence estimates are based on systematic assessments of the available data on incidence, prevalence, duration, and severity of a wide range of conditions, often relying on inconsistent, fragmented or partial data available from different studies. As a result, there are still substantial data gaps and uncertainties. Improving population-level information on the incidence, prevalence and health states associated with major health conditions remains a major priority for national and international health and statistical agencies.

Analyses of the *Global Burden of Disease* 2004 data found that of the nearly 6.5 billion of the world's population in 2004, an estimated 2.9% had severe disability and 15.3% had moderate or severe disability. This was generally the case around the world, though moderate levels of disability were more common in low-income and middle-income countries, especially in those aged 60 years and over. Thus, although the proportion of older people was greater in high-income countries, older people in these countries were relatively less disabled than their counterparts in low-income and middle-income countries. Disability was also more common among children in low-income and middle-income countries (see Chapter 2, Table 2.2).

When the major causes, globally, of disability are considered, adult onset hearing loss and refractive errors are the most common. Mental disorders such as depression, alcohol use disorders and psychoses such as bipolar disorder and schizophrenia also appear in the top 20 causes (see Table D.1). The pattern differs between the high-income countries, on the one hand, and middle-income and low-income countries, on the other, in that many more people in the latter group of countries experience disability associated with preventable causes, such as unintentional injuries and infertility arising from unsafe abortion and maternal sepsis. The data also highlight the lack of interventions in developing countries for easily treated conditions such as hearing loss, refractive errors and cataracts. Disability associated with unintentional injuries among younger people is far more common in low-income countries.

Table D.1. Prevalence of moderate and severe disability (in millions), by leading health condition associated with disability, and by age and income status of countries

	Health condition [b, c]	High-income countries [a] (with a total population of 977 million)		Low-income and middle-income countries (with a total population of 5 460 million)		World (population 6 437 million)
		0–59 years	60 years and over	0–59 years	60 years and over	All ages
1	Hearing loss [d]	7.4	18.5	54.3	43.9	124.2
2	Refractive errors [e]	7.7	6.4	68.1	39.8	121.9
3	Depression	15.8	0.5	77.6	4.8	98.7
4	Cataracts	0.5	1.1	20.8	31.4	53.8
5	Unintentional injuries	2.8	1.1	35.4	5.7	45.0
6	Osteoarthritis	1.9	8.1	14.1	19.4	43.4
7	Alcohol dependence and problem use	7.3	0.4	31.0	1.8	40.5
8	Infertility due to unsafe abortion and maternal sepsis	0.8	0.0	32.5	0.0	33.4
9	Macular degeneration [f]	1.8	6.0	9.0	15.1	31.9
10	Chronic obstructive pulmonary disease	3.2	4.5	10.9	8.0	26.6
11	Ischaemic heart disease	1.0	2.2	8.1	11.9	23.2
12	Bipolar disorder	3.3	0.4	17.6	0.8	22.2
13	Asthma	2.9	0.5	15.1	0.9	19.4
14	Schizophrenia	2.2	0.4	13.1	1.0	16.7
15	Glaucoma	0.4	1.5	5.7	7.9	15.5
16	Alzheimer and other dementias	0.4	6.2	1.3	7.0	14.9
17	Panic disorder	1.9	0.1	11.4	0.3	13.8
18	Cerebrovascular disease	1.4	2.2	4.0	4.9	12.6
19	Rheumatoid arthritis	1.3	1.7	5.9	3.0	11.9
20	Drug dependence and problem use	3.7	0.1	8.0	0.1	11.8

Notes: a. High-income countries are those with 2004 Gross National Income per capita of US$ 10 066 or more in 2004, as estimated by the World Bank (5).

b. GBD disability classes III and above.

c. Disease and injury associated with disability. Conditions are listed in descending order by global all-age prevalence.

d. Includes adult onset hearing loss, excluding that due to infectious causes; adjusted for availability of hearing aids.

e. Includes presenting refractive errors; adjusted for availability of glasses and other devices for correction.

f. Includes other age-related causes of vision loss apart from glaucoma, cataracts and refractive errors.

Source (3).

References

1. Murray CJL, Lopez AD, eds. *The Global Burden of Disease: a comprehensive assessment of mortality and disability from diseases, injuries and risk factors in 1990 and projected to 2020*, 1st ed. Cambridge, Harvard University Press, 1996.

2. Salomon JA, Murray CJL. Estimating health state valuations using a multiple-method protocol. In: Murray CJL et al., eds. *Summary measures of population health: concepts, ethics, measurement and applications*. Geneva, World Health Organization, 2002.

3. *The Global Burden of Disease, 2004 update*. Geneva, World Health Organization, 2008.

4. Mathers CD, Iburg KM, Begg S. Adjusting for dependent comorbidity in the calculation of healthy life expectancy. *Population Health Metrics*, 2006,4:4- doi:10.1186/1478-7954-4-4 PMID:16620383

5. *Data and statistics: country groups*. Washington, World Bank, 2004 (http://go.worldbank.org/D7SN0B8YU0, accessed 4 January 2010).

Technical appendix E

World Health Survey analysis for Chapter 3 – Health

A total of 51 countries were included in the analysis.

- High-income and high-middle-income countries (20): Bosnia and Herzegovina, Brazil, Croatia, Czech Republic, Dominican Republic, Estonia, Hungary, Kazakhstan, Latvia, Malaysia, Mauritius, Mexico, Namibia, the Russian Federation, Slovakia, Spain, South Africa, Turkey, United Arab Emirates, Uruguay.
- Low-income and low-middle-income countries (31): Bangladesh, Burkina Faso, Chad, China, Comoros, Congo, Côte d'Ivoire, Ecuador, Ethiopia, Georgia, Ghana, India, Kenya, Lao People's Democratic Republic, Malawi, Mali, Mauritania, Morocco, Myanmar, Nepal, Pakistan, Philippines, Paraguay, Senegal, Sri Lanka, Swaziland, Tunisia, Ukraine, Viet Nam, Zambia, Zimbabwe.

Countries were selected as follows. Starting with an initial 70 countries, 11 were excluded because of the absence of Pweight or Psweight: Australia, Austria, Belgium, Denmark, Germany, Greece, Guatemala, Italy, the Netherlands, Slovenia, and the United Kingdom of Great Britain and Northern Ireland. Eight countries were excluded for using short-form questionnaire: Finland, France, Ireland, Israel, Luxembourg, Norway, Portugal, and Sweden.

Estimates are weighted using *World Health Survey* post-stratified weights, when available (probability weights otherwise) and age-standardized. T-Tests are performed on results across disability status. Significant differences found between "disabled" and "not-disabled" are reported at 5%.

Glossary

Accessibility

Accessibility describes the degree to which an environment, service, or product allows access by as many people as possible, in particular people with disabilities.

Accessibility standards

A standard is a level of quality accepted as the norm. The principle of accessibility may be mandated in law or treaty, and then specified in detail according to international or national regulations, standards, or codes, which may be compulsory or voluntary.

Activity

In the ICF, the execution of a task or action by an individual. It represents the individual perspective of functioning.

Activity limitations

In the ICF, difficulties an individual may have in executing activities. An activity limitation may range from a slight to a severe deviation in terms of quality or quantity in executing the activity in a manner or to the extent that is expected of people without the health condition.

Affirmative action

The proactive recruitment of people with disabilities.

Appropriate technology

Assistive technology that meets people's needs, uses local skills, tools, and materials, and is simple, effective, affordable, and acceptable to its users.

Assessment

A process that includes the examination, interaction with, and observation of individuals or groups with actual or potential health conditions, impairments, activity limitations, or participation restrictions. Assessment may be required for rehabilitation interventions, or to gauge eligibility for educational support, social protection, or other services.

Augmentative and alternative communication

Methods of communicating that supplement or replace speech and handwriting – for example, facial expressions, symbols, pictures, gestures, and signing.

Assistive devices; also assistive technology

Any device designed, made or adapted to help a person perform a particular task. Products may be specially produced or generally available for people with a disability.

Barriers

Factors in a person's environment that, through their absence or presence, limit functioning and create disability – for example, inaccessible physical environments, a lack of appropriate assistive technology, and negative attitudes towards disability.

Body functions

In the ICF the physiological functions of body systems. Body refers to the human organism as a whole and this includes the brain. The ICF classifies body functions under several areas including mental functions, sensory functions and pain, voice and speech functions, and neuromusculoskeletal and movement-related functions.

Body structures

In the ICF the structural or anatomical parts of the body such as organs, limbs, and their components classified according to body systems.

Braille

A system of writing for individuals who are visually impaired that uses letters, numbers, and punctuation marks made up of raised dot patterns.

Capacity

A construct within the ICF that indicates the highest probable level of functioning that a person may achieve, measured in a uniform or standard environment: reflects the environmentally adjusted ability of the individual.

CBR (community-based rehabilitation)

A strategy within general community development for rehabilitation, equalization of opportunities, poverty reduction, and social inclusion of people with disabilities. CBR is implemented through the combined efforts of people with disabilities themselves, their families, organizations, and communities, and the relevant governmental and nongovernmental health, education, vocational, social, and other services.

CBR worker (community-based rehabilitation worker)

CBR workers may be paid employees or volunteers. They carry out a range of activities within CBR programmes including identification of people with disabilities, support for families, and referral to relevant services.

Condition – primary

A person's main health condition that may be associated with impairment and disability.

Condition – secondary

An additional health condition that arises from the increased susceptibility to a condition caused by the primary condition – though it may not occur in every individual with that primary condition.

Condition – co-morbid

An additional health condition that is independent of and unrelated to the primary health condition.

Conditional cash transfer

Cash payments to targeted eligible households conditional on measurable behaviour.

Contextual factors

Factors that together constitute the complete context of an individual's life, and in particular the background against which health states are classified in the ICF. There are two components of contextual factors: environmental factors and personal factors.

De-institutionalization

Refers to the transfer of people with disabilities or other groups from institutional care, to life in the community.

Digital divide

Refers to the gap between individuals, households, businesses, and geographic areas at different socioeconomic levels with regard to both their opportunities to access information and communication technologies and to their use of the Internet for a wide variety of activities.

Disability

In the ICF, an umbrella term for impairments, activity limitations, and participation restrictions, denoting the negative aspects of the interaction between an individual (with a health condition) and that individual's contextual factors (environmental and personal factors).

Disability discrimination

Any distinction, exclusion, or restriction on the basis of disability that has the purpose or effect of impairing or nullifying the recognition, enjoyment, or exercise on an equal basis with others, of all human rights and fundamental freedoms: includes denial of reasonable accommodation.

Disability management

Interventions and case management strategies used to address the needs of people with disabilities who had experience of work before the onset of disability. The key elements are often effective case management, supervisor education, workplace accommodation, and early return to work with appropriate supports.

Disabled people's organizations

Organizations or assemblies established to promote the human rights of disabled people, where most the members as well as the governing body are persons with disabilities.

Early intervention

Involves strategies which aim to intervene early in the life of a problem and provide individually tailored solutions. It typically focuses on populations at a higher risk of developing problems, or on families that are experiencing problems that have not yet become well established or entrenched.

Education – inclusive

Education which is based on the right of all learners to a quality education that meets basic learning needs and enriches lives. Focusing particularly on vulnerable and marginalized groups, it seeks to develop the full potential of every individual.

Education – special

Includes children with other needs – for example, through disadvantages resulting from gender, ethnicity, poverty, learning difficulties, or disability – related to their difficulty to learn or access education compared with other children of the same age. In high-income countries this category can also include children identified as "gifted and talented". Also referred to as special needs education and special education needs.

Enabling environments

Environments which support participation by removing barriers and providing enablers.

Environmental factors

A component of contextual factors within the ICF, referring to the physical, social, and attitudinal environment in which people live and conduct their lives – for example, products and technology, the natural environment, support and relationships, attitudes, and services, systems, and policies.

Equalization of opportunities

The process through which the various systems of society and the environment, such as services, activities, information, and documentation, are made available to all, particularly to persons with disabilities.

Facilitators

Factors in a person's environment that, through their absence or presence, improve functioning and reduce disability – for example, an accessible environment, available assistive technology, inclusive attitudes, and legislation. Facilitators can prevent impairments or activity limitations from becoming participation restrictions, since the actual performance of an action is enhanced, despite the person's problem with capacity.

Frail elderly

Older persons (usually over 75 years old) who have a health condition that may interfere with the ability to independently perform activities of daily living.

Functioning

An umbrella term in the ICF for body functions, body structures, activities, and participation. It denotes the positive aspects of the interaction between an individual (with a health condition) and that individual's contextual factors (environmental and personal factors).

Global Burden of Disease (GBD)

A measurement of impact of disease combining years of life lost to premature mortality plus years of life lost to time lived in states of less than full health, measured by disability-adjusted life-years.

Health

A state of well-being, achieved through the interaction of an individual's physical, mental, emotional, and social states.

Health conditions

In the ICF an umbrella term for disease (acute or chronic), disorder, injury, or trauma. A health condition may also include other circumstances such as pregnancy, ageing, stress, congenital anomaly, or genetic predisposition.

Health promotion

The process of enabling people to increase control over, and improve, their health.

Impairment

In the ICF loss or abnormality in body structure or physiological function (including mental functions), where abnormality means significant variation from established statistical norms.

Incidence

The number of new cases during a specified time period

Inclusive society

One that freely accommodates any person with a disability without restrictions or limitations.

Independent living

Independent living is a philosophy and a movement of people with disabilities, based on the right to live in the community but including self-determination, equal opportunities, and self-respect.

Informal care

Assistance or support given by a family member, friend, neighbour, or volunteer, without pay.

Informal economy

Economic activity that is neither taxed nor regulated by a government and not included in that government's gross national product.

Institution

Any place in which persons with disabilities, older people, or children live together away from their families. Implicitly, a place in which people do not exercise full control over their lives and their day-to-day activities. An institution is not defined merely by its size.

Intellectual impairment

A state of arrested or incomplete development of mind, which means that the person can have difficulties understanding, learning, and remembering new things, and in applying that learning to new situations. Also known as intellectual disabilities, learning disabilities, learning difficulties, and formerly as mental retardation or mental handicap.

International Classification of Functioning, Disability and Health (ICF)

The classification that provides a unified and standard language and framework for the description of health and health-related states. ICF is part of the "family" of international classifications developed by the World Health Organization.

Measure

In the ICF an activity or set of activities aimed at improving body functions, body structures, activities, and participation by intervening at the level of the individual, person, or society.

Mainstream services

Services available to any member of a population, regardless of whether they have a disability – for example, public transport, education and training, labour and employment services, housing, health and income support systems.

Margin of health

The level of vulnerability to health problems. For example, the risk of developing secondary conditions or the risk of experiencing health conditions earlier in life.

Mental health condition

A health condition characterized by alterations in thinking, mood, or behaviour associated with distress or interference with personal functions. Also known as mental illness, mental disorders, psychosocial disability.

Microfinance programmes

Small-scale funding for small business start-ups that can provide an alternative to formal employment.

Millennium Development Goals (MDGs)

Eight quantified targets, set out in the Millennium Declaration, for attainment by 2015, comprising end to poverty and hunger, universal education, gender equality, child health, maternal health, combating HIV/AIDS, environmental sustainability, and global partnership.

Mixed economy of care

A variety of suppliers from different sectors (public, private, voluntary, mixed) providing health care to one population

Morbidity

The state of poor health. Morbidity rate is the number of illnesses or cases of disease in a population.

Nongovernmental organization (NGO)

An organization, with no participation or representation by government, which works for the benefits of its members or of other members of the population, also known as a civil society organization.

Occupational therapy

Promoting health and well-being through occupation. The primary goal of occupational therapy is to enable people to participate in the activities of everyday life.

Occupational therapists achieve this outcome by enabling people to do things that will enhance their ability to participate, or by modifying the environment to better support participation.

Participation

In the ICF, a person's involvement in a life situation, representing the societal perspective of functioning.

Performance

A construct within the ICF that describes what individuals do in their current environment, including their involvement in life situations. The current environment is described using environmental factors.

Personal assistant

An individual who supports or assists a person with disability and is answerable to them directly.

Personal factors

A component of contextual factors within the ICF that relate to the individual – for example, age, gender, social status, and life experiences.

Physical and rehabilitation medicine doctors

Carry out services to diagnose health conditions, assess functioning and prescribe medical and technological interventions that treat health conditions and optimize functional capacity. Also known as physiatrists.

Physiotherapy

Provides services to individuals to develop, maintain, and maximize movement potential and functional ability throughout the lifespan. Also known as physical therapy.

Prevalence

All the new and old cases of an event, disease, or disability in a given population and time.

Prosthetist–orthotist

Provide prosthetic and orthotic care and other mobility devices aimed at improving functioning in people with physical impairments. Orthotic care involves external appliances designed to support, straighten or improve the functioning of a body part; prosthetic interventions involve an artificial external replacement for a body part.

Psychologist

A professional specializing in diagnosing and treating diseases of the brain, emotional disturbance, and behaviour problems, more often through therapy than medication.

Quality of life

An individual's perception of their position in life in the context of the culture and value systems in which they live, and in relation to their goals, expectations, standards, and concerns. It is a broad-ranging concept, incorporating in a complex way the person's physical health, psychological state, level of independence, social relationships, personal beliefs, and relationship to environmental factors that affect them.

Quota

In the context of employment, quota or reservation is an obligation to employ a fixed number or fixed proportion of people from a particular group.

Reasonable accommodation

Necessary and appropriate modification and adjustment not imposing a disproportionate or undue burden, where needed in a particular case, to ensure that persons with disabilities enjoy or exercise, on an equal basis with others, all human rights and fundamental freedoms.

Rehabilitation

A set of measures that assists individuals who experience or are likely to experience disability to achieve and maintain optimal functioning in interaction with their environment.

Reservation wage

The lowest wage at which a person is willing to work.

Risk factor

A risk factor is an attribute or exposure that is causally associated with an increased probability of a disease or injury.

Schools – inclusive

Children with disabilities attend regular classes with age-appropriate peers, learn the curriculum to the extent feasible, and are provided with additional resources and support depending on need.

Schools – integrated

Schools that provide separate classes and additional resources for children with disabilities, which are attached to mainstream schools.

Schools – special

Schools that provide highly specialized services for children with disabilities and remain separate from broader educational institutions; also called segregated schools.

Screen-reader software

Screen readers are a form of assistive technology potentially useful to people who are blind, visually impaired, illiterate, or have specific learning difficulties. Screen-readers attempt to identify and interpret what is being displayed on the screen and represent to the user with text-to-speech, sound icons, or a Braille output device.

Sheltered employment

Employment in an enterprise established specifically for the employment of persons with disabilities, but which may also employ nondisabled people.

Sign language interpreter

A sign-language interpreter is a person trained to interpret information from sign language into speech and vice versa. Sign languages vary across the world.

Social firm

A business set up to create employment for persons with disabilities or those who are otherwise disadvantaged in the labour market.

Social assistance

Noncontributory transfers targeted at the poor or vulnerable. These may include food or jobs instead of, or as well as, cash and may include compliance conditions (conditional cash transfers).

Social protection

Programmes to reduce deprivation arising from conditions such as poverty, unemployment, old age, and disability.

Social worker

Professional social workers restore or enhance the capacity of individuals or groups to function well in society, and help society accommodate their needs.

Specific learning disability

Impairments in information processing resulting in difficulties in listening, reasoning, speaking, reading, writing, spelling, or doing mathematical calculations – for example, dyslexia.

Speech and language therapy

Aimed at restoring people's capacity to communicate effectively and to swallow safely and efficiently.

Supported employment

Supported job placements providing the opportunity for integration in the mainstream workforce.

Therapy

The activities and interventions concerned with restoring and compensating for loss of function, and preventing or slowing deterioration in functioning in every area of a person's life.

Universal design

The design of products, environments, programmes, and services to be usable by all people, to the greatest extent possible, without the need for adaptation or specialized design.

Vocational rehabilitation and training

Programmes designed to restore or develop the capabilities of people with disabilities to secure, retain and advance in suitable employment – for example, job training, job counselling, and job placement services.

Index